NANOTECHNOLOGY IN MEDICINE AND BIOLOGY

Elsevier Series on Advanced Topics in Biomaterials

NANOTECHNOLOGY IN MEDICINE AND BIOLOGY

Edited by

HUINAN H. LIU

TOLOU SHOKUHFAR

SOUGATA GHOSH

ELSEVIER

Elsevier
Radarweg 29, PO Box 211, 1000 AE Amsterdam, Netherlands
The Boulevard, Langford Lane, Kidlington, Oxford OX5 1GB, United Kingdom
50 Hampshire Street, 5th Floor, Cambridge, MA 02139, United States

Library of Congress Cataloging-in-Publication Data
A catalog record for this book is available from the Library of Congress

British Library Cataloguing-in-Publication Data
A catalogue record for this book is available from the British Library

ISBN: 978-0-12-819469-0

For information on all Elsevier publications
visit our website at https://www.elsevier.com/books-and-journals

Publisher: Matthew Deans
Acquisitions Editor: Sabrina Webber
Editorial Project Manager: Fernanda A. Oliveira
Production Project Manager: Surya Narayanan Jayachandran
Cover Designer: Matthew Limbert

Typeset by STRAIVE, India

Contents

Contributors

Ankit A. Agrawal
Department of Pharmaceutical Sciences and Technology, Institute of Chemical Technology, Mumbai, Maharashtra, India

Aman Bajpai
Discipline of Chemistry, Indian Institute of Technology (IIT) Gandhinagar, Palaj, Gujarat, India

Rinti Banerjee
Nanomedicine Laboratory, Department of Biosciences and Bioengineering, Indian Institute of Technology Bombay, Powai, Mumbai, Maharashtra, India

Sudipta Basu
Discipline of Chemistry, Indian Institute of Technology (IIT) Gandhinagar, Palaj, Gujarat, India

Vaibhav N. Ghegade
Department of Pharmaceutical Sciences and Technology, Institute of Chemical Technology, Mumbai, Maharashtra, India

Sougata Ghosh
Department of Microbiology, School of Science, RK University, Rajkot, Gujarat, India; Department of Chemical Engineering, Northeastern University, Boston, MA, United States

Dhara Jajal
Charotar University of Science and Technology, Changa, Gujarat, India

Archana A. Kapse
Department of Pharmaceutical Sciences and Technology, Institute of Chemical Technology, Mumbai, Maharashtra, India

Radhika K. Kelkar
Department of Biotechnology Engineering, Kolhapur Institute of Technology's College of Engineering, Kolhapur, Maharashtra, India

Roshan Keshari
Nanomedicine Laboratory, Department of Biosciences and Bioengineering, Indian Institute of Technology Bombay, Powai, Mumbai, Maharashtra, India

Shruti Lohakare
Department of Pharmaceutical Sciences and Technology, Institute of Chemical Technology, Mumbai, Maharashtra, India

Susmit Mhatre
Department of Pharmaceutical Sciences and Technology, Institute of Chemical Technology, Mumbai, Maharashtra, India

Ebrahim Mostafavi
Stanford Cardiovascular Institute, Stanford, CA, United States; Department of Medicine, Stanford University School of Medicine, Stanford, CA, United States

Shamraja S. Nadar
Department of Chemical Engineering, Institute of Chemical Technology, Mumbai, Maharashtra, India

Anjali Pandya
Department of Pharmaceutical Sciences and Technology, Institute of Chemical Technology, Mumbai, Maharashtra, India

Neha P. Patil
Department of Biotechnology Engineering, Kolhapur Institute of Technology's College of Engineering, Kolhapur, Maharashtra, India

Pravin D. Patil
Department of Basic Science and Humanities, Mukesh Patel School of Technology Management and Engineering, SVKM's NMIMS University, Mumbai, Maharashtra, India

Runali Patil
Nanomedicine Laboratory, Department of Biosciences and Bioengineering; IIT Bombay-Monash Research Academy, Indian Institute of Technology Bombay, Powai, Mumbai, Maharashtra, India

Sadhana P. Patil
Department of Biotechnology Engineering, Kolhapur Institute of Technology's College of Engineering, Kolhapur, Maharashtra, India

Vandana B. Patravale
Department of Pharmaceutical Sciences and Technology, Institute of Chemical Technology, Mumbai, Maharashtra, India

Kaustubh A. Pawar
Department of Pharmaceutical Sciences and Technology, Institute of Chemical Technology, Mumbai, Maharashtra, India

Ajay N. Phirke
Department of Basic Science and Humanities, Mukesh Patel School of Technology Management and Engineering, SVKM's NMIMS University, Mumbai, Maharashtra, India

Pradnya V. Pise
Department of Biotechnology Engineering, Kolhapur Institute of Technology's College of Engineering, Kolhapur, Maharashtra, India

Sreeranjini Pulakkat
Department of Pharmaceutical Sciences and Technology, Institute of Chemical Technology, Mumbai, Maharashtra, India

Amarjitsing Rajput
Nanomedicine Laboratory, Department of Biosciences and Bioengineering, Indian Institute of Technology Bombay, Powai, Mumbai; Department of Pharmaceutics, Poona College of Pharmacy, Bharti Vidyapeeth Deemed University, Erandwane, Pune, Maharashtra, India

Poulomi Sengupta
Department of Chemistry, School of Science, Indrashil University, Rajpur, Gujarat, India

Sejal Shah
Department of Microbiology, School of Science, RK University, Rajkot, India

Sopan Shinde
Discipline of Chemistry, Indian Institute of Technology (IIT) Gandhinagar, Palaj, Gujarat, India

Tishya Srivastava
Department of Pharmaceutical Sciences and Technology, Institute of Chemical Technology, Mumbai, Maharashtra, India

Nanasaheb Thorat
Nuffield Department of Women's & Reproductive Health, Division of Medical Sciences, John Radcliffe Hospital, University of Oxford, Oxford, United Kingdom

Manishkumar S. Tiwari
Department of Chemical Engineering, Mukesh Patel School of Technology Management and Engineering, SVKM's NMIMS University, Mumbai, Maharashtra, India

Prashant Upadhaya
Department of Pharmaceutical Sciences and Technology, Institute of Chemical Technology, Mumbai, Maharashtra, India

Thomas J. Webster
Hebei University of Technology, Tianjin, China; Vellore Institute of Technology, Vellore, India

Preface

Nanotechnology has influenced every aspects of life, be it food, textiles, agriculture, environment, or health. The groundbreaking progress in the area of fabrication of the biomaterials with exotic shape, tunable size, and enhanced biocompatibility has revolutionized healthcare and medicine. It has helped to overcome the growing concerns of multidrug resistance in pathogens, adverse effects of drugs, and late diagnosis of diseases. On the contrary, nanotechnology-driven solutions have enhanced bioavailability of drugs and ensured targeted drugs' delivery and their triggered/sustained release. Moreover, nanotechnology is employed in designing sensors that can monitor the physiological levels of various metabolites and markers for early prediction of a disease and also in monitoring the efficiency of the administered drugs.

This book is the most comprehensive literature available for multivariate applications of nanotechnology particularly in the sectors of medicine and health. Novel multifunctionalized nanomaterials, included in this book, have immense potential for 3D and 4D bioprinting of tissues and organs. Various metals, metal oxides, and polymeric nanoparticles with their promising applications in both therapy and diagnosis are also elaborated most methodically with detailed underlying mechanism. Various nanostructures, introduced here, emphasize their significant role in revolutionizing therapy and diagnosis (theranostics) against cancerous, infectious, cardiovascular, autoimmune, and neurodegenerative diseases. Also various parameters of nanovectors used for drug delivery and theranostic applications are discussed in detail followed by their targeting mechanisms and their off-target toxicities.

Another notable aspect of this book is the rich collection of nanomaterials for tissue repair and regeneration. Polymer-, ceramic-, and metal-based biomaterials and their composites for hard tissue repair are included. Further, collagen, chitosan, silk, poly-ε-caprolactone, poly(L-lactic acid), poly(lactic-*co*-poly(glycolic acid), and several other polymer-based nanobiomaterials for soft tissue engineering are also discussed in depth.

Tissue-specific drug delivery with higher bioavailability and enhanced action is another challenge. Hence, this book also includes nanoparticles, polymeric nanoparticles, and lipid-based drug delivery systems. Overcoming the hydrophobic barriers using the lipid-based drug delivery systems such as liposomes, nanostructured lipid carriers, and solid lipid nanoparticles is another attractive aspect of this book. Nanoscaffolds help in the cell delivery, adhesion, and proliferation of stem cells that are employed in regenerative medicine. This ensures rapid healing of wounded tissues and faster postsurgical recovery. The role of nanotechnology for designing several implants with high biocompatibility, antimicrobial resistance, and modified surface properties are also covered. The authors of this book are involved in the state-of-the-art developments in the area of nanomedicine and have presented the information furnished in the respective chapter out of their vast experience and command in the fields.

Lastly, we believe that this would be the ideal textbook for nanomedicine courses in various graduate courses and PhD programs with courses in subjects like Biotechnology, Medicine, Instrumentation, Biophysics, Nanotechnology, Biomechanics, and Chemical Engineering. It would provide an excellent introduction with basic and applied knowledge about the principles of nanotechnology, bioprinting, drug delivery, tissue engineering, regenerative medicine, bioimaging, and nanoinspired implants to the beginner, intermediate, and advanced undergraduate, graduate, and postgraduate students.

Considering the enormous responsibility, we all have to ensure human health and safety; we consider this book a top priority. This book essentially highlights the advances and prospects on nanomedicine as next-generation therapeutics.

Huinan H. Liu
Tolou Shokuhfar
Sougata Ghosh

CHAPTER 1

Nanobiomaterials for three-dimensional bioprinting

Sougata Ghosh[a,b], Ebrahim Mostafavi[c,d], Nanasaheb Thorat[e], and Thomas J. Webster[f,g]

[a]Department of Microbiology, School of Science, RK University, Rajkot, Gujarat, India
[b]Department of Chemical Engineering, Northeastern University, Boston, MA, United States
[c]Stanford Cardiovascular Institute, Stanford, CA, United States
[d]Department of Medicine, Stanford University School of Medicine, Stanford, CA, United States
[e]Nuffield Department of Women's & Reproductive Health, Division of Medical Sciences, John Radcliffe Hospital, University of Oxford, Oxford, United Kingdom
[f]Hebei University of Technology, Tianjin, China
[g]Vellore Institute of Technology, Vellore, India

1.1 Introduction

Tissue engineering has witnessed tremendous advances owing to a detailed understanding of physiological and biochemical processes at the nanoscale. Thus nanotechnology has been actively involved in the augmentation and innovation of healthcare. The widely used medical processes for addressing bone, cartilage, and nerves injuries involve surgical methods that are not only painful but also possess poor healing capacity for delicate structures. One of the most attractive alternative advances is harnessing the body's adult stem cell population for repairing and regenerating tissues (O'Brien et al., 2015).

As the success of stem cell therapy largely depends on the cellular microenvironment and nanoenvironment, classical scaffold-based tissue engineering has been developed that can effectively mimic natural biological environments, tissue structure, and function. Various metals, metal-alloys, graphene, carbon nanotubes, ceramics, and polymer-based biomaterials have been developed with high biocompatibility for the fabrication of implants (Kale et al., 2017; Ghosh et al., 2018; Ghosh, 2019). This innovative approach not only enables healthy and rapid restoration and regeneration, but it also helps in the maintenance of the implanted construct and simultaneously facilitates the integration of natural tissue with the tissue-engineered implant (Wang et al., 2020; Xie et al., 2020).

Three-dimensional (3D) techniques seem to be one of the most efficient manufacturing technologies that can be employed for the rationale

Nanotechnology in Medicine and Biology
https://doi.org/10.1016/B978-0-12-819469-0.00003-4

engineering of biomimetic constructs which are compatible with the complex extracellular matrix (ECM) structure, mechanical, chemical, and morphological properties of the specific tissue that is undergoing treatment (Zhu et al., 2018). The conventional approaches for developing 3D scaffolds include phase separation, freeze drying, porogen leaching, and electrospinning. However, these techniques have several drawbacks, such as limited control over scaffold geometry, pore size and distribution, pore interconnectivity, as well as internal channel construction. Further, these limitations compromise nutrient transportation, cell migration, and survival, especially in the core of the scaffold.

In view of this background, O'Brien et al. (2015) suggested key characteristics that should be concurrently employed for successful tissue emulation and regeneration: (1) possess sufficient mechanical strength and material degradation rate; (2) be able to modulate a 3D cellular microenvironment; (3) encourage cellular adhesion, proliferation, and tissue formation; and (4) enable adequate nutrient and waste exchange.

In this chapter, we discuss the fabrication of highly ordered scaffold microarchitectures by recent advances in modalities of 3D printing that include inkjet bioprinting, bioplotting, fused-deposition modeling (FDM), selective laser sintering (SLS), and stereolithography. Further, applications of 3D printing offer great precision and control over the internal architecture for repair and regeneration of bone, cartilage and osteochondral, neural, and vascular tissues have been elaborated. Finally, the scope of ultramodern four-dimensional (4D) printing technologies with their promises for modulating neural stem cell behavior is discussed.

1.2 Inkjet bioprinting

Inkjet is a printing technology where ink droplets are ejected on paper and can be of two types that include a continuous inkjet printing system and an on-demand inkjet printing. However, for bioprinting, bioinks are used, which is usually a solution with suspended cells, biomaterials, drugs and/or proteins or deoxyribonucleic acid (DNAs). Direct printing involves biomaterials that are printed with cells mixed in bioink together while indirect printing uses biomaterials is prepared first where cells are seeded and cultured.

Kim et al. (2010) reported inkjet printing mediated fabrication methods of various patterns of poly(lactic-*co*-glycolic acid) (PLGA) on a polystyrene (PS) substrate. Later, human adipose-derived stem cells (hASCs), isolated from subcutaneous adipose tissue, were seeded on the PLGA-patterned PS substrate. Stable attachment of the hASCs followed by efficient proliferation up to confluency within the PLGA patterns was promising.

Pati et al. (2014) developed a technique for the bioprinting of cell-laden constructs with novel decellularized extracellular matrix (dECM) bioinks that was able to provide an optimized microenvironment conducive to the 3D growth of structured tissue. Extracellular matrices were derived from cartilage, heart, and adipose tissues that were initially decellularized. The tissues were treated chemically and enzymatically to obtain the novel bioinks. The appropriate source material facilitated the creation of a proper microenvironment for the target cells. Thus the decellularized ECM obtained from heart tissue, for instance, is a quite ideal biomaterial for culturing cardiomyocytes. Fig. 1.1 depicts the 3D open porous structures of dECMs with a polycaprolactone (PCL) framework that were fabricated using a multihead tissue/organ building system (MtoBS). It is important to note that the cartilage and adipose tissue constructs were printed by depositing the cell-laden dECM pregel following fabrication of the PCL framework (Fig. 1.1A, C, D). A line width of 200 nm in the PCL framework of cartilage tissues provided more load-bearing support, while line widths of 100 nm for adipose tissue constructs reduced the stiffness.

1.3 Bioplotting

Bioplotting is another method of 3D printing where either tubes or spheroids of biomaterials are extruded from a syringe to obtain layered structures which are then cured using radiation, a chemical reaction, or solidification with time. Occasionally, bioplotting modalities are associated with several syringes containing multiple cell types to ensure efficient and convenient integration of cells derived from multiple tissue types in the final construct. Thus bioplotting is ideal for fabrication of co-cultured scaffolds and tissue/organ-like constructs. Relatively, viscous biomaterials are preferred for bioplotting as the physical and chemical properties of materials is a key determinant for maximum resolution. The major advantages of bioplotting include a requirement of lower cell numbers and a broad spectrum of material selection. However, the bioink required for bioplotting must be a liquid material, which is a major drawback for tissue reconstructions involving high mechanical strength (O'Brien et al., 2015).

Bioplotting was applied for tissue engineering to provide a functional de novo living valve replacement that could effectively integrate with host tissue (O'Brien et al., 2015). Initially, hybrid hydrogels were developed

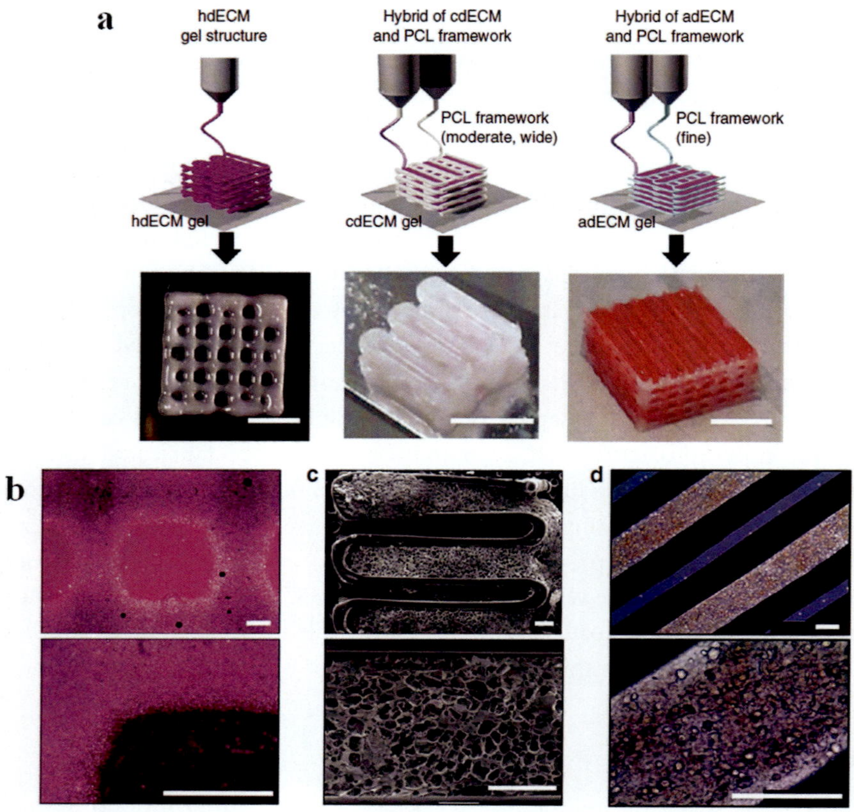

Fig. 1.1 Printing process of particular tissue constructs with dECM bioink. (A) Heart tissue construct was printed with only the heart dECM (hdECM). Cartilage and adipose tissues were printed with the cartilage dECM (cdECM) and the adipose dECM (adECM), respectively, and in combination with a PCL framework (scale bar, 5 mm). (B) Representative microscopic images of the hdECM construct (scale bar, 400 mm). (C) SEM images of a hybrid structure of cdECM with a PCL framework (scale bar, 400 mm). (D) Microscopic images of the cell-printed structure of adECM with a PCL framework (scale bar, 400 mm). *(Reprinted with permission from Pati, F., Jang, J., Ha, D.H., Kim, S.W., Rhie, J.W., Shim, J.H., Kim, D.H., Cho, D.W., 2014. Printing three-dimensional tissue analogues with decellularized extracellular matrix bioink. Nat. Commun. 5, 3935. Copyright © 2014 Springer Nature.)*

using methacrylated hyaluronic acid (Me-HA) and methacrylated gelatin (Me-Gel), and heart valve conduits were bioprinted that contained encapsulated human aortic valvular interstitial cells (HAVIC) as seen in Fig. 1.2. Upon an increase of Me-Gel concentration, the stiffness of the conduits was reduced, viscosity was enhanced, cell spreading was facilitated, and the HAVIC fibroblastic phenotype was maintained better. Although the relative concentrations of Me-Gel and Me-HA influenced the bioprinting accuracy, careful optimization resulted in fabrication of the trileaflet valve with an

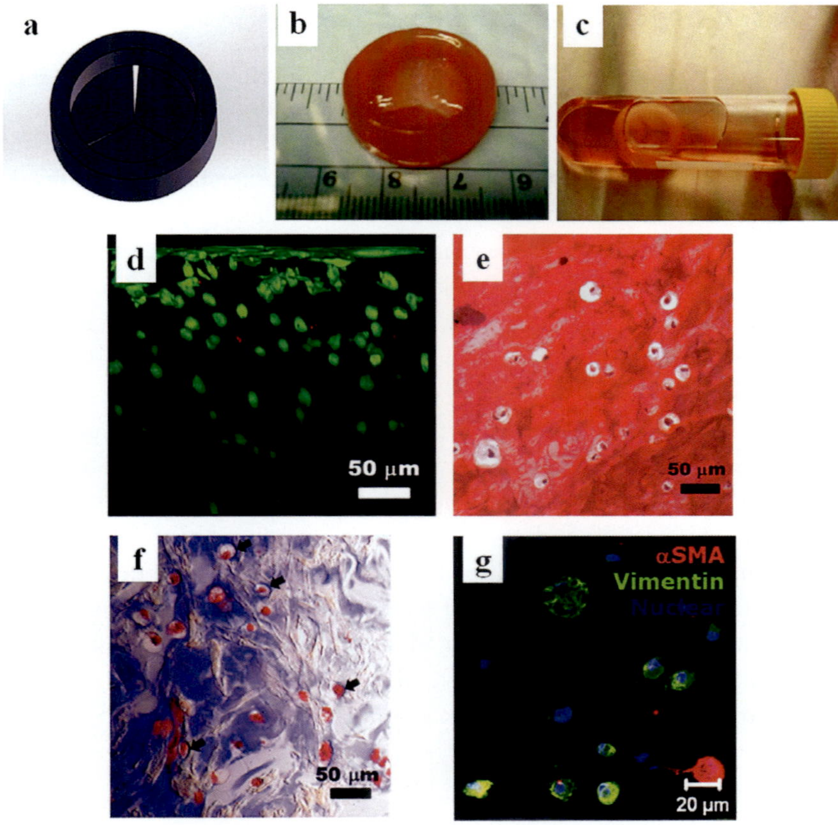

Fig. 1.2 Bioprinting of heart valve conduits with the encapsulation of HAVIC within the leaflets: (A) heart valve model designed by Solidworks; (B) as-printed valve conduit; (C) the bioprinted valve conduit kept intact after a 7-day static culture in a culture tube; (D) cross-sectional view of a Live/Dead image showed high cell viability from the surface to a >300-μm depth; (E, F) histological staining of the bioprinted leaflets after a 7-day culture. (E) Safranin-O staining was used to stain the GAGs red, which also stained the Me-HA within the hydrogel red. (F) Masson's Trichrome staining was used to stain collagen blue, which also stained the Me-Gel within the hydrogel blue. The arrow shows the newly secreted collagen around the HAVIC, indicating the remodeling process; (G) representative image of immunohistochemical staining for αSMA (green) and vimentin (red), and Draq 5 counter-staining for cell nuclei (blue). *(Reprinted with permission from Duan, B., Kapetanovic, E., Hockaday, L.A., Butcher, J.T., 2014. Three-dimensional printed trileaflet valve conduits using biological hydrogels and human valve interstitial cells. Acta Biomater. 10, 1836–1846. Copyright © 2013 Acta Materialia Inc. Published by Elsevier Ltd.)*

accurate shape and desirable properties. Significantly, HAVIC encapsulated within bioprinted heart valves were highly viable and could effectively remodel the initial matrix by collagen and glyosaminoglycan deposition. Thus bioplotting can be one of the most powerful tools for de novo living valve replacements (Duan et al., 2014).

1.4 Fused-deposition modeling

In this 3D printing technology, a melted thermoplastic is deposited in thin layers on a flat surface, and eventually, a model is built layer by layer. FDM is one of the oldest, most inexpensive, rapid, and a well-standardized method for the fabrication of scaffolds for musculoskeletal applications. As the molten thermoplastic lacks mechanical strength, it is difficult to replicate geometries with sharp overhanging structures, or long, unsupported spans within the scaffold. The resolution of FDM-generated structures is dependent on the nozzle diameter, properties of the materials, and mechanical positioning of the extrusion end of the printing nozzle (O'Brien et al., 2015).

Schantz et al. (2005) reported the application of FDM for developing polymer-ceramic scaffolds using novel polycaprolactone-calcium phosphate (PCL/CaP) matrices. These structures were characterized by a honeycomb-like design and complete interconnectivity of the pores as illustrated in Fig. 1.3A. On seeding human mesenchymal stem cells (MSCs) with the fibrin glue into PCL/CaP scaffolds and culturing for periods of up to eight weeks, enhanced cellular adhesion, proliferation and osteogenic differentiation were observed (Fig. 1.3B and C). The PCL/CaP scaffolds showed up to a 27-fold increase in degradation compared with pristine PCL scaffolds.

1.5 Selective laser sintering

SLS is a higher resolution alternative to FDM that employs a long wavelength laser or high-energy light source to fuse beads of material together, one layer at a time. In this method, the layer of beads is deposited by fusing each bead to a solid structure with laser-associated heating. The process is repeated to develop a 3D design. Alternatively, high-energy electron beams can also be used to melt beads of metal into a fully functioning prototype. SLS is a promising technique for developing size-controlled constructs for rigid tissues, such as bone. Thus, SLS is more suitable for hard tissues of a single material type, such as osteogenic scaffolds or supporting structures for tissues within the body (O'Brien et al., 2015).

Duan et al. (2010) reported the application of SLS for fabricating 3D nanocomposite scaffolds based on calcium phosphate (Ca–P)/poly(hydroxybutyrate-*co*-hydroxyvalerate) (PHBV) and carbonated hydroxyapatite (CHAp)/poly(L-lactic acid) (PLLA) nanocomposite

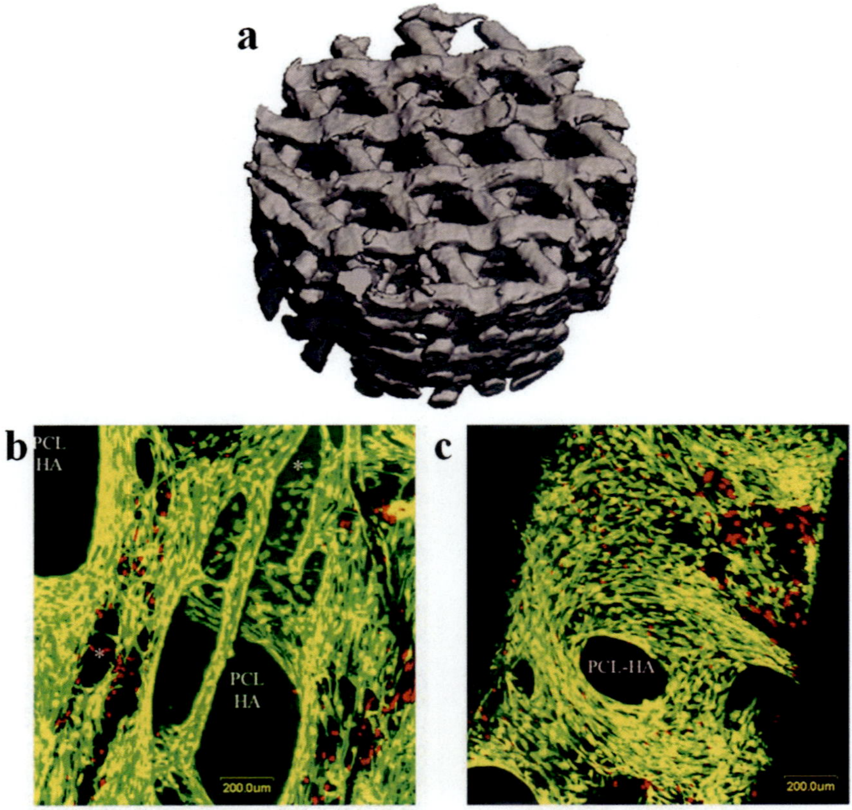

Fig. 1.3 (A) PCL-CaP scaffold architecture observed under microcomputed tomography. Characterization of cell proliferation and viability on the PCL-CaP scaffold. (B) Viable cells are stained with fluorescence diacetate (FDA, green stain), while the nuclei of apoptotic cells and cytoplasm of dead cells are counterstained with propidium iodide (PI, red stain). Optical sectioning was performed with a confocal laser microscope and superimposed images are shown (both original magnification ×10). A dense cellular network can be observed after 4 weeks in culture, covering the bars and struts of the scaffold with only a few spaces in the pores left open (stars). (C) After 8 weeks, the remaining spaces are filled up completely. A slight increase in nonviable and apoptotic cells (red) is noticed. *(Reprinted with permission from Schantz, J., Brandwood, A., Hutmacher, D.W., Khor, H.L., Bittner, K., 2005. Osteogenic differentiation of mesenchymal progenitor cells in computer designed fibrin-polymer-ceramic scaffolds manufactured by fused deposition modeling. J. Mater. Sci: Mater. Med. 16, 807–819. Copyright © 2005 Springer Science + Business Media, Inc.)*

microspheres. The scaffolds exhibited an interconnected porous structure that facilitated the attachment of osteoblastic SaOS-2 cells. The cells were remarkably viable, displaying a normal morphology and phenotype after 3 and 7 days of culture on all scaffolds, as seen in Fig. 1.4. A significant improvement in cell proliferation and alkaline

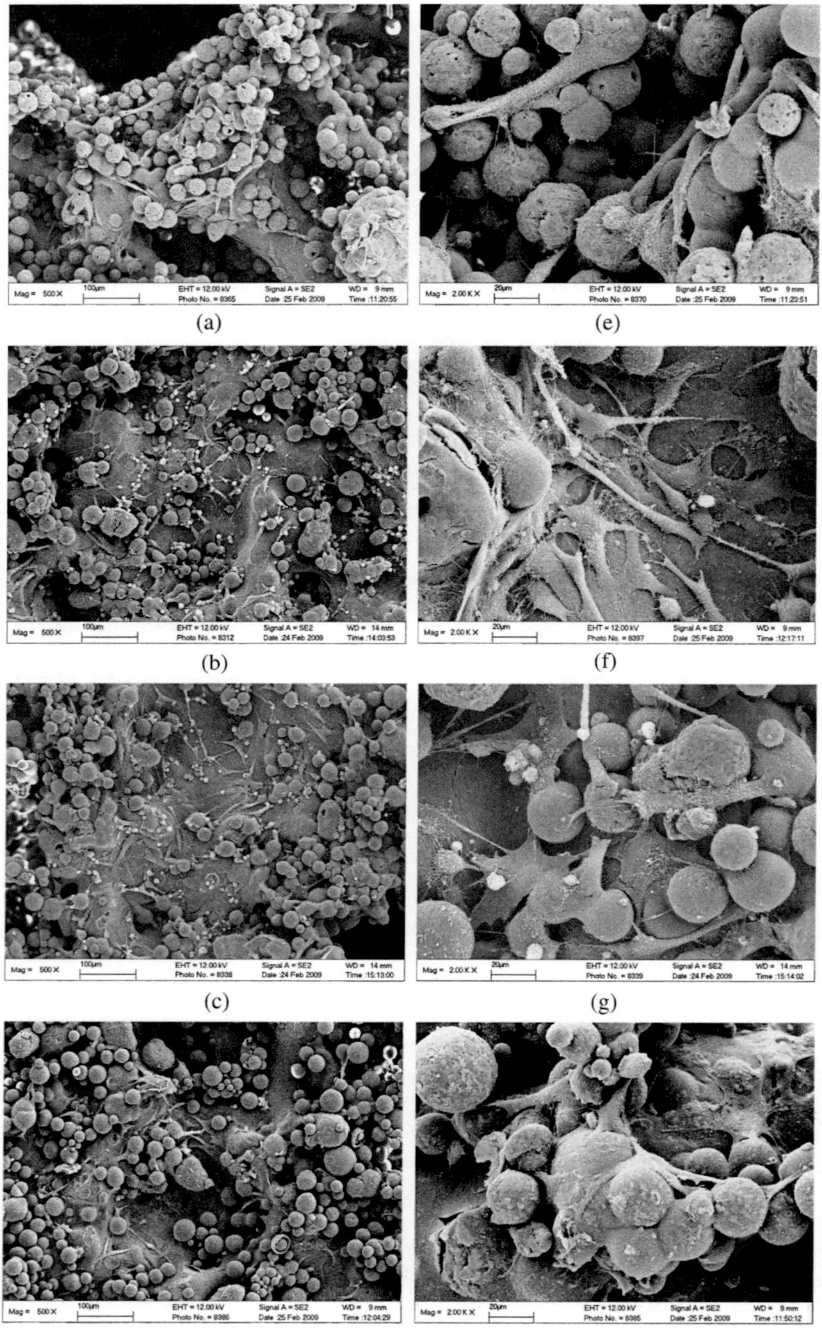

Fig. 1.4 SEM images of sintered scaffolds with a magnification of ×500. (A) PHBV; (B) Ca-P/PHBV; (C) PLLA; and (D) CHAp/PLLA. Morphology of SaOS-2 cells cultured on different scaffolds for 7 days with a magnification ×2000. (E) PHBV; (F) Ca-P/PHBV; (G) PLLA; and (H) CHAp/PLLA. *(Reprinted with permission from Duan, B., Wang, M., Zhou, W.Y., Cheung, W.L., Li, Z.Y., Lu, W.W., 2010. Three-dimensional nanocomposite scaffolds fabricated via selective laser sintering for bone tissue engineering. Acta Biomater. 6, 4495–4505. Copyright © 2010 Acta Materialia Inc. Published by Elsevier Ltd.)*

phosphatase activity was observed for the Ca-P/PHBV scaffolds, whereas the CHAp/PLLA nanocomposite scaffolds exhibited a similar level of cell response compared with PLLA polymer scaffolds. Hence, SLS-assisted development of nanocomposite scaffolds can not only extend a biomimetic environment for osteoblastic cell attachment, but also facilitate cell proliferation and differentiation that can be promising for bone tissue engineering applications.

1.6 Stereolithography

In SL, light is used for crosslinking polymeric materials to develop geometrically patterned layers of a 3D construct. A laser and a directed mirror array are employed for projecting patterned light onto the surface of a resin-containing vat, followed by curing of the resin. SL is advantageous as it offers rapid fabrication of high resolution constructs from which the uncured resin is removed. SL provides an effective and precise reconstruction of tissue morphology which is ideal for designing various biomimetic and bioactive nanomaterial scaffolds. Fig. 1.5 illustrates 3D-printed structures made out of a biodegradable UV-cured resin fabricated via SL. The biomaterial was composed of commercial polyurethane resin as an oligomer, trimethylolpropane trimethacrylate (TEGDMA) as a reactive diluent, and phenylbis (2,4,6-trimethylbenzoyl)-phosphine oxide (Irgacure 819) as a photoinitiator. The 3D-printed structures exhibited a tensile strength of 68 MPa. Further, the flexural strength and modulus can reach 115 MPa and 5.8 GPa, respectively. Additionally, graphene-reinforced nanocomposites were fabricated using a solvent-free method that could be molded into porous bone structures (a jawbone with a square architecture and a sternum with a round architecture) and a gyroid scaffold for bone tissue engineering (Feng et al., 2019).

1.7 3D printing for complex tissue and organ regeneration

Recent advances have enabled 3D bioprinting to engineer living organs, which is a comprehensive and integrative approach for the precise positioning of multiple cell types with high density to mimic their natural counterparts. A successful clinical implant facilitates the growth and development of functional complex tissues with appropriate vasculature and neural networks. The bioprinting techniques mentioned in the earlier section have the potential to fabricate patient-specific complex structures. The success rate of complex tissue/organ bioprinting depends on three important parameters.

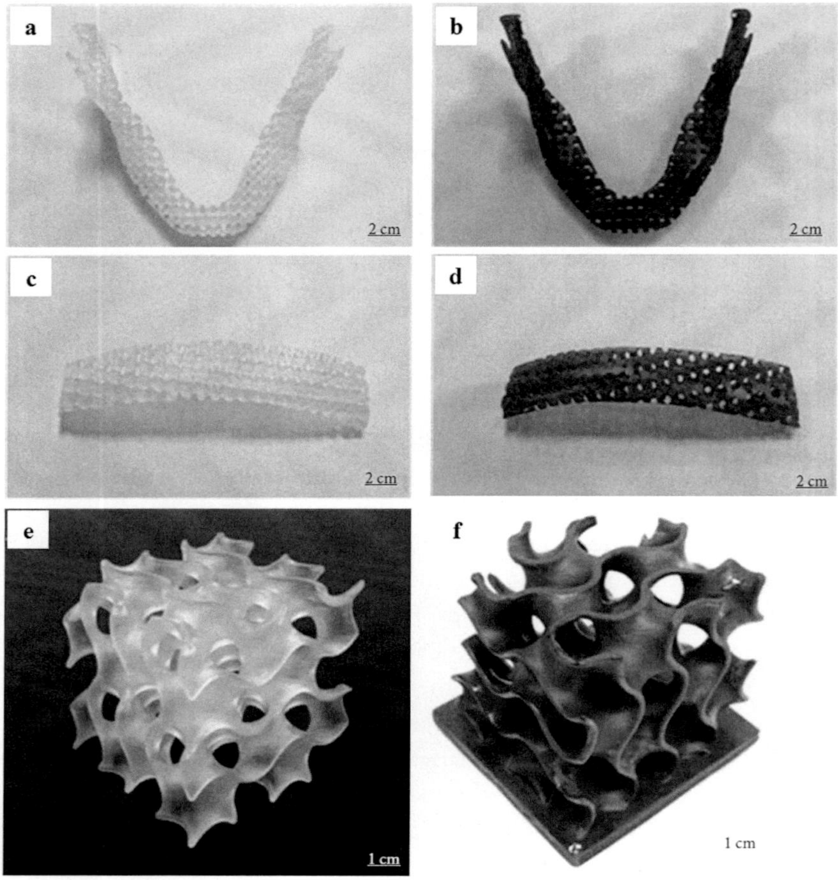

Fig. 1.5 Images of (A) pure UV-cured resin and (B) graphene-reinforced nanocomposite jawbone with a square architecture; (C) pure UV-cured resin and (D) graphene-reinforced nanocomposite sternum with a round architecture; (E) pure UV-cured resin; and (F) graphene-reinforced nanocomposite gyroid scaffold for bone tissue engineering. *(Reprinted from Feng, Z., Li, Y., Hao, L., Yang, Y., Tang, T., Tang, D., Xiong, W., 2019. Graphene-reinforced biodegradable resin composites for stereolithographic 3D printing of bone structure scaffolds. J. Nanomater. 2019, Article ID 9710264.)*

First, cell viability needs to be taken into account which is majorly affected by the time of the printing process. A prolong printing technique can severely compromise the viability of fragile cells. Second is mass transport and mechanical stimulation, where the cells are directly encapsulated in the bioinks in the printing process or are postseeded onto the printed constructs. During this process, it is essential to supplement them with nutrients and oxygen, which will ensure not only viability but also the functionality of the cells when associated with the constructs. Third, construct maturation should ensure that the cells must be able to proliferate with appropriate cell-cell interactions, secrete their own matrix components, perform natural biological functions, and integrate into the host tissue (Cui et al., 2017). In this section, we present recent developments for complex tissue and organ bioprinting.

1.7.1 Bone

Bone with distinct hierarchical organizational levels is considered to be one of the most complex heterogeneous tissue with unique structural and mechanical properties. Continuous remodeling makes bone a dynamic structure under various physiological conditions. Bone is highly vascularized as the transverse channel connects it to blood vessels in the periosteum. Migration of MSCs to the site of repair followed by osteogenic differentiation and osseointegration are crucial for bone healing. It is important to note that biomolecules are released from the ECM, which leads to remodeling during bone regeneration. In view of this background, structural, and functional details should be carefully considered while fabricating 3D-bioprinted bone-biomimetic constructs (Ashammakhi et al., 2019).

Kang et al. (2016) reported an integrated tissue-organ printer (ITOP) that could fabricate stable, human-scale tissue constructs of any shape. Cell-laden hydrogels mixed with biodegradable polymers were printed in integrated patterns on sacrificial hydrogels, which offer better mechanical stability. The efficient diffusion of nutrients to the printed cells was assured by rational incorporation of microchannels into the tissue constructs. An engineered mandible fragment with identical size and shape to the human counterpart was fabricated for facial reconstruction after traumatic injury as depicted in Fig. 1.6. Mandible bone defects have an arbitrary shape. Initially, data from computed tomography (CT) scan of a human mandible defect in combination with Mimics software was used to produce a computer-aided design (CAD) model of the portion with the defect, with dimensions of 3.6 cm × 3.0 cm × 1.6 cm (Fig. 1.6A). Human amniotic fluid-derived stem cells (hAFSCs) were selected for bioprinting, which shows an ability to differentiate into osteogenic lineages in appropriate media. The dispensing paths of a cell-laden hydrogel, a mixture of PCL and tricalcium phosphate (TCP), and Pluronic F127 was determined (Fig. 1.6B). PCL/TCP and hAFSCs mixed with the composite hydrogel were then printed in a type I pattern with a Pluronic F127 temporary support as illustrated in Fig. 1.6C. Interestingly, cell viability was found to be almost 91% after one day in the

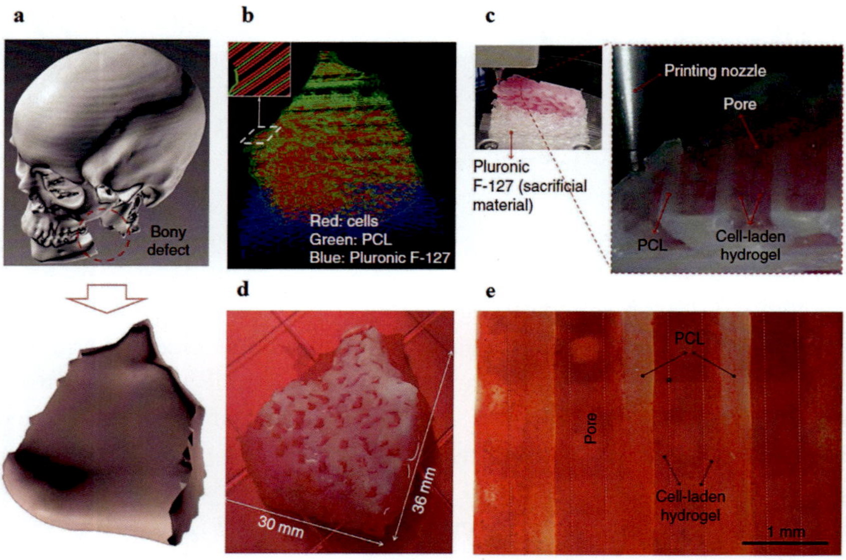

Fig. 1.6 Mandible bone reconstruction. (A) A 3D CAD model recognized a mandible bony defect from human CT image data. (B) A visualized motion program was generated to construct a 3D architecture of the mandible bone defect using CAM software developed by our laboratory. Lines of green, blue, and red colors indicate the dispensing paths of PCL, Pluronic F-127 and cell-laden hydrogel, respectively. (C) A 3D printing process using the integrated organ printing system. The image shows patterning of a layer of the construct. (D) Photograph of the 3D-printed mandible bone defect construct, which was cultured in osteogenic medium for 28 d. (E) Osteogenic differentiation of hAFSCs in the printed construct was confirmed by Alizarin Red S staining, indicating calcium deposition. *(Reprinted with permission from Kang, HW., Lee, S.J., Ko, I.K., Kengla, C., Yoo, J.J., Atala, A., 2016. A 3D bioprinting system to produce human-scale tissue constructs with structural integrity. Nat. Biotechnol. 34, 312–319. Copyright © 2016, Nature Publishing Group, a division of Macmillan Publishers Limited. All Rights Reserved.)*

3D-printed bone structures. Superior osteogenic differentiation was observed on the 28th day as seen in Fig. 1.6D that also exhibited calcium deposition in the hAFSC-laden hydrogel after Alizarin Red S staining as observed in Fig. 1.6E.

Another study demonstrated the maturation of the bioprinted bone using an in vivo calvarial bone reconstruction model (Kang et al., 2016). Like an earlier case, initially, rat calvarial bone constructs were fabricated in a circular shape (8-mm diameter × 1.2-mm thickness) with hAFSCs. The constructs were then cultured in osteogenic media for 10 days followed by implantation in a calvarial bone defect region of Sprague Dawley rats. After 5 months newly formed vascularized bone tissue were observed throughout the implants, including the central portion, with no sign of necrosis. Mature bone (red) and osteoid (blue) formation was indicated on modified Tetrachrome staining while large blood vessel formation within newly formed bone tissue throughout the bioprinted bone constructs, including the central portion was demonstrated by Von Willebrand factor (vWF) immunostaining.

Byambaa et al. (2017) reported an extrusion-based direct-writing bioprinting strategy for the fabrication of microstructured bone-like tissue constructs containing a perfusable vascular lumen. Perfusable blood vessels inside the bioprinted construct were created by printing a central cylinder with a 5% gelatin methacryloyl (GelMA) hydrogel at low methacryloyl substitution (GelMALOW). Further, cell-laden cylinder elements made of a GelMA hydrogel loaded with silicate nanoplatelets was developed for the induction of osteogenesis, as seen in Fig. 1.7. Initially, individual rods with desired chemical and physical properties were fabricated, which were then integrated to build large and complex architectures with specific microniches. The cylinders then collectively formed pyramidal constructs which were composed of 28 rods. A fluorescent dye, sulforhodamine 101 (Texas Red) cadaverine, was incorporated within the gel. 3D-printed rods with four different compositions (in terms of GelMA mass fraction, cell-laden composition, silicate nanoplatelets concentration, and VEGF-content) were used to fabricate bone tissue constructs with a specific and predefined architecture. The HUVECs and hMSCs loaded into the internal cylinder could migrate to and proliferate on the inner surface of this channel while the perfusable channel itself functions as a central blood vessel in a cell-laden construct. Interestingly, silicate nanoplatelets in the outer layers of the construct and the sustained perfusion of the osteogenic medium triggered the differentiation of the encapsulated hMSCs into bone tissue while the VEGF gradient provided the ideal chemical microenvironment for osteogenic differentiation and/or vascularization.

1.7.2 Cartilage and osteochondral tissue

ITOP was also reported to be efficient at fabricating cartilage tissue constructs using ear cartilage reconstruction that was comprised of a complex shape identical to human-sized external ears (Kang et al., 2016). The framework of an auricle consisting of a single piece of cartilage with a complicated geometry of ridges was initially designed using a CT image of an ear. Further, the motion program was developed to print a chondrocyte-laden hydrogel, PCL and Pluronic F-127. The source of the cells used for

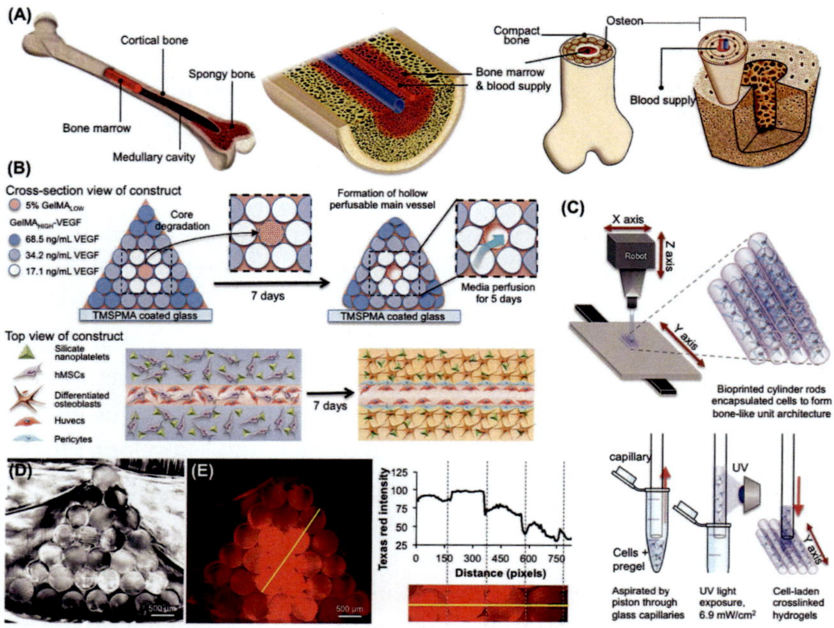

Fig. 1.7 Fabrication of a bone mimetic 3D architecture containing osteogenic and vasculogenic niches. (A) Schematic illustration of a complex bone tissue structure. (B) Illustration of the bioprinting strategy for fabricating a complex bone tissue architecture. A perfusable vascular lumen lined with HUVECs that can be fabricated within a pyramidal bioprinted construct by arranging individual rods of VEGF-functionalized GelMA bioinks with different mechanical strength. The hMSCs-laden three outer layers of cylinders were loaded with silicate nanoparticles to induce osteogenic differentiation of hMSCs into bone tissue. VEGF was covalently conjugated into the three outer layers of the cylindrical hydrogels. The concentrations of conjugated VEGF were determined with ELISA to be 17.1, 34.2, and 68.5 ng mL^{-1}. (C) A scheme of the 3D printing procedure of independent cell-laden cylinders using an automatized and computer-controlled bioprinter. (D) Cross-section image of the pyramidal bioprinted construct. (E) Chemical conjugation of a gradient sulforhodamine 101 (Texas Red) cadaverine onto –COOH-modified GelMA-bioprinted fibers. The fluorescence intensity was directly proportional to the conjugated amount of the fluorescent dye. *(Reprinted with permission from Byambaa, B., Annabi, N., Yue, K., Santiago, G.T., Alvarez, M.M., Jia, W., Kazemzadeh-Narbat, M., Shin, S.R., Tamayol, A., Khademhosseini, A., 2017. Bioprinted osteogenic and vasculogenic patterns for engineering 3D bone tissue. Adv. Healthcare Mater. 6, 1,700,015. Copyright © 2017 WILEY-VCH Verlag GmbH & Co. KGaA, Weinheim.)*

this osteochondral bioprinting was from rabbit ear chondrocytes. After mixing the cells with the composite hydrogel, human ear-shaped cartilage constructs were bioprinted with dimensions of 3.2 cm × 1.6 cm × 0.9 cm. Significantly high cell viability of 91% ± 8% was noted on day 1 after printing while after 5 weeks, the constructs exhibited the production of a new cartilaginous matrix. The microchannels in the constructs facilitated the formation of a new viable cartilaginous matrix throughout the entire ear constructs. The cells in the newly formed tissues exhibited a morphological identity similar to native ear cartilage that was characterized by cells located within typical chondrocyte lacunae, surrounded by a cartilaginous matrix.

In vivo maturation properties of the printed ear constructs were checked by implanting them in the dorsal subcutaneous space of athymic mice that were retrieved after 1 and 2 months. Interestingly, the shape of the 3D-printed constructs was well maintained, with notable cartilage formation. High glycosaminoglycan (GAG) content, vascularization, endothelial cell marker expression, and superior biomechanical properties were identical to the native rabbit ear cartilage.

3D-printed osteochondral tissue can be a powerful regenerative therapy as the osteochondral interface of an arthritic joint is notoriously difficult to repair due to its extremely poor regenerative capacity and complex stratified architecture. Castro et al. (2015) generated 3D printing biomimetic nanocomposite scaffolds for improved osteochondral tissue regeneration. This was achieved by developing two biologically inspired nanomaterials comprised of (1) osteoconductive nanocrystalline hydroxyapatite (nHA) (primary inorganic component of bone) and (2) core-shell poly(lactic-*co*-glycolic) acid (PLGA) nanospheres encapsulated with chondrogenic transforming growth-factor β1 (TGF-β1) for sustained delivery. With the help of a novel table-top stereolithography 3D printer and the nano-ink (i.e., nHA + nanosphere + hydrogel), a porous and highly interconnected osteochondral scaffold with hierarchical nano-to-micro structure and spatiotemporal bioactive factor gradients was generated. This novel osteochondral scaffold remarkably facilitated the adhesion, proliferation, and osteochondral differentiation of human bone marrow-derived MSCs.

1.7.3 Neural tissue

Biomaterial inks composed of hydrogels, thermoplastic, and thermoset polyesters and composite are used for the fabrication of nerve conduits using 3D bioprinting for perfect repair or replacement of a damaged peripheral nerve which was otherwise a formidable clinical challenge. Table 1.1 presents various 3D-printed scaffolds for neural tissue engineering that provided transitional three-dimensional support for cell attachment, migration, proliferation, as well as assist the nerve reconstruction in long distance nerve defects, which can reach a length of 4 cm or even longer (Yu et al., 2020). Incorporation of carbon nanotubes (CNTs) in the scaffolds not only

Table 1.1 Bioprinted cells and bioactive molecules for nerve tissue engineering

Cell	Bioactive molecule	Material	Printing resolution	Cell density (cells/mL)	Cell viability	Printing method	Application
Schwann cells	–	Alginate/HA	353 ± 7 μm	5.2×10^5	92.3%	Bioplotting	Good structural integrity and long-term cell viability
PC12 cell; RSC96 cell	NGF	GelMA/chitosan	545 ± 61 μm	–	97.1% ± 3.69%	Bioplotting	Enhance 3D neurite outgrowth and elongation
Schwann cells; NG108–15 cells	–	–	60 μm	2×10^5	89%–92%; 86%–96%	Inkjet	Neurite outgrows faster and earlier
Schwann cells	–	Gelatin/sodium alginate	160 μm	2×10^6	91.87% ± 0.55%	Extrusion	Improve cell adhesion and related factor expression
NSCs	–	PU hydrogel	250 μm	4×10^6	~80%	FDM	Promote the recovery of traumatic brain injury in zebrafish
NSCs	VEGF	Collagen hydrogel/fibroin Gel	700 μm	1×10^6	93.23% ± 3.77%	Inkjet	Support cellular proliferation and migration over time
Human fibroblasts	Forkhead box D3	PU hydrogel	410 μm	1×10^6	65%	Extrusion	Human fibroblasts could be reprogrammed into neural crest stem-like cells
NSCs	–	Graphene/PU hydrogel	410 μm	4×10^6	> 60%	Extrusion	NSCs had a tendency to differentiate toward glial and neuronal lineages
iPSCs	–	GelMA/gelatin/fibroin gel	200 μm	1×10^7	> 75%	Extrusion	Differentiate and extend axons throughout microscale scaffold channels
GMSCs	–	–	400–500 μm	–	~90%	Kenzan method	Promote rat facial nerve regeneration

Reprinted from Yu, X., Zhang, T., Li, Y., 2020. 3D printing and bioprinting nerve conduits for neural tissue engineering. Polymers 12, 1637. (Open Access).

modify their surface properties but also enhance the interaction between neural cells and biomaterials. CNTs promote superior electrical conductivity and provide a nanoscale architecture identical to the natural neural environment.

Lee et al. (2018) reported amine functionalized multiwalled carbon nanotubes (MWCNTs) incorporated in poly(ethylene glycol) diacrylate (PEGDA) polymer hydrogels for enhancing electrical properties as well as nanofeatures on the surface of the neural scaffold. The tunable porous structure of the scaffolds was attributed to the stereolithography 3D printing. On incorporation of 0.1% MWCNT into the scaffolds, the average total neurite length significantly increased by 113% over the control scaffold. The NE-4C cell lines efficiently differentiated into neurons with appropriate inducing factors after 4 days of culture associated with the 3D bioprinted neural scaffolds. Furthermore, a biphasic pulse stimulation with a 500 μA current promoted neuronal maturity as quantified through protein expression.

Zhang et al. (2018) reported the promise of 3D bioprinted scaffold-free neural constructs using human gingiva-derived mesenchymal stem cells (GMSCs) to bridge facial nerve defects in rats. Initially, GMSCs spheroids were collected and assembled into a 9×9 mm square needle-array 3.2 mm in length on each side in the software designed configuration and were allowed to fuse into 3D-tubular structures as illustrated in Fig. 1.8. Then, these scaffold-free neural constructs were allowed to mature in a bioreactor for 7–10 days, and a stable, suturable 3D-nerve construct with a diameter of 2.0 mm was generated as seen in Fig. 1.8A. The aligned nerve like structures appeared that expressed both the neuronal marker β-tubulin III and Schwann cell marker S-100β as observed in Fig. 1.8B and C. The 3D-bioprinted neural grafts were further transplanted into segmental defects of the buccal branch (BB) of the facial nerve of rats. Significant levels of nerve remodeling and regeneration were observed with higher facial palsy scores at 7 weeks after transplantation. Further, nerve stimulation in the vibrissa muscles indicated effective compound muscle action potential (CAMP) recovery 12 weeks after transplantation.

1.7.4 Vascular tissue

The vascular system plays a vital role for connecting all parts of the body and transport of nutrients, respiratory gases, waste materials, and hormones. However, malfunction of the vascular system is associated with tissue overgrowth (e.g., angiogenesis in cancer) as well as cell death and necrosis. Also, vascular abnormalities are often observed in age-related cardiovascular, neurovascular, and musculoskeletal diseases.

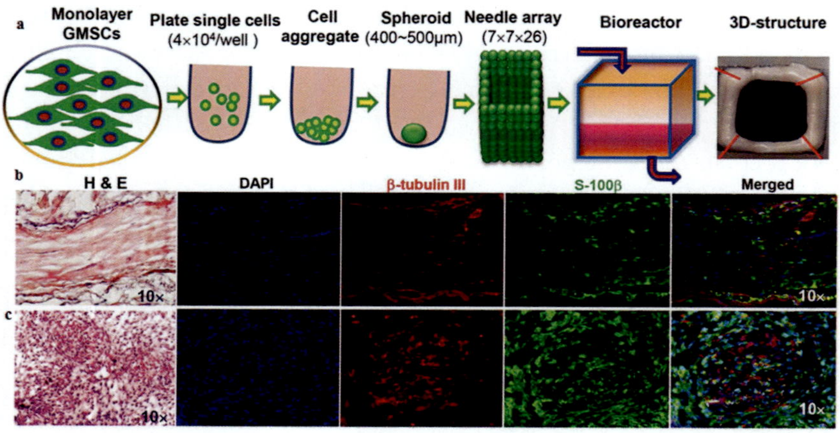

Fig. 1.8 3D bioprinting scaffold-free nerve constructs from GMSC spheroids. (A) Procedures for 3D bioprinting scaffold-free nerve constructs from GMSC spheroids. (B) Longitudinal section of 3D bioprinted nerve constructs. H&E staining (the left panel); immunofluorescence staining with β-tubulin III and S-100β primary antibodies. (C) Transverse section of 3D bioprinted nerve constructs. H&E staining (the left panel); immunofluorescence staining with β-tubulin III and S-100β primary antibodies. Cell nuclei were counterstained by DAPI (blue). Scale bars: 200 μm. Data are representative of two independent experiments. *(Reprinted with permission from Zhang, Q., Nguyen, P.D., Shi, S., Burrell, J.C., Cullen, D.K., Le, A.D., 2018. 3D bio-printed scaffold-free nerve constructs with human gingiva derived mesenchymal stem cells promote rat facial nerve regeneration. Sci. Rep. 8, 6634. Copyright © 2018.)*

Lee et al. (2014) created a functional in vitro vascular channel with perfused open lumens using only cells and biological matrices employing 3D bioprinting. The fabricated vasculature exhibited an intact, confluent endothelium lining, presenting barrier function for both plasma protein and high molecular weight dextran molecule. The fluidic vascular channel supported the viability of the tissue up to 5 mm in distance at 5 million cells/mL density under physiological flow conditions. Significantly, under static-cultured conditions, vascular channels showed active angiogenic sprouting from the vessel surface. However, this phenomenon was inhibited under steady physiological flow.

In another study, Kolesky et al. (2016) reported a cell-laden 3D bioprinting technique to develop vascularized tissues that exceeded 1 cm in thickness and can be perfused on a chip for long time periods (> 6 weeks). In this approach, the parenchyma, stroma, and endothelium were integrated into a single thick tissue by co-printing multiple inks composed of human mesenchymal stem cells (hMSCs) and human neonatal dermal fibroblasts (hNDFs) within a customized extracellular matrix (gelatin-fibrin) alongside the embedded vasculature. Further, the structure was subsequently lined with human umbilical vein endothelial cells (HUVECs). Under a 3D culture condition, the gelatin-fibrin matrix supported HUVECs, hNDFs, and hMSCs where the endothelial cells expressed vascular endothelial-cadherin (VE-Cad). HNDFs and hMSCs showed superior proliferation that facilitated them to spread on this matrix surface in bulk. High-printed cell viability (95%) was noticed that was dependent on gelatin processing. A stable vasculature was observed when a simple tissue construct composed of two parallel channels embedded within a fibroblast cell-laden matrix was printed as depicted in Fig. 1.9. The channels were lined with HUVECs, perfused with growth media that resulted in the formation of a confluent monolayer that lined each blood vessel as observed in Fig. 1.9A. After 6 weeks of active perfusion, the endothelial cells not only maintained their phenotype but also expressed specific markers such as CD31, von Willebrand factor (vWF), and VE-Cad as seen in Fig. 1.9B and C. Lumen formation was also observed and it was confirmed that the perfusable vasculature critically supported living tissues thicker than 1 mm over long time periods.

1.7.5 Organs

Printing surgical models for preoperative planning and constructing personalized prostheses for patients have become much more convenient due to advancements in 3D printing technologies. However, the ultimate goal is to develop functional human organs and tissues. This can address the challenges of organ transplantation due to the lack of organ donors and life-long immunosuppression. In due course, the first synthetic trachea, and other human tissues were successfully printed including skin, liver, neuronal tissue, muscle-tendon units, and cartilage. Also, living heart valves were fabricated using this bioprinting technology. 3D-printed aortic sleeves took 9 h to print 6.3-cm long and 2-mm thick graft at a reduced cost compared with commercially available stents. Researchers from the University of Michigan, USA, successfully implanted a bioresorbable 3D printed tracheal splint fabricated using microextrusion bioprinting in a child with severe tracheobronchomalacia. Japan has introduced custom-made facial bones that were manufactured using ink-jet 3D printing. This is more effective care in maxillofacial surgery in patients with mandibular hypoplasia, micrognathia, or microsomia. In the Netherlands, an entire jaw and skull reconstruction was conducted using tailor-made 3D-printed implants fabricated by the Dutch company Xiloc Medical B.V. Recently, a 3D-printed vertebral body C2 was implanted in a 12-year old boy after the surgical removal of a rare

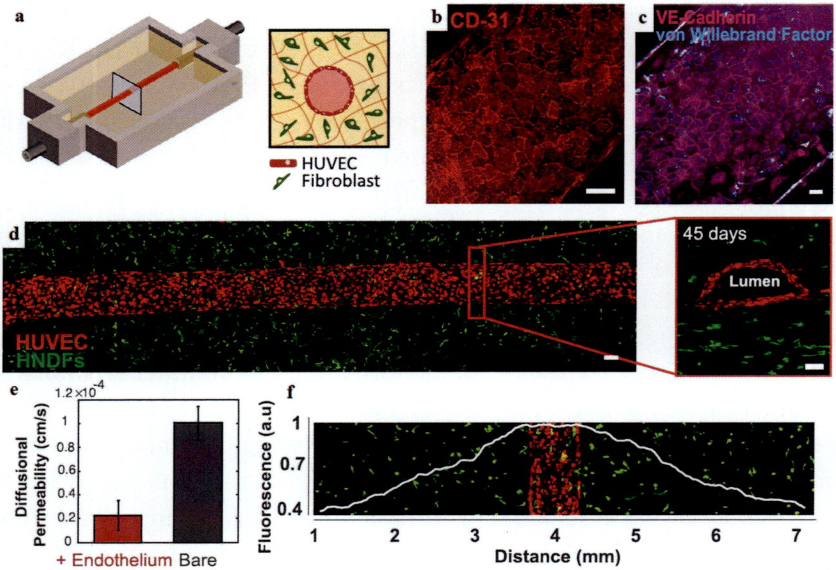

Fig. 1.9 Three-dimensional vascularized tissues remain stable during long-term perfusion. (A) Schematic depicting a single HUVEC-lined vascular channel supporting a fibroblast cell-laden matrix and housed within a 3D perfusion chip. (B, C) Confocal microscopy image of the vascular network after 42 d, CD-31 (red), vWF (blue), and VE-Cadherin (magenta). (Scale bars: 100 μm). (D) Long-term perfusion of HUVEC-lined (red) vascular network supporting an HNDF laden (green) matrix shown by top-down (left) and cross-sectional confocal microscopy at 45 d (Right). (Scale bar: 100 μm). (E) Quantification of barrier properties imparted by the endothelial lining of channels, demonstrated by reduced diffusional permeability of FITC-dextran. (F) GFP-HNDF distribution within the 3D matrix shown by fluorescent intensity as a function of distance from the vasculature. *(Reprinted with permission from Kolesky, D.B., Homan, K.A., Skylar-Scott, M.A., Lewis, J.A., 2016. Three-dimensional bioprinting of thick vascularized tissues. PNAS. 113(12), 3179–3184.)*

musculoskeletal malignant neoplasm Ewing's sarcoma. This proved to be a life-saving cervical spine reconstruction strategy. In view of the background, 3D-printed organs with structural and functional identity with the native organs can prove to be a boon toward personalized precision surgical strategy (Radenkovic et al., 2016).

1.8 4D printing

An advanced next-generation bioprinting technique, termed 4D printing, allows for the structural and/or functional reprogramming of printed scaffolds or implants under external stimuli. Compared with conventional bioprinting, 4D printing is ideal for fabricating dynamic structures using nanobiomaterials for biomedical applications.

Cui et al. (2019) reported a 4D-printed brain model using a novel near-infrared (NIR) light responsive nanocomposite with dynamic and remote-controlled transforming properties. The shape memory polymers (SMP) used for bioprinting included a rigid epoxy monomer (bisphenol A diglycidyl ether, BDE), an aliphatic diamine crosslinker [poly(propylene glycol) bis(2-aminopropyl) ether, PBE], and a crosslinking modulator (decylamine, DA). Further, graphene nanoplatelets (6–8 nm thick × 5 μm wide) were incorporated into an epoxy ink system that remarkably increased the tensile modulus of the nanocomposites indicating reinforcement effects. Parameters like mechanical stirring, sonication time, storage time, and graphene concentration may also influence the dispersion and reaggregation of graphene in epoxy mixtures. The NIR-responsive photothermal property of the nanocomposites was attributed to the graphene content even at a lower concentration (0.5%),

A 4D-printed brain model was fabricated using NE-4C neural stem cells (NSCs) for the neural tissue construct. For this, initially a 3D tissue construct was temporarily fixed to a flat shape followed by seeding of the NSCs on the flat surface of the construct which was eventually cultured for several days. Superior neural differentiation was observed in the cell-laden construct after 2 weeks which was associated with the expression of neuron-specific Class III β-tubulin (TuJ1) and microtubule-associated protein 2 (MAP2), and some astrocytes detected by glial fibrillary acidic protein (GFAP). Hence, 4D printing of neural scaffolds can have potential biomedical applications as neurodegenerative therapeutics. Although the currently popular forms of 4D printing are polyjet printing and syringe printing, all other 3D printing platforms definitely have strong potential to contribute to the future of 4D printing (Miao et al., 2017).

1.9 Conclusion and future perspectives

The emergence of 3D printing techniques has revolutionized the healthcare sector. A wide range of bioprinting modalities and biocompatible nanomaterials can be combined to make an appropriate strategy suitable for the desired application. A broad spectrum of biomaterials ranging from metals and metallic alloys to ceramics and polymers can be used in bioinks in combination with biological components such as cells, proteins, and growth factors.

Although 3D printing has shown promising applications in healthcare, it is still in its infancy owing to certain challenges. After grafting of 3D-printed constructs in the body, limited vascularization is a serious drawback. Hence, a rational selection of the graft position in close proximity to existing blood vessels may prove to be beneficial. More porous bioprinted constructs are more useful and can be connected by microvascular surgery to facilitate the steady supply of nutrients to the embedded cells. Further, 3D printing can have a most promising outcome for the surgical correction of cartilage-associated defects as cartilage is an histologically simple and avascular tissue.

3D-printed complex vasculature structurally and functionally identical to native blood vessels undoubtedly has the potential to revolutionize healthcare. However, organ-specific 3D printing of a vascular network is still at the stage of prototyping and validation. Nanotechnology along with computational modeling and chemical engineering may collectively form a multidisciplinary approach for developing personalized 3D printed synthetic organs at an affordable cost. Finally, the chemical properties of the biomaterial, biocompatibility of the bioink, durability of the constructs, risk of implant failure, leaching or degradation of the implanted constructs, and overall safety behind using a bioprinted implant must be carefully investigated before introducing 3D-printed composites in patients.

Acknowledgments

Dr. Sougata Ghosh acknowledges the Department of Science and Technology (DST), Ministry of Science and Technology, Government of India and Jawaharlal Nehru Centre for Advanced Scientific Research, India, for funding under the Postdoctoral Overseas Fellowship in Nano Science and Technology (Ref. JNC/AO/A.0610.1(4) 2019-2260 dated August 19, 2019). Dr. Ebrahim Mostafavi would like to acknowledge the support from the National Institute of Biomedical Imaging and Bioengineering (5T32EB009035).

References

Ashammakhi, N., Hasan, A., Kaarela, O., Byambaa, B., Sheikhi, A., Gaharwar, A.K., Khademhosseini, A., 2019. Advancing frontiers in bone bioprinting. Adv. Healthcare Mater. 8, 1801048.

Byambaa, B., Annabi, N., Yue, K., Santiago, G.T., Alvarez, M.M., Jia, W., Kazemzadeh-Narbat, M., Shin, S.R., Tamayol, A., Khademhosseini, A., 2017. Bioprinted osteogenic and vasculogenic patterns for engineering 3D bone tissue. Adv. Healthcare Mater. 6, 1700015.

Castro, N.J., O'Brien, J., Zhang, L.G., 2015. Integrating biologically inspired nanomaterials and table-top stereolithography for 3D printed biomimetic osteochondral scaffolds. Nanoscale 7, 14010–14022.

Cui, H., Nowicki, M., Fisher, J.P., Zhang, L.G., 2017. 3D bioprinting for organ regeneration. Adv. Healthcare Mater. 6, 1601118.

Cui, H., Miao, S., Esworthy, T., Lee, S.J., Zhou, X., Hann, S.Y., Webster, T.J., Harris, B.T., Zhang, L.G., 2019. A novel near-infrared light responsive 4D printed nanoarchitecture with dynamically and remotely controllable transformation. Nano Res. 12, 1381–1388.

Duan, B., Wang, M., Zhou, W.Y., Cheung, W.L., Li, Z.Y., Lu, W.W., 2010. Three-dimensional nanocomposite scaffolds fabricated via selective laser sintering for bone tissue engineering. Acta Biomater. 6, 4495–4505.

Duan, B., Kapetanovic, E., Hockaday, L.A., Butcher, J.T., 2014. Three-dimensional printed trileaflet valve conduits using biological hydrogels and human valve interstitial cells. Acta Biomater. 10, 1836–1846.

Feng, Z., Li, Y., Hao, L., Yang, Y., Tang, T., Tang, D., Xiong, W., 2019. Graphene-reinforced biodegradable resin composites for stereolithographic 3D printing of bone structure scaffolds. J. Nanomater. Article ID 9710264.

Ghosh, S., 2019. Mesoporous silica based nano drug delivery system synthesis, characterization and applications. In: Mohapatra, S.S., Ranjan, S., Dasgupta, N., Mishra, R.K., Thomas, S. (Eds.), Nanocarriers for Drug Delivery. Elsevier Inc., Amsterdam, Netherlands, pp. 285–317.

Ghosh, S., Sanghavi, S., Sancheti, P., 2018. Metallic biomaterial for bone support and replacement. In: Balakrishnan, P., Sreekala, M.S., Thomas, S. (Eds.), Fundamental Biomaterials: Metals. vol. 2. Woodhead Publishing Series in Biomaterials, Woodhead Publishing, pp. 139–165.

Kale, S.N., Kitture, R., Ghosh, S., Chopade, B.A., Yakhmi, J.V., 2017. Nanomaterials as enhanced antimicrobial agents/activity enhancer for transdermal applications: a review. In: Grumezescu, A.M. (Ed.), Antimicrobial Architectonics from Synthesis to Applications. Elsevier Inc. Amsterdam, Netherlands, pp. 279–321.

Kang, H.W., Lee, S.J., Ko, I.K., Kengla, C., Yoo, J.J., Atala, A., 2016. A 3D bioprinting system to produce human-scale tissue constructs with structural integrity. Nat. Biotechnol. 34, 312–319.

Kim, J.D., Choi, J.S., Kim, B.S., Choi, Y.C., Cho, Y.W., 2010. Piezoelectric inkjet printing of polymers: stem cell patterning on polymer substrates. Polymer 51, 2147–2154.

Kolesky, D.B., Homan, K.A., Skylar-Scott, M.A., Lewis, J.A., 2016. Three-dimensional bioprinting of thick vascularized tissues. Proc. Natl. Acad. Sci. U. S. A. 113 (12), 3179–3184.

Lee, V.K., Kim, D.Y., Ngo, H., Lee, Y., Seo, L., Yoo, S.S., Vincent, P.A., Dai, G., 2014. Creating perfused functional vascular channels using 3D bio-printing technology. Biomaterials 35, 8092–8102.

Lee, S.J., Zhu, W., Nowicki, M., Lee, G., Heo, D.N., Kim, J., Zuo, Y.Y., Zhang, L.G., 2018. 3D printing nano conductive multi-walled carbon nanotube scaffolds for nerve regeneration. J. Neural Eng. 15, 016018.

Miao, S., Castro, N., Nowicki, M., Xia, L., Cui, H., Zhou, X., Zhu, W., Lee, S.J., Sarkar, K., Vozzi, G., Tabata, Y., Fisher, J., Zhang, L.G., 2017. 4D printing of polymeric materials for tissue and organ regeneration. Mater Today (Kidlington) 20 (10), 577–591.

O'Brien, C.M., Holmes, B., Faucett, S., Zhang, L.G., 2015. Three-dimensional printing of nanomaterial scaffolds for complex tissue regeneration. Tissue Eng. Part B Rev. 21 (1), 103–114.

Pati, F., Jang, J., Ha, D.H., Kim, S.W., Rhie, J.W., Shim, J.H., Kim, D.H., Cho, D.W., 2014. Printing three-dimensional tissue analogues with decellularized extracellular matrix bioink. Nat. Commun. 5, 3935.

Radenkovic, D., Solouk, A., Seifalian, A., 2016. Personalized development of human organs using 3D printing technology. Med. Hypotheses 87, 30–33.

Schantz, J., Brandwood, A., Hutmacher, D.W., Khor, H.L., Bittner, K., 2005. Osteogenic differentiation of mesenchymal progenitor cells in computer designed fibrin-polymer-ceramic scaffolds manufactured by fused deposition modeling. J. Mater. Sci. Mater. Med. 16, 807–819.

Wang, Y., Gao, M., Wang, D., Sun, L., Webster, T.J., 2020. Nanoscale 3D bioprinting for osseous tissue manufacturing. Int. J. Nanomedicine 15, 215–226.
Xie, Z., Gao, M., Lobo, A.O., Webster, T.J., 2020. 3D bioprinting in tissue engineering for medical applications: the classic and the hybrid. Polymers (Basel). 12 (8), 1717.
Yu, X., Zhang, T., Li, Y., 2020. 3D printing and bioprinting nerve conduits for neural tissue engineering. Polymers 12, 1637.
Zhang, Q., Nguyen, P.D., Shi, S., Burrell, J.C., Cullen, D.K., Le, A.D., 2018. 3D bio-printed scaffold-free nerve constructs with human gingiva derived mesenchymal stem cells promote rat facial nerve regeneration. Sci. Rep. 8, 6634.
Zhu, W., Webster, T.J., Zhang, L.G., 2018. How can 3D printing be a powerful tool in nanomedicine? Nanomedicine (Lond.) 13 (3), 251–253.

CHAPTER 2

Nanobiomaterials for drug delivery and theranostics

Aman Bajpai[a,*], Sopan Shinde[a,*], and Sudipta Basu[a]
[a]Discipline of Chemistry, Indian Institute of Technology (IIT) Gandhinagar, Palaj, Gujarat, India

2.1 Introduction

Since ancient time, there have been diverse medicinal traditions used by physicians worldwide. Over the generations, till the present day, these traditions have been significantly renovated to tackle diseases and illness. Although old traditions have been modified, nearly 25% of new bioactive compounds are derived from natural resources based on conventional knowledge and practices. In the recent years, natural products are widely screened for treating major life tethering diseases including Cancer, Diabetes, Neurodegenerative Disorders (Alzheimer's and Parkinson's diseases) and Human Immunodeficiency Virus (HIV). This is mainly because the natural products as drug candidates possess exceptional benefits, such as minimal toxicity and side effects, and desirable therapeutic potential. However, poor solubility, poor absorption in the body, in vivo stabilization, biocompatibility and a lack of selectivity eventually throttle the complete annihilation of the disease. Consequently, despite the success in preclinical studies, clinical trials of many of these drug candidates were terminated due lack of reaching the anticipated efficacy in patients.

To overcome these problems, the US Food and Drug Administration (FDA) in 2004 took an initiative to modernize the traditional drug development path to new medical products (Pene et al., 2009). Since then, substantial novel approaches have been developed to construct the sustained release drug formulations as the delivery systems for targeting specific body parts and improving drug efficacy. In modern medical practices, these innovative approaches take advantage of the distinctive characteristics of nanoscale biomaterials to accommodate the therapeutic drug and imaging agent in a single carrier of nanometer size utilized for imaging, diagnosis, drug delivery,

* These authors contributed equally.

Nanotechnology in Medicine and Biology
https://doi.org/10.1016/B978-0-12-819469-0.00002-2

and tissue regeneration. In this chapter, we discuss the development of nanoscale materials as the next-generation therapeutic for cancer treatment.

Cancer is the second major evolutionary health issue globally with inferior diagnosis and higher mortality rates. According to the GLOBOCAN 2018 statistics, this cancer burden was raised to 18.1 million new cases and 9.6 million deaths worldwide. Traditional chemotherapy approaches used to treat many cancers are limited by a lack of specificity leading to a low accumulation of the active drug to the tumor sites causing several off-target toxic effects. Advances in nanotechnology have brought multifunctional platforms for improved cancer diagnostic techniques to provide early detection attainment, target-specific drug delivery, therapy, and reducing the adverse off-target effect of the therapeutic drugs. Though significant progress has been made in the arena, several of those drug delivery systems are associated with undesirable side effects due to improper pharmacokinetics and pharmacodynamics that limit their effectiveness in the clinic.

In this chapter, we highlight the drug delivery and theranostic application of selective self-assembled and synthetic nanobiomaterials engineered from organic and inorganic moieties for cancer treatment. We further discuss the design principles, toxicity profiles, drug delivery, and therapeutic applications of the nanomaterials developed in the past two decades. Moreover, we extend our discussion toward the emerging approaches and challenges for the development of next-generation nanomaterials for improved therapeutic outcomes.

2.2 Design parameters of nanomedicine for drug delivery and theranostics

An essential aspect in nanomedicine development is controlled drug release at the site of action or disease site. The design and synthesis of nanovectors that can transport the drug selectively or specifically to a target zone is a complex process and influenced by various factors. All of these factors as listed in Fig. 2.1 essentially have to be balanced against each other. Therefore, to develop an ideal nanomedicine with desirable pharmaceutical significance (e.g., ease of administration and stability), an extensive understanding of biochemical interactions in the body from the beginning of the dose given until reaching the target site is crucial. There are some essential rationales that an ideal nanomedicine design must meet to exert its effective potential for clinical applications. These underlying rationale include the following (Soares et al., 2018): (1) knowledge of key components (of both

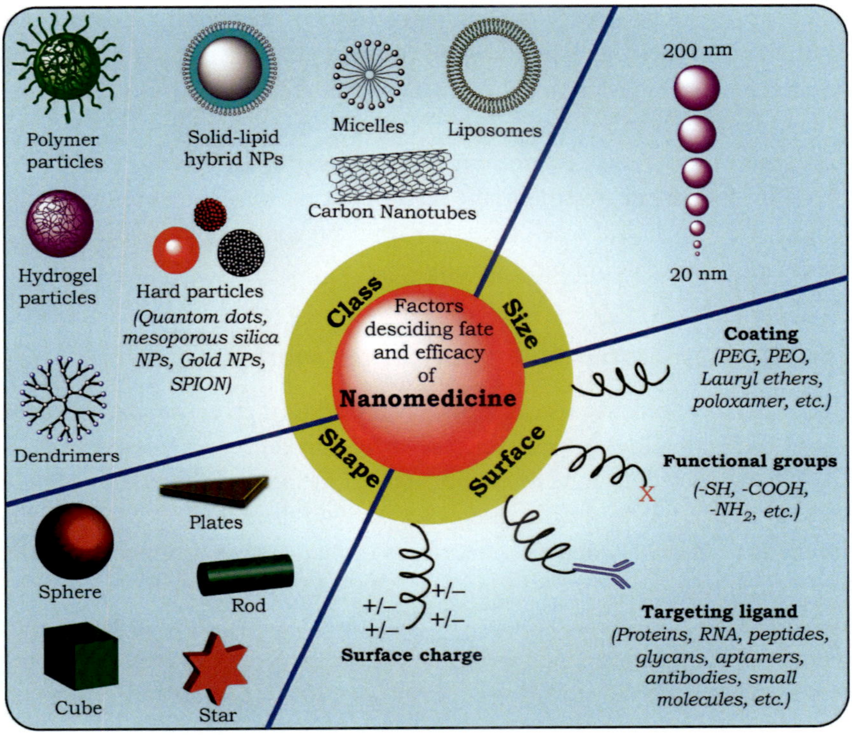

Fig. 2.1 Parameters deciding the fate and efficacy of nanomedicine used for cancer treatment.

the nanobiomaterial and target site) and understanding of their interactions; (2) identifying the key features and their relationship to performance; (3) proper pharmacokinetics (i.e., extended retention time in the blood and also in different body fluids), and pharmacodynamics (i.e., ability to accumulate cancerous tissue for an appropriate period after overcoming biological barriers); (4) worthy features such as safety, efficacy, and capability to produce a sterile form; and (5) acceptable pharmaceutical features (i.e., stability, storage, and ease of administration).

The major concern of nanomedicine is its accumulation in the tumor site without affecting the noncancerous tissue. An efficacy of nanomedicine depends on the biocompatibility of the material used in the preparation, the prolonged circulation period to recognize the cancer tissue and accumulate there, and finally it should be readily excretable from the body by the renal system. The shape, size, surface charge, and surface chemistry are the important parameters of the biomaterial-based drug delivery systems which decide their fate in the biological milieu (Toy et al., 2014). These parameters are variable depending on the type of cancer being treated and the therapeutic agents to be delivered. Once entered into the bloodstream, a nanomaterial will be recognized as a foreign body by the immune cells and may result in the multilevel immune defense against it (Zolnik et al., 2010). Therefore for cancer treatment, the nanomedicine should be engineered in such a form that it will reach the target after preventing or having minimal interactions with the immune system.

2.3 Targeted drug delivery for cancer therapy

In the early 20th century, German physician Paul Ehrlich envisioned the concept of drug targeting by proposing the "magic bullet" concept (Valent et al., 2016). The targeted drug delivery and targeted therapy are the two frequently used but unlike terms in drug discovery. Targeted drug delivery refers to the strategy that selectively delivers the drug to the target zone irrespective of the drug administration method (Torchilin, 2000). On the other hand, targeted cancer therapy refers to the treatment that uses an active drug to target specific proteins and genes which are actively responsible for the cancer cell proliferation, angiogenesis, and survival of tumor cells (Gerber, 2008; Mimeault et al., 2008; Strebhardt and Ullrich, 2008). Apparently, for targeted drug delivery traversing physiological barriers, we need different drug delivery systems as dependent on the drug administration route selected. Herein, we highlight the "passive" and "active" targeting mechanisms for intravenously administered nanomedicine for delivering anticancer therapeutic agents.

2.3.1 Passive targeting

In passive targeting, nanocarriers are preferentially accumulated at tumor affected areas through fenestrated capillaries into the tumor interstitium and cells by passive diffusion as depicted in Fig. 2.2. This is due to an enhanced permeability and retention (EPR) effect caused by physiological changes in the tumor microenvironment. The EPR effect is the primary gold standard for using nanoparticles in cancer treatment. Unlike the tight endothelial junctions seen in normal vasculature, the tumor tissues have leaky vasculature allowing the nanocarriers to easily enter and accumulate at the tumor site to a greater extent than that of normal tissue (Jain and Stylianopoulos, 2010). Enhanced vascular permeability allows the easy extravasation of the larger particles (with a size range of 10–500 nm) and their accumulation in the interstitial space. Once the drug-encapsulated

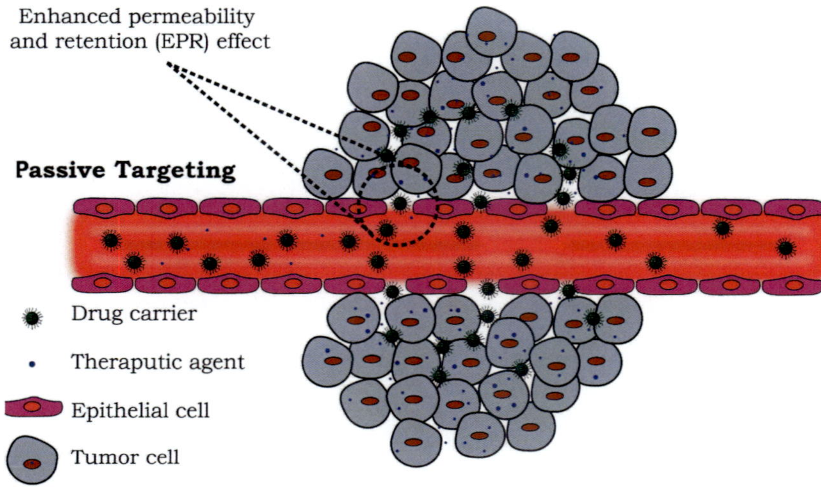

Fig. 2.2 Passive targeting: Nanocarrier carrying a therapeutic agent delivered to tumor mass through the enhanced permeability and retention (EPR) effect.

nanocarrier evades from the immune response, after prolonged circulation, their accumulation is decided by the size, surface charge, and targeting ligand attached on the surface. Depending on the tumor type, the cut-off size of porosity of the vasculature varies between 10 and 800 nm. However, as evident from the in vitro and in vivo experimental trials, nanocarriers with the size of 30–200 nm are the best for efficient extravasation with better tumor retention capability (Chamseddine et al., 2018; Hickey et al., 2015; Jain and Stylianopoulos, 2010; Torchilin, 2005). Also, to escape from filtration by the renal excretion, apart from the size > 10 nm, the preferred charge on the nanoparticle surface should be neutral or negative (Gullotti and Yeo, 2009). The modification of the nanocarrier surface with various hydrophilic spacers such as poly(ethylene glycol) (PEG) or poly(ethylene oxide) (PEO), poloxamer, lauryl ethers, polysorbate, etc. avoids uptake by the mononuclear phagocytes and thereby improves blood circulation time and extravasation.

Though a prolonged circulation period significantly improves the extravasation of a nanocarrier by passive diffusion, the passive targeting may not be effective in all tumors due to certain limitations: (1) the targeting effect is highly dependent on the degree of tumor vascularization and angiogenesis which is term dependent on the type and status of the tumors and (2) most solid tumors have high interstitial fluid pressure. This limits the efficient uptake and homogeneous distribution of drug-loaded nanocarriers by a passive mechanism (Heldin et al., 2004). To overcome these challenges, active targeting of nanomaterials specifically into tumor tissues has emerged as an efficient strategy.

2.3.2 Active targeting

It is essential to significantly increase the quantity of drug delivered to the disease site than that of passively targeted nanovectors to achieve improved therapeutic efficiency and reduce adverse effects. Active drug targeting involves the conjugation of the nanocarrier surface with a suitable targeting ligand so that the encapsulated drug is exclusively delivered to the target site by crossing the biological barriers. Examples of targeting molecules include antibodies, ligands, peptides, nucleic acids, and small molecules that bind directly to a complimentary receptor overexpressed on a tumor-cell surface or on vascular cells while limiting its access to normal cells. The binding affinity of the ligand to the overexpressed receptor influences the penetration of the nanocarrier to the tumor site by overcoming the heterogeneous intensity of the EPR effect. The active targeting strategy can be executed in two distinguished cell targets: (i) tumor cell targeting and (ii) vascular (i.e., tumoral endothelium) targeting as shown in Fig. 2.3.

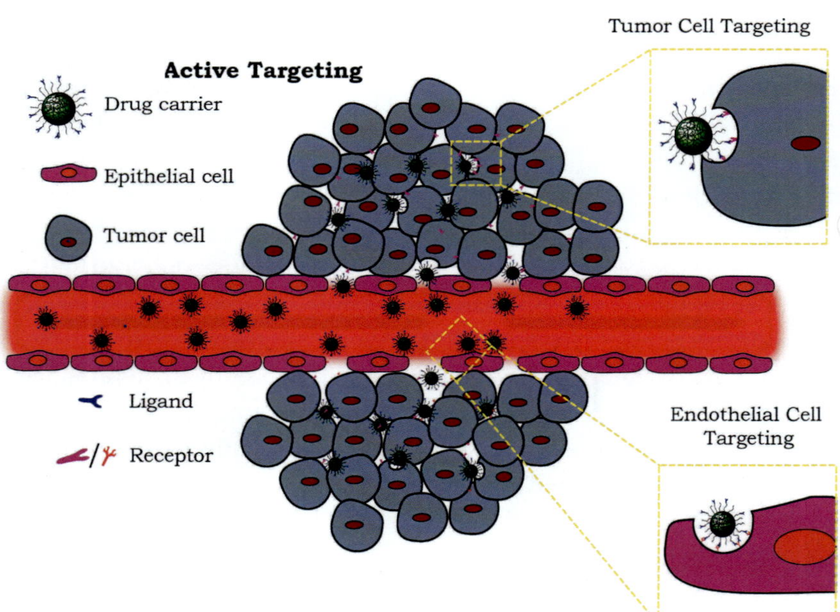

Fig. 2.3 Active targeting mechanism: interaction among the ligand grafted on nanocarrier surface and overexpressed receptors on tumor cells and vascular cells enhances the carrier uptake.

2.3.2.1 Tumor cell targeting

The internalization-inclined transmembrane receptors overexpressed on the cancer cell surface have a direct influence on the uptake of drug-loaded nanocarriers functionalized/decorated with the complementary ligand. In addition to enhanced tumor accumulation (EPR effect), actively targeted nanocarriers are responsible for the intensified internalization into tumor cells. This is the base of the development of nanocarriers targeted to endocytosis-prone surface receptor accountable for the improved efficacy of cancer therapy. It is noteworthy that the higher density of targeting ligands on nanocarriers have a direct impact on the specific cell binding and hence internalization of nanoparticles into the tumor cell. High-density ligand/receptor interactions results in the increased concentration of therapeutic drugs in an intracellular microenvironment, and thus simultaneously improving therapeutic efficacy (Attia et al., 2019). Therefore, the choice of an appropriate targeting ligand is an essential criterion for the active targeting, because it determines the nanocarrier's ability to target cancer cells.

2.3.2.2 Vascular targeting (anti-angiogenesis)

The initial work on vascular targeting was reported in 1923; however, the concept got attention in 1971 when Judah Folkman suggested that the prevention of new vessel sprouts from piercing into a neoplasm (so-called "anti-angiogenesis") can inhibit tumor growth (Folkman, 1971). A tumor needs to develop new vessels (the process termed as an angiogenetic switch) for blood supply to allocate itself with nutrients and oxygen as well as to eliminate metabolic waste products. Therefore, cutting off the tumor supply by inhibiting the vascularization can abate cancer cells from food and oxygen with consequent hypoxia and necrosis (Lammers et al., 2008). This is the base for developing a nanocarrier drug delivery system actively targeted to tumor endothelial cells. In this strategy, nanocarriers decorated with the ligands bind to and obstruct the preexisting angiogenic blood vessels, thereby cutting the tumor's blood and oxygen supply to cause tumor cell death from extensive hemorrhagic necrosis. Endothelial cells are heritably more stable than the tumor cells, hence, less likely to undergo mutations developing resistance to anti-angiogenetic therapy (Kerbel, 1991). Therefore, instead of targeting the tumor cells, targeting the endothelial cells forming tumor vessels is more advantageous. Further, the different phenotype of endothelial cells involved in angiogenesis than the endothelial cells of normal vasculature provides an additional benefit to anti-angiogenetic therapy (Augustin et al., 1994; Kerbel, 1991; Ran and Thorpe, 2002). The common targets aimed at tumor neovasculature include integrins ($\alpha_{2b}\beta_3$, $\alpha_v\beta_3$, and $\alpha_5\beta_1$) and aminopeptidase-*N* (CD13). These targets are recognized by numerous cyclic and linear derivatives of the oligopeptides RGD (arginyl-glycyl-aspartic acid) and NGR (asparaginyl-glycylargininic acid), respectively (Lammers et al., 2008).

2.4 Toxicity of nanobiomaterials

The major setback of using nanomaterials is the unwanted toxicity associated with the nanovector itself or its degradation products, caused by disadvantageous interactions with biological entities. The toxicity of nanoparticles sometimes may not have an immediate impact on human health but can cause long-term side effects. The long-term toxic effects of certain nanoparticles are a subject of many controversies and several studies are still under process for assessing their consequences. Although numerous nanovectors are being developed, only a few have reached to the preclinical and clinical trials due to the lack of in-depth study of nanomaterials interactions with biological entities. Over the past decade, plenty of research has been performed to understand the causes of toxicity of various nanomaterials. It has been observed that, immediately on administration, nanoparticles start interacting with their contiguous environment. The nature of these interactions is contingent on their physicochemical properties such as the shape, size, and surface chemistry of nanoparticles (Kim et al., 2012; Sukhanova et al., 2018). Depending on these properties, nanoparticles can enter into the intercellular spaces or can cross the intracellular barriers (Guarnieri et al., 2014; Hadrup et al., 2015; Siegrist et al., 2019). Many cytotoxic studies revealed that nanomaterials subjected to type, dose, and incubation time show their involvement in reactive oxygen species (ROS) generation, disruption of membrane functionality and cellular barriers, DNA mutations and sometimes in dysfunction of cellular metabolism.

The harmful effects related to the physical and chemical nature of nanovectors do not necessarily discourage their use for therapeutic purposes. The nanovectors that show simultaneous biocompatibility and target-specific/selective delivery of therapeutic agents are often used for the clinical purposes provided by their optimal dose. Further, the surface modifier such as PEG can significantly reduce the toxic effects of pristine nanoparticles which otherwise harm the organism (Yan et al., 2011).

2.5 Biodegradable nanomaterials used in controlled drug delivery and imaging

Although numerous theranostic nanoparticles of sizes between 1 and 1000 nm have been developed, very few are usable for cancer therapies at clinical levels due to certain complications such as poor biocompatibility, bioavailability, biodegradability, and stability. These nanoplatforms can be synthesized from a wide variety of materials mainly categorized into organic and inorganic nanoparticles based on their composition.

2.5.1 Organic and polymer-based nanocarriers

2.5.1.1 Liposomes

Liposomes were discovered by Alec Bangham in the 1960s and are unilamellar or multilamellar vesicles consisting of single or multiple aquatic compartments. Since their discovery, liposome-based nanocarriers are widely utilized by several pharmaceutical industries and are deemed to be the most successful carrier system for drug delivery and theranostics applications. Liposomes can be constructed using natural or synthetic amphiphilic phospholipids and cholesterol. These are the most widely used nanoplatforms for delivering therapeutic agents (e.g., doxorubicin, paclitaxel, Galbanic acid) and imaging probes (e.g., TPE-BICOOH, IR780, Cy5.5) due to their biocompatibility and capability to encapsulate both hydrophobic/lipophilic and hydrophilic molecules. The hydrophobic drug molecules and/or imaging probes are entrapped in the hydrophobic tails of the lipid core while the hydrophilic molecules are encapsulated in inner aquatic compartments. Depending on the method of preparation (i.e., sonication, stirring, extrusion, microfluidification, or electroformation) and composition, the liposome sizes varying between 50 and 450 nm have been utilized for drug delivery applications. The advantages of using the liposomes as a drug carrier are as follows: (i) the protection of the drug from the naturally occurring phenomenon such as enzymatic degradation and immunologic inactivation; (ii) low toxicity due to its high biocompatibility as their membrane structure is similar to the cell membranes; and (iii) prolonged blood circulation period (Daraee et al., 2016).

The liposomal properties vary significantly owing to their composition (Kneidl et al., 2014). Therefore, based on the composition, liposomes are categorized into four types as depicted in Fig. 2.4.

(1) *The conventional liposomes:* These lysosomes are formed from phospholipids which can be either cationic or anionic with natural cholesterol as

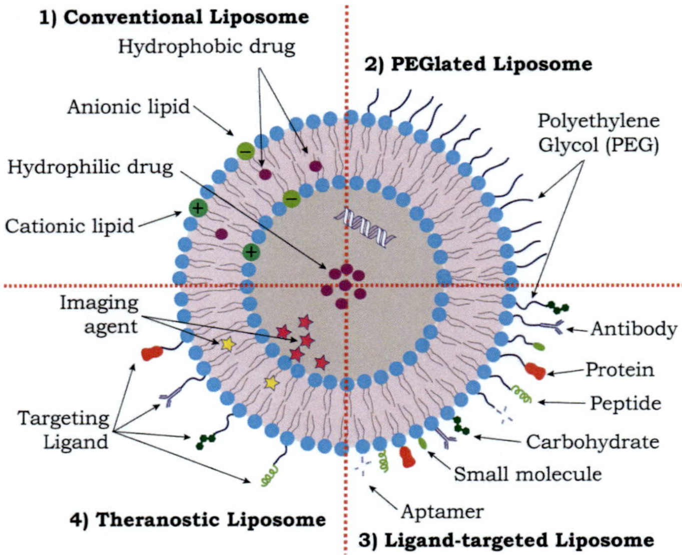

Fig. 2.4 Representative liposome types for drug delivery and theranostic applications.

the additive. The type of phospholipid used influences the surface charge of the liposome and fluidity of the bilayer membrane. The surface charge also contributes to the stability of the liposome and their localization in tumors. The addition of cholesterol into the phospholipid bilayer decreases the fluidity of the liposome membrane and increases its in vitro/in vivo stability. The neutral liposomes are less stable and generally have a tendency to aggregate. Therefore, neutral liposomes preferentially localize in the solid tumors based on the EPR effect and mostly release the cargo in the extracellular environment. On the other hand, liposomes with a more positive potential preferentially target the angiogenic vessels and, thus, have a potentially enhanced antitumor effect (Zhao et al., 2011).

(2) *PEGylated liposomes*: Lipids modified with PEG, that is, PEGylated lipids, are used as one of the components of the liposomal membrane. PEG is a hydrophilic polymer that provides a steric barrier on a liposome surface, providing extra stability to liposomes. Hence, PEGylated liposomes evade uptake by the immune cells, thereby extending blood circulation time.

(3) *Ligand-targeted liposomes*: Targeting ligands such as peptides, antibodies, and carbohydrates are either directly attached to the liposome surface or to the end of PEG chains linked on the liposome surface.

(4) *Theranostic liposome*: It is a consolidated version of the former three types of liposomes and generally comprises a targeting, an imaging, and a therapeutic element (Sercombe et al., 2015). The additive phospholipids or molecules can be incorporated during the liposomal formulations to achieve the discharge of cargo triggered by a certain stimulus (e.g., temperature, pH, enzymes, and light). For example, incorporated lysolipids that form stabilized defects at the phase transition temperature is utilized in ThermoDox, a liposome formulation in clinical trials for the treatment of hepatocellular carcinoma (Needham and Dewhirst, 2001). This ThermoDox utilizes the lysolipid thermally sensitive liposome (LTSL) technology for entrapping doxorubicin and releases it selectively at 41.3°C. Doxil (PEGylated liposomal doxorubicin), Myocet (non-PEGylated liposomal doxorubicin), and DaunoXome (PEGylated liposomal doxorubicin/daunorubicin) are the clinically approved liposome-based formulations. These formulations contain doxorubicin or daunorubicin in the aqueous core for the treatment of metastatic breast cancer and acute myeloid leukemia (Fassas and Anagnostopoulos, 2005; Hofheinz et al., 2005).

2.5.1.2 Biodegradable polymer-based nanocarriers

Polymeric-based nanocarriers are the distinct nanoscale drug delivery platforms obtained by the assembly of biodegradable polymers. The biodegradable polymers used for vaccine formulations are either obtained from natural sources, such as, protein-based polymers (e.g., albumin, collagen, and gelatin) (Verma et al., 2018) and polysaccharides (e.g., chitosan, dextran, agarose, hyaluronic acid, alginate, cyclodextrin, starch, and cellulose) or chemically synthesized from biodegradable polymers such as PEG, poly-(lactic-*co*-glycolic acid) (PLGA), poly(lactic acid) (PLA), polycarbonate, polycarbolactone, and poly(acrylic acid) to name a few (Wang et al., 2014b). In polymer-based formulations, the theranostic agents are tagged to the polymer matrix by covalent bonding or noncovalent interactions such as electrostatic interactions [e.g., positively charged fluorescent dye, tris(2,2-bi-pyridyl)dichlororuthenium(*II*)hexahydrate and negatively charged silica matrix] and by means of hydrophobic interactions. The important advantages of using the drug delivery platforms formulated using biodegradable biopolymers include the stabilization of therapeutic agents, sustained delivery, and steady release rate. Additionally, the biodegradable polymers, such as poly(glycolic acid), PLGA, polylactide (PLA), and gelatin, can be completely broken down to reduce their toxicity (BaoLin and Ma, 2014; Panyam and

Labhasetwar, 2003; Sung and Kim, 2020). PLGA is an extensively investigated polymer for formulating the biodegradable nanoparticles due to their low toxicity, biocompatibility, and biodegradability with tissue cells. This US FDA-approved polymer has tunable mechanical properties and a broad erosion time (Makadia and Siegel, 2011). Besides the targeted drug delivery and biocompatibility to accumulate the drug to the cancerous tissue, polymeric nanocarriers could also be utilized as optical imaging probes in cancer diagnosis by incorporating imaging probes into the polymeric nanocarriers (Perumal et al., 2019). Polymeric nanocarriers offer control on physical phenomena like size, shape, and surface functionalization. The functionalization of polymeric or other nonpolymeric nanoplatforms (e.g., liposomes, quantum dots, and dendrimers) with PEG offers advantages of increasing surface area for functionalization, preventing aggregation, evading phagocytosis, providing great stability, prolonging blood circulation time, improving biodistribution, and greater bioavailability of the nanoparticles. Currently, several of the US FDA-approved NPs are coated with PEG (Otsuka et al., 2003; Paszkiewicz et al., 2020).

Protein-based polymeric formulations show exceptional properties in the field of nanomedicine. These nanocarriers are non-toxic, can be degraded by enzymatic actions, are easily metabolizable, and possess good biocompatibility (Lee et al., 2016; Zhang et al., 2018). Additionally, protein nanoparticles have been known to provoke a weak or negligible immune response (Lohcharoenkal et al., 2014). Albumin is a major plasma protein that biologically functions as a transporter of various proteins. It has a determinative edge over other nanomaterials in the field of nanomedicine. The presence of amino and carboxylic groups on surfaces of albumin nanoparticles facilitates covalent binding of targeting ligands and other surface modifications. Apart from that, albumin nanoparticles are easy to prepare with a high drug loading capacity, and have a long half-life in circulating plasma (Elzoghby et al., 2012). Abraxane (ABI-007), a paclitaxel albumin-stabilized nanoparticle formulation, was the first FDA-approved commercialized nab-technology based product that revealed significant benefits for the cure of metastatic breast cancer, non-small cell lung cancer (NSCLC), and pancreatic cancer (Gradishar, 2006). Several other nab-technology based nanoformulations, such as nab-docetaxel (ABI-008) and nab-paclitaxel/rituximab-coated nanoparticles (AR160) have already entered into clinical trials for cancer therapy. Recently, Lu and coworkers (Gao et al., 2019) have developed theranostic albumin-bound BPBBT nanoparticles. The payload, BPBBT, is a D-A-D NIR-II probe with both aggregation-induced emission (AIE) and

Twisted intramolecular charge transfer (TICT) characteristics when bound to the human serum albumin (HSA). The BPBBT NPs showed promising results with accurate and high-resolution intraoperative NIR-II fluorescence images from an orthotopic mouse colon tumor with a capability to detect invisible metastatic tumor lesions of sizes as small as 0.5 mm × 0.3 mm. Additionally, the NIR-II image-guided photothermal therapy (PTT) using BPBBT particles showed complete curing of mice exhibiting colon cancer, without recurrence in 30 days and 100% survival rates. On the contrary, the mice receiving no PTT (treated with PBS only) and conventional PTT had severe tumor recurrence and survival of up to a maximum of 22 and 25 days, respectively.

Polymeric micelles are spherical or globular shape nanocarriers used for the delivery of poorly water-soluble therapeutics. These supramolecular nanostructures (10–100 nm) are obtained by an entropically favored self-assembly of amphiphilic block copolymers in an aqueous medium, resulting in a hydrophobic core stabilized by a hydrophilic shell above their critical micelle concentration (CMC) and critical micelle temperature (CMT) (Yokoyama et al., 1998). Hydrophobic drugs and/or imaging agents are entrapped in the hydrophobic core which behaves as a reservoir. On the other hand, the hydrophilic shell protects the hydrophobic core and keeps the drug-loaded micelle from rapid clearance. Micelles formed from the PEG-*b*-poly(*d*,*l*-lactic acid) (PEG-PLA) is used for the solubilization of hydrophobic compounds. Paclitaxel loaded in PEG-PLA (Genexol-PM) is the first commercialized polymeric micelle formulation used to treat metastatic breast cancer (Kim et al., 2004). The acute dose-toxicity of Genexol-PM was significantly lower than that of the conventional Chremophor EL paclitaxel drug formulation. Following the approval of Genexol-PM, several other polymeric micelles based formulations have entered clinical trials (Table 2.1). In NC-6300, the covalent conjugation of doxorubicin (DOX) to the carboxylic acid groups in PEG-*b*-p(*b*-Asp) via a hydrolysable hydrazine linker allows the triggered release of DOX in response to pH stimulus ($pH < 5.0$).

2.5.1.3 Dendrimers

Dendrimers are highly branched three-dimensional globular nanostructures which are defined by three unique components: (1) the central core, (2) the interior branched structure, made up of repetitive units (generations) attached with the central core, and (3) the periphery with surface functional groups (e.g., -COOH, -COONa, $-NH_2$, and -OH). With increased

Table 2.1 Polymeric micelles formulations as drug carrier under clinical investigation.

Name	Polymer	Payload	Application	Clinical status	Reference NCT Number
NK012	PEG-Pglu	7-ethyl-10-hydroxy-camptothecin	Small-cell lung cancer	Phase II	NCT00951613
			Refractory solid tumors	Phase I	NCT00542958
			Metastatic colorectal cancer	Phase I	NCT01238939
			Metastatic triple-negative breast cancer	Phase I	NCT01238939
NC-6004	PEG-Pglu	Cisplatin	Pancreatic cancer	Phase III	NCT02043288
			Squamous cell carcinoma of the head and neck (SCCHN)	Phase I/II	NCT03109158
				Phase II	NCT03771820
			Locally advanced and metastatic pancreatic cancer	Phase I/II	NCT00910741
			Head and neck neoplasms	Phase I/II	NCT02817113
			Solid tumors	Phase I	NCT02240238
NK105	PEG-PAPB	Paclitaxel	Metastatic breast cancer	Phase III	NCT01644890
Nanoxel M	PEG-PLA	Docetaxel	Non-muscle-invasive bladder cancer	Phase III	NCT02982395
			Head and neck squamous cell carcinoma	Phase II	NCT02639858
NC-4016	PEG-Pglu	Oxaliplatin	Advanced solid tumor or lymphoma	Phase I	NCT03168035
BIND-014	PEG-PLA	Docetaxel	Advanced or metastatic cancer	Phase I	NCT01300533
			KRAS-positive or squamous cell nonsmall-cell lung cancer	Phase II	NCT02283320
			Nonsmall-cell lung cancer	Phase II	NCT01792479
			Urothelial carcinoma, Cholangiocarcinoma, cervical cancer, SCCHN	Phase II	NCT02479178
			Metastatic castration-resistant prostate cancer	Phase II	NCT01812746
NC-6300	PEG-*b*-p(b-Asp)	Doxorubicin	Solid tumor, soft tissue sarcoma, metastatic sarcoma, sarcoma	Phase I/II	NCT03168061

generations, dendrimers possess more compact, dense, and globular structure than that of lower generations. In nanomedicine research, dendrimers have emerged as a competitive excipient having multifunctional surfaces offering a drug delivery platform for both the hydrophobic and hydrophilic drug candidates as represented in Fig. 2.5. The branched interior structure with void spaces offers the noncovalent interactions such as hydrophobic interactions and hydrogen bonding, which stabilize the hydrophobic therapeutic molecule in the dendritic structure. On the other hand, the apparent surface groups on the periphery can be covalently conjugated with the targeting ligands (e.g., folic acid conjugated PAMAM dendrimer NPs) (Amreddy et al., 2018), imaging probes (Shi et al., 2008), and therapeutic agents for selective or specific targeting, diagnosis (Svenson and Tomalia, 2005), and cancer treatment, respectively (Kalva et al., 2015).

A great number of dendrimers have been synthesized with structural differences used in biomedical applications, including poly(amidoamines) (PAMAM) (Tomalia et al., 1985), polypropyleneimines (PPI) (Wörner and

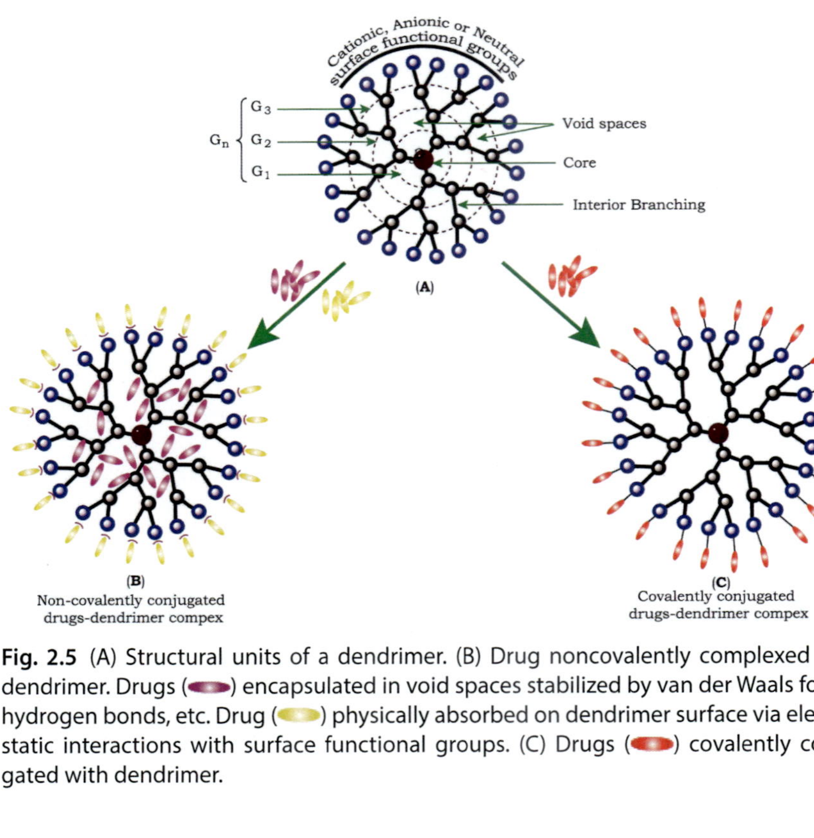

Fig. 2.5 (A) Structural units of a dendrimer. (B) Drug noncovalently complexed with dendrimer. Drugs (purple) encapsulated in void spaces stabilized by van der Waals forces, hydrogen bonds, etc. Drug (yellow) physically absorbed on dendrimer surface via electrostatic interactions with surface functional groups. (C) Drugs (red) covalently conjugated with dendrimer.

Mülhaupt, 1993), polyamides or polypeptides (Spetzler and Tam, 1995), polyester (Frechet, 1994) dendrimers. The surface functional groups determine the pharmacokinetics of dendrimer nanoparticles. Also, the toxicity of the dendrimer has been observed to be dependent on terminal functional groups. The densely positively charged dendrimer can strongly interact with the negatively charged cell membrane, which ultimately leads to lysis of the cell. For example, dendrimers with positively charged surface groups (such as amines) demonstrate dose-dependent toxicity (Kimura and Ogura, 2001). For this reason, positively charged surfaces are often coated with neutral molecules such as acetyl groups, heparin, poly(ethylene oxide) (PEO) otherwise named as PEG chains to improve their biocompatibility (Hong et al., 2004). As an example, Szoka and coworkers reported a polyester-based dendrimer-PEO-doxorubicin conjugate that caused complete DOX-insensitive C-26 tumor regression and 100% survival of BALB/c mice bearing C-26 colon carcinomas over a 60 day experiment. The antitumor efficacy of dendrimer-PEO-doxorubicin relates satisfactorily with the FDA-approved Doxil (Lee et al., 2006). The stimuli-controlled delivery strategy by incorporating the stimuli-sensitive groups in dendrimer structure enables the release of payloads from dendrimer nanoparticles in response to a specific trigger represents the attractive strategy for targeted therapy (Wang et al., 2016). For example, Nigam et al. reported drug carriers for thermally activated cancer chemotherapy by developing generation 2 (G2) PAMAM dendrimer-conjugated iron oxide nanoparticles loaded with doxorubicin (DOX) for the treatment of cervical cancer (Nigam and Bahadur, 2017). Other examples of stimuli-responsive dendrimer-based drug delivery nanosystems for cancer treatment are listed in Table 2.2.

2.5.2 Inorganic nanobiomaterials for drug delivery and imaging

2.5.2.1 Carbon-based nanomaterials

Carbon-based nanomaterials (CBNs) exhibit unique characteristics that have been widely exploited in various biomedical applications, including imaging, biosensing, drug delivery, tissue engineering, diagnosis, and cancer therapy. The extensive surface area, aspect ratio, and chemical purity of sp^2-carbon nanomaterials render them an ideal candidate for drug delivery and theranostics (Cha et al., 2013; Yang et al., 2013). The sp^2-CNBs have defined structures that include zero-dimensional (0D) fullerenes, one-dimensional (1D) carbon nanotubes (CNTs), and two-dimensional (2D) graphenes as most typical examples in this class of nanovectors (Liu and

Table 2.2 Stimuli-responsive dendrimer-based nanovectors as drug carriers for cancer treatment.

Gn-Dendrimer	Surface modification	Responsiveness	Payload	References
G4-PAMAM	PEG	Redox	Doxorubicin	Hu et al. (2014)
G4-PAMAM	PEG	Redox and pH	Doxorubicin	Hu et al. (2016)
G4-PAMAM	PEG-chitosan-folic acid	pH	pDNA	Wang and Yang (2018)
G3.5-PAMAM	2-(*N,N*-dimethylamino) ethyl acrylate	Redox and pH	Letrozole	Nguyen et al. (2017)
G4-PBAE	PEG-chitosan-folic acid	pH and temperature	Doxorubicin	Shen et al. (2011)
G3-Peptide	PEG-(Gly-Phe-Leu-Gly)	Enzyme (Cathepsin B)	Doxorubicin	Zhang et al. (2014a)
G3-Peptide	PEG-(Gly-Phe-Leu-Gly)	Enzyme (Cathepsin B)	Gemcitabine	Zhang et al. (2017)

Liang, 2012). The hollow interior structures of fullerene and CNTs provide the space for the encapsulation of a biomedical payload; and in CNTs and graphene, the attachment of drugs to the π-electron rich surface can be achieved by π-π stacking interactions. CBNs can be further functionalized chemically to make them more suitable for biological targeting, to improve solubility and biocompatibility, as well as for multifunctional applications including imaging and therapy.

(i) Fullerenes

These carbon allotropes have hollow cage-like structures formed by the bonding among the pentagon and hexagon shapes. Since the discovery of Buckminsterfullerene (C60) in 1985, fullerenes have been studied as a key nanostructured material in nanomedicines. Because of their small sizes (< 100 nm), fullerene-based nanodrugs can easily diffuse through the leaky tumor vasculature and accumulate at the tumor site. The main obstacle of using naked fullerene as nanomedicine is its poor water solubility and hence poor biocompatibility. However, many studies have reported to overcome this problem by supramolecular approaches (i.e., by forming the inclusion complexes of fullerenes with the cyclodextrins or calixarenes) as well as by direct functionalization of fullerenes with, for example, amino acid, carboxylic acid, polyhydroxy groups, amphiphilic polymers, and chemotherapeutics (Mendes et al., 2013). The chemically functionalized fullerenes such as polyhydroxy fullerenes (PHF, also called as fullerenols or fullerols) and carboxy fullerenes (CF) were found to be heated to their ignition temperature on exposure to low-intensity near-infrared region (NIR) light ($<10W/cm^2$). Krishna et al. exploited the photoacoustic and photothermal properties of PHP for noninvasive imaging and treatment of cancer. Photothermal ablation experiments were conducted in vivo. PHP nanoparticles were injected into the tumors of mice followed by subsequent exposure to the 785 nm, 500 mW, and continuous-wave NIR laser for 10 min. A rapid shrinkage (by 32%) in a cross-sectional area of the tumor was observed within 2 h of postirradiatoin (Krishna et al., 2010). AC60-based nanoparticles with "off-on" states were synthesized by conjugating the DOX on amine functionalized fullerene via a ROS sensitive thioketal linker (C60-DOX NPs). Subsequently, C60-DOX NPs were coated with Distearoyl-sn-glycero-3-phosphoethanolamine-PEG-CNGRCK2HK3HK11 (DSPE-PEG-NGR), providing the (C60-DOX-NGR NPs) with excellent stability in physiological conditions and active tumor-targeting ability. In in-vivo experiments, the "off" to "on" state of C60-DOX-NGR was remotely controlled by irradiating the tumor with a 532 nm laser. Both the release of DOX and ROS generation was achieved at the same time in the "on sate," thereby, it performed a combined photodynamic and chemotherapy in tumors as depicted in Fig. 2.6 (Shi et al., 2016). Similarly, chemically modified fullerenes (C60-IONP-PEG-FA) were also used as multifunctional nanoplatforms with active tumor targeting and magnetic-targeted abilities. C60-IONP-PEG-FA showed excellent PDT and RTT (radiofrequency thermal therapy) efficacies indicating their potential for cancer theranostic applications (Shi et al., 2014).

Fullerenes with an appropriate metal atom/ion entrapped inside the hollow core, so-called "metallofullerenes" were used as contrast agents in magnetic resonance imaging (MRI). Most of the paramagnetic metallofullerenes complexes prepared by entrapping gadolinium (Gd) not only for its ability to enhance the contrast of magnetic resonance images considerably but also to prevent leakage of Gd (III) in vivo, thereby reducing its potential toxicity (Zhang et al., 2014b). Various Gd@Cn ($n=60$ or 82) derivatives have been developed using specific chemical alterations and are currently being explored for imaging and cancer therapy purposes (Han et al., 2018; Leconte et al., 2007; Mikawa et al., 2001; Mody et al., 2009).

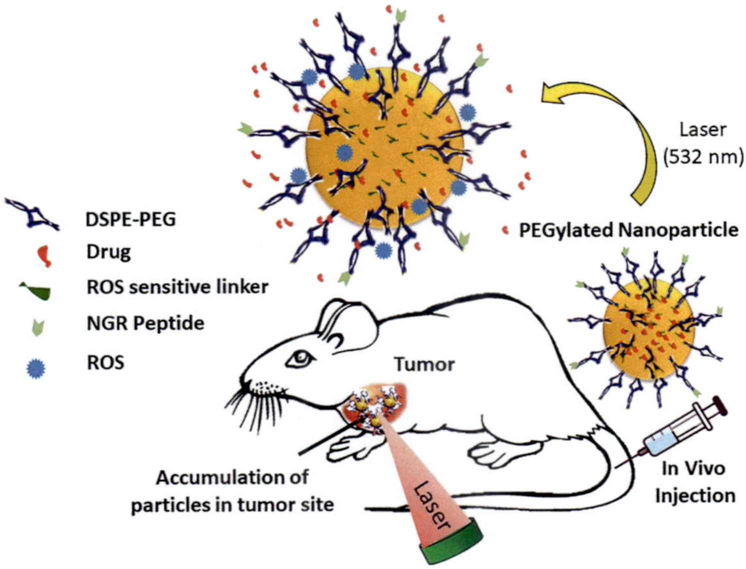

Fig. 2.6 Schematic illustration of the light-induced spatial and temporal switching of the "off to on" state of C60-DOX-NGR NPs in 4T1 tumor-bearing mouse.

(ii) Carbon nanotubes

CNTs are hollow cylinder-shaped structures, having potential as an emerging and promising excipient for biosensing, drug delivery and theranostic applications. Based on the number of layers, CNTs are categorized into single-walled CNTs (SWCNTs) and multiwall CNTs (MWCNTs). The large aspect ratio, high electron mobility, chemical stability and sensitivity make them exceptionally fit for biosensing and drug delivery applications. Therapeutic drugs are either encapsulated intrinsically, that is, in the hollow cavity or chemically conjugated (via a covalent or noncovalent bonding) on the surface of CNTs (Maiti et al., 2019) as represented in Fig. 2.7. Due to poor solubility and high aggregation tendency, pristine CNTs form aggregates in an aqueous medium and lead to potential cytotoxicity. However, the functionalization of the surface of CNTs with appropriate chemical entities, such as PEG-coated CNTs, can reduce their aggregation tendency and improve the circulation time, thereby reducing the cytotoxicity. Moreover, the targeting groups linked to the surface-functionalized CNTs allow target-specific delivery of a therapeutic payload (Lay et al., 2011). Numerous examples of surface-modified SWCNTs have already been developed by researchers worldwide for drug delivery and theranostic applications. For example, Rusling et al. developed a PEGlated SWNTs

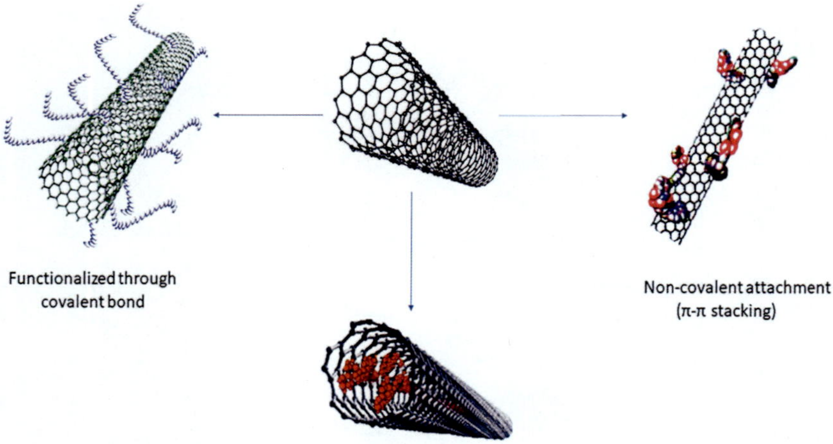

Fig. 2.7 Functionalized CNT for biomedical purposes.

that overcome the overt SWCNTs, causing a high dispersion of nanotube excipient for the anticancer drug cisplatin in mice. PEG-SWCNTs loaded with an anticancer drug, cisplatin, along with the attached epidermal growth factor (EGF) as a targeting ligand for a targeted therapeutic combination successfully inhibited the growth of squamous cell tumors in mice (Bhirde et al., 2010). SWNTs hold potential as a theranostic agent because of its photoluminescence in the 1000–1400 nm region and ability to generate substantial amounts of heat on excitation with NIR light (700–1100 nm). These characteristics are highly useful not only for in vivo tumor imaging but also for photothermal and photodynamic ablation of tumors (Moon et al., 2009; Murakami, 2017; Wang et al., 2014a).

(iii) Graphene and graphene oxide

Graphene is one of the most considered nanoparticles in the field of drug delivery because of its unique physical and chemical properties. Graphene is composed of a two-dimensional single-layered sp^2-hybridized carbon with a honeycomb-like structure (Yang et al., 2016). It has a high thermal conductivity and high mechanical strength, with an unusually high optical transparency. Because of its unique properties, graphene offers new interesting viewpoints in nanomedicine for the improvement of chemotherapy and theranostic systems (Pei et al., 2020).

Graphene oxide (GO) is a well-known derivative of graphene. It has multiple functional groups like hydroxyl, carboxyl, carbonyl, and epoxide on its surfaces which provides excellent water solubility, biocompatibility, and help in carrying multiple drugs which is basic for the conveyance of anticancer medications. Generally, nano-GO are of the size 20–100 nm (Pei et al., 2020). The photothermal impact of the nanomolecules is identified with the size of the atom. It has been found that the photothermal impact of the material turns out to be less with the increasing size of the nanoparticles.

Graphene oxide nanomolecules with PEG have become the "brilliant norm" for surface functionalization in biomedical and designing applications. PEG on the surface of the graphene oxide can improve the biocompatibility and hydrophilicity of the nano-GO particles (Plachá and Jampilek, 2019).

2.5.2.2 Gold nanoparticles

Gold nanoparticles (GNPs) emerged as one of the most vibrant agents for theranostics. GNPs perform various functions such as drug carrier, photothermal agent, and radiosensitizer. Gold commonly exists either in the Au (I) or Au (III) oxidation state, whereas GNPs exist in nonoxidized state Au(0). Several techniques have been used to synthesize GNPs, some of them are chemical, electrochemical, and thermal methods. The preparation of GNPs using chemical methods requires two steps in the first step gold complex as $HAuCl_4$ is reduced by reducing agents such as citric acid, formaldehyde, and borohydrides. Then, in the second step, stabilizing agents are added such as phosphorus ligands, oxygen-based ligands, nitrogen-based ligands, and trisodium citrate dihydrate to avoid aggregation in the particles (Herizchi et al., 2016).

GNPs can be synthesized in a wide range of sizes with different surface functionalities. Their adjustability in size and surface makes them an excellent candidate for the drug delivery system. In a study, platinum-bonded DNA-AuNPs were delivered into the cancer cell, the reduced pH of the intercellular space supported the reductive release of cisplatin from the system. Pt-DNA-AuNPs ended up being more powerful than cisplatin in killing cancer cells (Brown et al., 2010). The size of the GNPs ranged from 1 to 100 nm with various morphologies, such as nanorods, nanospheres, and nanocages, with versatile thermal and optical properties. It has various applications in imaging and therapy which is shown in Fig. 2.8.

Regular-sized GNPs are used as an agent for computed tomography (CT) as it has a high atomic number and a high X-ray absorption coefficient. The high absorption X-ray coefficient makes GNPs a good agent

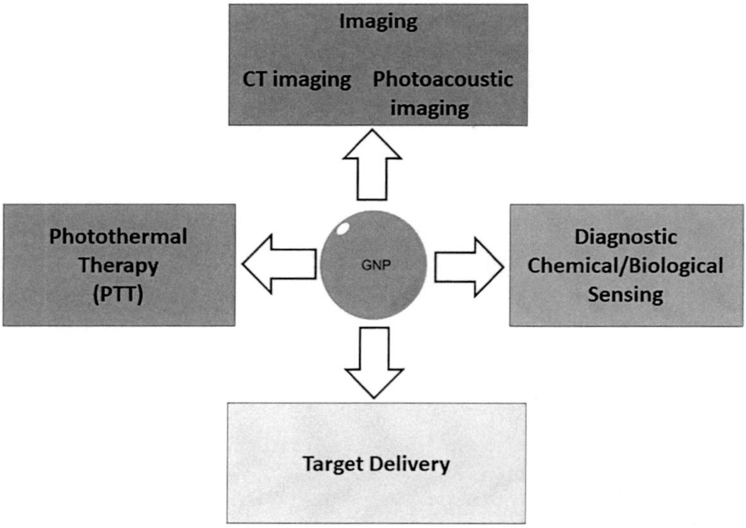

Fig. 2.8 Properties of gold nanoparticles for cancer therapy and theranostics.

for radiotherapy. Gold nanoparticles have also been explored for the photocontrolled release of drugs. Agasti et al. have used gold nanoparticles for the photocontrolled release of the anticancerous drug paclitaxel, as they observed the controlled release of anticancer drug paclitaxel under low-power photoirradiation in physiological conditions (Vivero-Escoto et al., 2009).

GNPs scatter light so strongly that they can be brighter than the chemical fluorophores. Moreover, they do not photobleach so they can be easily detected at low concentration. This property of GNPs can be used for intracellular tracking in dark field optical microscopy.

Studies showed that GNPs can be used for photothermal therapy (PTT). They absorb the light from the NIR which excites the protons to its higher energy level and displays a photo killing effect (Jain et al., 2012). GNPs accumulate specifically at the tumor site which improves radiotherapy and reduces its impact on the neighboring normal cells.

2.5.2.3 Magnetic nanoparticles

Metal-based nanoparticles which have a magnetic core and are capable of MRI detection have been proven as a good source of detecting cancer at an early stage, and they can also monitor tumor response to the therapy and hence can be a good theranostics agent. Some of the most commonly used metals for designing magnetic nanoparticles (MNPs) are iron, cobalt, nickel, and manganese (Williams and Corr, 2013). The size and shape of the MNPs can be controlled during the synthesis steps. The iron nanoparticle is an example of a MNP. It can be a synthesized by chemical and physical methods. In the chemical method, Fe^{2+} and Fe^{3+} states of iron are co-precipitated in an aqueous solution resulting in the formation of Fe_3O_4 and Fe_2O_3 or a mixture of both. During the synthesis of these nanoparticles, it is very important to prevent them from oxidation. To achieve that, the synthesis of nanoparticles has been conducted under inert conditions. These iron nanoparticles are then coated with PEG, polypeptides, and gelatin to prevent them from the self-assembly of iron nanoparticles (Yigit et al., 2012).

MNPs provide specificity and high toxicity toward cancer cells. The study conducted by Haam and associates, by using magnetic nanocrystals and a chemotherapeutic drug (DOX), encapsulated them in a multifunctional magneto-polymeric nanohybrid (MMPNs). The study outcomes indicated that the combination of the chemotherapeutic drug with magnetic nanocrystals in MMNP, showed a significant decrease in tumor growth in mice grafted with breast cancer.

Despite several benefits of using MNPs in cancer therapy, there are some problems associated with it. For example, MNPs get aggregated in the blood once injected intravenously, thereby causing blood vessels to block. To overcome the problem, some specific polymer-coated MNPs have been developed as shown in Fig. 2.9. Various MNPs have been designed by coating them with suitable polymers for magnetic hyperthermia. To provide the prolonged circulation time for these particles, a PEG-DSPE-Cy5.5 (DSPE = distearoyl-phosphoethanolamine) lipid coating has been found to

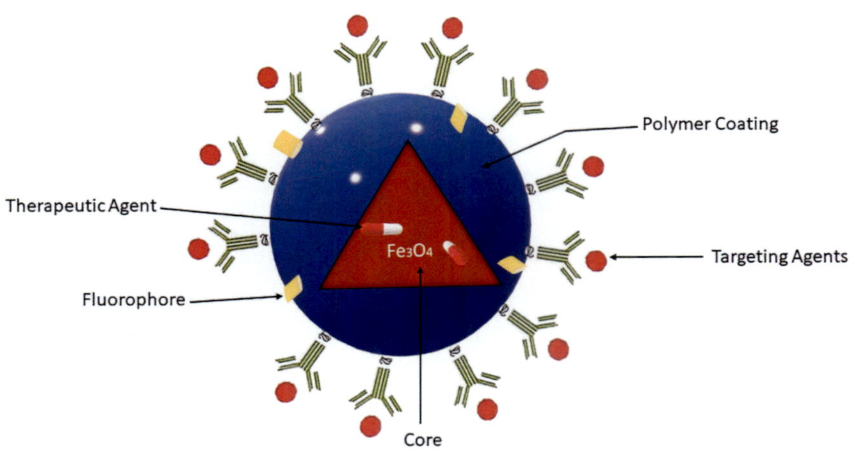

Fig. 2.9 Functionalized magnetic nanoparticle structure.

be useful. This lipid film coating on the top of the particles provides stability from the external environment. Another problem of using MNPs for therapy and theranostics is its toxicity. The use of metal as a core component for MNPs may make them toxic. Using toxic materials for therapy over a long period of time is an inefficient idea. These nanoparticles may create an adverse effect on cell viability, cell proliferation, and various other biological mechanisms. During therapy, these nanoparticles accumulate within the organ which may lead to several other disorders. Therefore, pure metals like cobalt, cadmium, and zinc are not suitable for biomedical purposes, while iron-oxide-based or titanium-based nanoparticles are considered for biomedical purposes because of their less toxicity and biocompatibility (Jiang et al., 2019).

In general, these MNPs contain magnetic material that resides at the core of the particle which is covered by either organic moieties (polymers or liposomes) or inorganic moieties (such as silica) along with therapeutic agents (anticancer drugs). Further, a protective lipid covering is used for the protection of the particle before reaching the infected area, where it can accumulate because of the EPR effect (Yoo et al., 2011).

2.5.2.4 Quantum dots

Quantum dots (QDs) are semiconductor particles a few nanometers in size because of which they show distinct optical and electronic properties compared with larger size particles. QDs absorb light at the near-infrared region which makes them suitable for fluorescence imaging in animal models. By the absorption of light from the UV region, the electrons from quantum dots get excited to their higher energy state and when it comes back to its ground state it releases energy in the form of light.

With the increasing demand for developing nanomaterials having properties of both drug carriers and imaging the diseased tissues at the same platform, QD have emerged as the most convenient nanoplatform for cancer therapy and theranostics. The various biomedical applications of quantum dots are listed in Fig. 2.10. QDs show an intense bright fluorescence which makes them suitable for diagnosis, whereas their chemical and physical properties make them suitable for drug delivery (Matea et al., 2017).

QDs can be prepared by two general methods: (1) colloidal-based synthesis and (2) lithography-based synthesis. In the colloidal-based synthesis, the semiconductor precursor such as indium is added under vigorous stirring and high temperatures to the solvent which has molecules that will coordinate to the surface of the QDs particles. On the other hand, in the

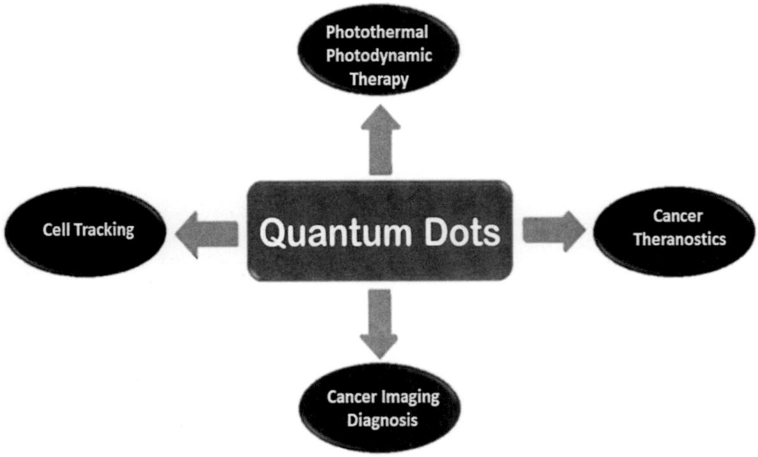

Fig. 2.10 Biomedical applications of quantum dots.

lithography-based method, a high-resolution focused beam of the electron is used that draws the customized design on the surface of the polymeric compound (Chomoucka et al., 2009).

QDs are composed of cadmium, lead, mercury, silver, and copper as heavy metals, which increase their toxicity profile. Cadmium is known to inhibit DNA, RNA, and proteins synthesis, and it can also break down the DNA strands. In vivo studies show that quantum dots get accumulated in the lungs resulting in lung injury and inflammation. Roberts et al. explained that most cadmium containing QDs become persevered in the lungs during postexposure to QDs among rodents, while some are stored in the airway. These deposited particles are however hard to clear from lungs (Roberts et al., 2013). To use them clinically, it is important to generate a minimum toxicity profile to reduce toxicity and improve biocompatibility in QDs so that they are functionalized by biocompatible molecules or polymers at the surface (Al-Jamal and Kostarelos, 2012).

2.5.2.5 Mesoporous silica nanoparticles

Mesoporous silica nanoparticles (MSNs) are nanosized mesoporous silica, which have unique features like stability, adjustable pores, and large surface area making them suitable for loading various anticancerous drugs. They contain pores with a diameter ranging from 2 to 50 nm. MSNs have an external and internal surface that can be selectively functionalized with different organic and inorganic groups. These nanoparticles can encapsulate a large range of therapeutic agents such as proteins, peptides, small molecules, without making any chemical modification as they can accumulate into the pores of MSNs. MSNs can also be used as theranostic agents since many bioimaging dyes can also be loaded into the pores of MSNs. MSNs are considered as efficient nanocarriers for therapeutic agents because they have high storage capacity, controlled release properties, and target specific delivery (Manzano and Vallet-Regí, 2020). Owing to the presence of polar groups (like Si-OH and Ti-OH), MSNs are hydrophilic in nature and improve the solubility of hydrophobic drugs to improve their bioavailability and absorption.

Interestingly, MNPs can be encapsulated into MSN along with chemotherapeutic drugs to improve chemotherapeutic results. Most MSNs can be used for hyperthermia therapy which can reduce cancer cells viability (Zhou et al., 2018).

MSNs are composed of amorphous metal oxides and can be prepared by a sol-gel method where a surfactant is used as a template for a structure designing agent. This process involves hydrolysis and condensation of silicon oxide under catalytic conditions.

The toxicity of MSNs is dependent on their size and administration route. An in vitro study of MSNs in SHSY5Y cells and bone marrow cells revealed that at low doses, there was no toxic effect observed while at higher doses, substantial toxicity was observed (Shivendra et al., 2018).

2.6 Conclusion and future perspectives

The application of nanotechnology in medicine started with cancer therapy and eventually branched out for other disease treatments. Advancements in nanotechnology and materials science has implicated that nanomaterial-based formulations are the new wave of clinical research. The continuous progressive evolution in nanomedicine research has introduced potential tools for cancer diagnosis, cancer treatment, and cancer management. In this book chapter, we highlighted the diversity of various organic and inorganic nanoparticles that have been clinically used or have the potential to be used as a nanocarrier to improve the efficacy of cancer treatment overcoming various challenges faced by traditional chemotherapy. Nanomaterials have empowered the therapeutic outcome of biologicals and synthetic drugs by delivering them selectively to the target site and thereby reducing the toxic effect which otherwise would be caused due to nonspecific drug delivery. A distinctive attribute of multifunctional theranostic nanoparticles has allowed clinicians to offer improved therapeutic effectiveness and guarantees as a nonsurgical technique for tumor obliteration using combination therapies. The multifunctional theranostic nanoparticles can detect malignant cells (active targeting), tumor location and size in the body (real-time in vivo imaging), and tumor ablation with minimal or no harm to normal tissues via stimuli-responsive therapy (e.g., PDT, PTT, and RTT). Ground-breaking advancements of theranostic nanoparticles hold the potential to be transformed into the clinic due to their tumor specificity, improved biocompatibility, and less complexity.

In the most recent couple of decades, significant progress has been observed in nanoparticle-based cancer therapy. Despite that, there are plenty of challenges and unreciprocated questions such as stability and lack of understanding in vivo behavior of nanoformulations and the reasons for in vivo toxicity effects are major setbacks for their clinical progression. Most of the nanoformulations developed in the recent years have been studied in vitro for their efficacy which eventually misses the complexity of nanocarrier-cell interactions in vivo. To this end, it is of high priority to examine the pharmacological, toxicological, and immunological properties of nanoparticles in vivo utilizing appropriate animal models. Many theranostic particles are obtained by complex preparation and purification methods which further increases their production cost. Hence, despite appreciable potential as cancer theranostics in clinical practice, this results in discontinuation from the market (e.g., Ontek, FDA-approved diphtheria toxin-based recombinant fusion toxin has been discontinued from the market because of production problems related to the bacterial expression system with problematic purification). Therefore, development of approaches which can reduce production complexity is essential. There are only a few nanoformulations approved for cancer treatment in clinical practice, and most of them are based on passive targeting (EPR). However, considering the urge of targeting nanoparticles to the tumor for a more specific delivery, several ongoing clinical trials for cancer treatment are focused on active targeting mechanisms. At this stage, further advancements in nanomedicine can be anticipated for next-generation nanotheranostics capable for improved cancer management strategies.

References

Al-Jamal, W.T., Kostarelos, K., 2012. Quantum-dot toxicity. In: Bhushan, B. (Ed.), Encyclopedia of Nanotechnology. Springer Netherlands, Dordrecht, pp. 2197–2200.

Amreddy, N., Babu, A., Panneerselvam, J., Srivastava, A., Muralidharan, R., Chen, A., Zhao, Y.D., Munshi, A., Ramesh, R., 2018. Chemo-biologic combinatorial drug delivery using folate receptor-targeted dendrimer nanoparticles for lung cancer treatment. Nanomedicine 14 (2), 373–384.

Attia, M.F., Anton, N., Wallyn, J., Omran, Z., Vandamme, T.F., 2019. An overview of active and passive targeting strategies to improve the nanocarriers efficiency to tumour sites. J. Pharm. Pharmacol. 71 (8), 1185–1198.

Augustin, H.G., Kozian, D.H., Johnson, R.C., 1994. Differentiation of endothelial cells: analysis of the constitutive and activated endothelial cell phenotypes. Bioessays 16 (12), 901–906.

BaoLin, G., Ma, P.X., 2014. Synthetic biodegradable functional polymers for tissue engineering: a brief review. Sci. China Chem. 57 (4), 490–500.

Bhirde, A.A., Patel, S., Sousa, A.A., Patel, V., Molinolo, A.A., Ji, Y., Leapman, R.D., Gutkind, J.S., Rusling, J.F., 2010. Distribution and clearance of PEG-single-walled carbon nanotube cancer drug delivery vehicles in mice. Nanomedicine 5 (10), 1535–1546.

Brown, S.D., Nativo, P., Smith, J.-A., Stirling, D., Edwards, P.R., Venugopal, B., Flint, D.J., Plumb, J.A., Graham, D., Wheate, N.J., 2010. Gold nanoparticles for the improved anticancer drug delivery of the active component of Oxaliplatin. J.Am. Chem. Soc. 132 (13), 4678–4684.

Cha, C., Shin, S.R., Annabi, N., Dokmeci, M.R., Khademhosseini, A., 2013. Carbon-based nanomaterials: multifunctional materials for biomedical engineering. ACS Nano 7 (4), 2891–2897.

Chamseddine, I.M., Frieboes, H.B., Kokkolaras, M., 2018. Design optimization of tumor vasculature-bound nanoparticles. Sci. Rep. 8 (1), 17768.

Chomoucka, J., Drbohlavova, J., Adam, V., Kizek, R., Hubalek, J., 2009. Synthesis of glutathione-coated quantum dots, 2009. In: 32nd International Spring Seminar on Electronics Technology,. 13–17 May 2009.

Daraee, H., Etemadi, A., Kouhi, M., Alimirzalu, S., Akbarzadeh, A., 2016. Application of liposomes in medicine and drug delivery. Artif. Cells Nanomed. Biotechnol. 44 (1), 381–391.

Elzoghby, A.O., Samy, W.M., Elgindy, N.A., 2012. Albumin-based nanoparticles as potential controlled release drug delivery systems. J. Control. Release 157 (2), 168–182.

Fassas, A., Anagnostopoulos, A., 2005. The use of liposomal daunorubicin (DaunoXome) in acute myeloid leukemia. Leuk. Lymphoma 46 (6), 795–802.

Folkman, J., 1971. Tumor angiogenesis: therapeutic implications. N. Engl. J. Med. 285 (21), 1182–1186.

Frechet, J.M., 1994. Functional polymers and dendrimers: reactivity, molecular architecture, and interfacial energy. Science 263 (5154), 1710–1715.

Gao, S., Wei, G., Zhang, S., Zheng, B., Xu, J., Chen, G., Li, M., Song, S., Fu, W., Xiao, Z., Lu, W., 2019. Albumin tailoring fluorescence and photothermal conversion effect of near-infrared-II fluorophore with aggregation-induced emission characteristics. Nat. Commun. 10 (1), 2206.

Gerber, D.E., 2008. Targeted therapies: a new generation of cancer treatments. Am. Fam. Physician 77 (3), 311–319.

Gradishar, W.J., 2006. Albumin-bound paclitaxel: a next-generation taxane. Expert Opin. Pharmacother. 7 (8), 1041–1053.

Guarnieri, D., Sabella, S., Muscetti, O., Belli, V., Malvindi, M.A., Fusco, S., De Luca, E., Pompa, P.P., Netti, P.A., 2014. Transport across the cell-membrane dictates nanoparticle fate and toxicity: a new paradigm in nanotoxicology. Nanoscale 6 (17), 10264–10273.

Gullotti, E., Yeo, Y., 2009. Extracellularly activated nanocarriers: a new paradigm of tumor targeted drug delivery. Mol. Pharm. 6 (4), 1041–1051.

Hadrup, N., Sharma, A.K., Poulsen, M., Nielsen, E., 2015. Toxicological risk assessment of elemental gold following oral exposure to sheets and nanoparticles—a review. Regul. Toxicol. Pharmacol. 72 (2), 216–221.

Han, Z., Wu, X., Roelle, S., Chen, C., Schiemann, W.P., Lu, Z.-R., 2018. Author correction: targeted gadofullerene for sensitive magnetic resonance imaging and risk-stratification of breast cancer. Nat. Commun. 9 (1), 153.

Heldin, C.-H., Rubin, K., Pietras, K., Östman, A., 2004. High interstitial fluid pressure—an obstacle in cancer therapy. Nat. Rev. Cancer 4 (10), 806–813.
Herizchi, R., Abbasi, E., Milani, M., Akbarzadeh, A., 2016. Current methods for synthesis of gold nanoparticles. Artif. Cells Nanomed. Biotechnol. 44 (2), 596–602.
Hickey, J.W., Santos, J.L., Williford, J.-M., Mao, H.-Q., 2015. Control of polymeric nanoparticle size to improve therapeutic delivery. J. Control. Release 219, 536–547.
Hofheinz, R.-D., Gnad-Vogt, S.U., Beyer, U., Hochhaus, A., 2005. Liposomal encapsulated anti-cancer drugs. Anticancer Drugs 16 (7), 691–707.
Hong, S., Bielinska, A.U., Mecke, A., Keszler, B., Beals, J.L., Shi, X., Balogh, L., Orr, B.G., Baker, J.R., Banaszak Holl, M.M., 2004. Interaction of poly(amidoamine) dendrimers with supported lipid bilayers and cells: hole formation and the relation to transport. Bioconjug. Chem. 15 (4), 774–782.
Hu, W., Cheng, L., Cheng, L., Zheng, M., Lei, Q., Hu, Z., Xu, M., Qiu, L., Chen, D., 2014. Redox and pH-responsive poly (amidoamine) dendrimer–poly (ethylene glycol) conjugates with disulfide linkages for efficient intracellular drug release. Colloids Surf. B. Biointerfaces 123, 254–263.
Hu, W., Qiu, L., Cheng, L., Hu, Q., Liu, Y., Hu, Z., Chen, D., Cheng, L., 2016. Redox and pH dual responsive poly(amidoamine) dendrimer-poly(ethylene glycol) conjugates for intracellular delivery of doxorubicin. Acta Biomater. 36, 241–253.
Jain, R.K., Stylianopoulos, T., 2010. Delivering nanomedicine to solid tumors. Nat. Rev. Clin. Oncol. 7 (11), 653–664.
Jain, S., Hirst, D.G., O'Sullivan, J.M., 2012. Gold nanoparticles as novel agents for cancer therapy. Br. J. Radiol. 85 (1010), 101–113.
Jiang, Z., Shan, K., Song, J., Liu, J., Rajendran, S., Pugazhendhi, A., Jacob, J.A., Chen, B., 2019. Toxic effects of magnetic nanoparticles on normal cells and organs. Life Sci. 220, 156–161.
Kalva, N., Parekh, N., Ambade, A.V., 2015. Controlled micellar disassembly of photo- and pH-cleavable linear-dendritic block copolymers. Polym. Chem. 6 (38), 6826–6835.
Kerbel, R.S., 1991. Inhibition of tumor angiogenesis as a strategy to circumvent acquired resistance to anti-cancer therapeutic agents. Bioessays 13 (1), 31–36.
Kim, T.-Y., Kim, D.-W., Chung, J.-Y., Shin, S.G., Kim, S.-C., Heo, D.S., Kim, N.K., Bang, Y.-J., 2004. Phase I and pharmacokinetic study of Genexol-PM, a Cremophor-free, polymeric micelle-formulated paclitaxel, in patients with advanced malignancies. Clin. Cancer Res. 10 (11), 3708.
Kim, T.-H., Kim, M., Park, H.-S., Shin, U.S., Gong, M.-S., Kim, H.-W., 2012. Size-dependent cellular toxicity of silver nanoparticles. J. Biomed. Mater. Res. A 100A (4), 1033–1043.
Kimura, H., Ogura, Y., 2001. Biodegradable polymers for ocular drug delivery. Ophthalmologica 215 (3), 143–155.
Kneidl, B., Peller, M., Winter, G., Lindner, L.H., Hossann, M., 2014. Thermosensitive liposomal drug delivery systems: state of the art review. Int. J. Nanomedicine 9, 4387–4398.
Krishna, V., Singh, A., Sharma, P., Iwakuma, N., Wang, Q., Zhang, Q., Knapik, J., Jiang, H., Grobmyer, S.R., Koopman, B., Moudgil, B., 2010. Polyhydroxy fullerenes for non-invasive Cancer imaging and therapy. Small 6 (20), 2236–2241.
Lammers, T., Hennink, W.E., Storm, G., 2008. Tumour-targeted nanomedicines: principles and practice. Br. J. Cancer 99 (3), 392–397.
Lay, C.L., Liu, J., Liu, Y., 2011. Functionalized carbon nanotubes for anticancer drug delivery. Expert Rev.Med. Devices 8 (5), 561–566.
Leconte, Y., Veintemillas-Verdaguer, S., Morales, M.P., Costo, R., Rodríguez, I., Bonville, P., Bouchet-Fabre, B., Herlin-Boime, N., 2007. Continuous production of water dispersible carbon–iron nanocomposites by laser pyrolysis: application as MRI contrasts. J. Colloid Interface Sci. 313 (2), 511–518.
Lee, C.C., Gillies, E.R., Fox, M.E., Guillaudeu, S.J., Fréchet, J.M.J., Dy, E.E., Szoka, F.C., 2006. A single dose of doxorubicin-functionalized bow-tie dendrimer cures mice bearing C-26 colon carcinomas. Proc. Natl. Acad. Sci. U. S. A. 103 (45), 16649–16654.

Lee, E.J., Lee, N.K., Kim, I.-S., 2016. Bioengineered protein-based nanocage for drug delivery. Adv. Drug Deliv. Rev. 106, 157–171.
Liu, Z., Liang, X.-J., 2012. Nano-carbons as theranostics. Theranostics 2 (3), 235–237.
Lohcharoenkal, W., Wang, L., Chen, Y.C., Rojanasakul, Y., 2014. Protein nanoparticles as drug delivery carriers for Cancer therapy. Biomed. Res. Int. 2014, 180549.
Maiti, D., Tong, X., Mou, X., Yang, K., 2019. Carbon-based nanomaterials for biomedical applications: a recent study. Front. Pharmacol. 9, 1401.
Makadia, H.K., Siegel, S.J., 2011. Poly lactic-co-glycolic acid (PLGA) as biodegradable controlled drug delivery carrier. Polymers 3 (3), 1377–1397.
Manzano, M., Vallet-Regí, M., 2020. Mesoporous silica nanoparticles for drug delivery. Adv. Funct. Mater. 30 (2), 1902634.
Matea, C.T., Mocan, T., Tabaran, F., Pop, T., Mosteanu, O., Puia, C., Iancu, C., Mocan, L., 2017. Quantum dots in imaging, drug delivery and sensor applications. Int. J. Nanomedicine 12, 5421–5431.
Mendes, R.G., Bachmatiuk, A., Büchner, B., Cuniberti, G., Rümmeli, M.H., 2013. Carbon nanostructures as multi-functional drug delivery platforms. J. Mater. Chem. B 1 (4), 401–428.
Mikawa, M., Kato, H., Okumura, M., Narazaki, M., Kanazawa, Y., Miwa, N., Shinohara, H., 2001. Paramagnetic water-soluble Metallofullerenes having the highest Relaxivity for MRI contrast agents. Bioconjug. Chem. 12 (4), 510–514.
Mimeault, M., Hauke, R., Batra, S.K., 2008. Recent advances on the molecular mechanisms involved in the drug resistance of cancer cells and novel targeting therapies. Clin. Pharmacol. Ther. 83 (5), 673–691.
Mody, V.V., Nounou, M.I., Bikram, M., 2009. Novel nanomedicine-based MRI contrast agents for gynecological malignancies. Adv. Drug Deliv. Rev. 61 (10), 795–807.
Moon, H.K., Lee, S.H., Choi, H.C., 2009. In vivo near-infrared mediated tumor destruction by Photothermal effect of carbon nanotubes. ACS Nano 3 (11), 3707–3713.
Murakami, T., 2017. Photodynamic action of single-walled carbon nanotubes. Chem. Pharm. Bull. 65 (7), 629–636.
Needham, D., Dewhirst, M.W., 2001. The development and testing of a new temperature-sensitive drug delivery system for the treatment of solid tumors. Adv. Drug Deliv. Rev. 53 (3), 285–305.
Nguyen, T.L., Nguyen, T.H., Nguyen, C.K., Nguyen, D.H., 2017. Redox and pH responsive poly (Amidoamine) dendrimer-heparin conjugates via disulfide linkages for Letrozole delivery. Biomed. Res. Int. 2017, 8589212.
Nigam, S., Bahadur, D., 2017. Dendrimer-conjugated iron oxide nanoparticles as stimuli-responsive drug carriers for thermally-activated chemotherapy of cancer. Colloids Surf. B. Biointerfaces 155, 182–192.
Otsuka, H., Nagasaki, Y., Kataoka, K., 2003. PEGylated nanoparticles for biological and pharmaceutical applications. Adv. Drug Deliv. Rev. 55 (3), 403–419.
Panyam, J., Labhasetwar, V., 2003. Biodegradable nanoparticles for drug and gene delivery to cells and tissue. Adv. Drug Deliv. Rev. 55 (3), 329–347.
Paszkiewicz, S., Irska, I., Piesowicz, E., 2020. Environmentally friendly polymer blends based on post-consumer glycol-modified poly(ethylene terephthalate) (PET-G) foils and poly(ethylene 2,5-Furanoate) (PEF): preparation and characterization. Materials 13 (12), 2673.
Pei, X., Zhu, Z., Gan, Z., Chen, J., Zhang, X., Cheng, X., Wan, Q., Wang, J., 2020. PEGylated nano-graphene oxide as a nanocarrier for delivering mixed anticancer drugs to improve anticancer activity. Sci. Rep. 10 (1), 2717.
Pene, F., Courtine, E., Cariou, A., Mira, J.-P., 2009. Toward theragnostics. Crit. Care Med. 37(Suppl. 1):S50–S58.
Perumal, V., Sivakumar, P.M., Zarrabi, A., Muthupandian, S., Vijayaraghavalu, S., Sahoo, K., Das, A., Das, S., Payyappilly, S.S., Das, S., 2019. Near infra-red polymeric nanoparticle based optical imaging in Cancer diagnosis. J. Photochem. Photobiol. 199, 111630.

Plachá, D., Jampilek, J., 2019. Graphenic materials for biomedical applications. Nanomaterials 9 (12), 1758.
Ran, S., Thorpe, P.E., 2002. Phosphatidylserine is a marker of tumor vasculature and a potential target for cancer imaging and therapy. Int. J. Radiat. Oncol. Biol. Phys. 54 (5), 1479–1484.
Roberts, J.R., Antonini, J.M., Porter, D.W., Chapman, R.S., Scabilloni, J.F., Young, S.-H., Schwegler-Berry, D., Castranova, V., Mercer, R.R., 2013. Lung toxicity and biodistribution of cd/se-ZnS quantum dots with different surface functional groups after pulmonary exposure in rats. Part. Fibre Toxicol. 10 (1), 5.
Sercombe, L., Veerati, T., Moheimani, F., Wu, S.Y., Sood, A.K., Hua, S., 2015. Advances and challenges of liposome assisted drug delivery. Front. Pharmacol. 6, 286.
Shen, Y., Ma, X., Zhang, B., Zhou, Z., Sun, Q., Jin, E., Sui, M., Tang, J., Wang, J., Fan, M., 2011. Degradable dual pH- and temperature-responsive Photoluminescent dendrimers. Chem. A Eur. J. 17 (19), 5319–5326.
Shi, X., Wang, S.H., Swanson, S.D., Ge, S., Cao, Z., Van Antwerp, M.E., Landmark, K.J., Baker Jr., J.R., 2008. Dendrimer-functionalized shell-crosslinked iron oxide nanoparticles for in-vivo magnetic resonance imaging of tumors. Adv. Mater. 20 (9), 1671–1678.
Shi, J., Wang, L., Gao, J., Liu, Y., Zhang, J., Ma, R., Liu, R., Zhang, Z., 2014. A fullerene-based multi-functional nanoplatform for cancer theranostic applications. Biomaterials 35 (22), 5771–5784.
Shi, J., Wang, B., Wang, L., Lu, T., Fu, Y., Zhang, H., Zhang, Z., 2016. Fullerene (C60)-based tumor-targeting nanoparticles with "off-on" state for enhanced treatment of cancer. J. Control. Release 235, 245–258.
Shivendra, C., Geetha, M., Pravir, K., Rashmi, K.A., 2018. Cellular toxicity of mesoporous silica nanoparticle in SHSY5Y and BMMNCs cell. Pharm. Nanotechnol. 6 (4), 245–252.
Siegrist, S., Cörek, E., Detampel, P., Sandström, J., Wick, P., Huwyler, J., 2019. Preclinical hazard evaluation strategy for nanomedicines. Nanotoxicology 13 (1), 73–99.
Soares, S., Sousa, J., Pais, A., Vitorino, C., 2018. Nanomedicine: principles, properties, and regulatory issues. Front. Chem. 6, 360.
Spetzler, J.C., Tam, J.P., 1995. Unprotected peptides as building blocks for branched peptides and peptide dendrimers. Int. J. Pept. Protein Res. 45 (1), 78–85.
Strebhardt, K., Ullrich, A., 2008. Paul Ehrlich's magic bullet concept: 100 years of progress. Nat. Rev. Cancer 8 (6), 473–480.
Sukhanova, A., Bozrova, S., Sokolov, P., Berestovoy, M., Karaulov, A., Nabiev, I., 2018. Dependence of nanoparticle toxicity on their physical and chemical properties. Nanoscale Res. Lett. 13 (1), 44.
Sung, Y.K., Kim, S.W., 2020. Recent advances in polymeric drug delivery systems. Biomater. Res. 24 (1), 12.
Svenson, S., Tomalia, D.A., 2005. Dendrimers in biomedical applications—reflections on the field. Adv. Drug Deliv. Rev. 57 (15), 2106–2129.
Tomalia, D.A., Baker, H., Dewald, J., Hall, M., Kallos, G., Martin, S., Roeck, J., Ryder, J., Smith, P., 1985. A new class of polymers: starburst-dendritic macromolecules. Polym. J. 17 (1), 117–132.
Torchilin, V.P., 2000. Drug targeting. Eur. J. Pharmacol. 11, S81–S91.
Torchilin, V.P., 2005. Recent advances with liposomes as pharmaceutical carriers. Nat. Rev. Drug Discov. 4 (2), 145–160.
Toy, R., Peiris, P.M., Ghaghada, K.B., Karathanasis, E., 2014. Shaping cancer nanomedicine: the effect of particle shape on the in vivo journey of nanoparticles. Nanomedicine (Lond.) 9 (1), 121–134.
Valent, P., Groner, B., Schumacher, U., Superti-Furga, G., Busslinger, M., Kralovics, R., Zielinski, C., Penninger, J.M., Kerjaschki, D., Stingl, G., Smolen, J.S., Valenta, R., Lassmann, H., Kovar, H., Jäger, U., Kornek, G., Müller, M., Sörgel, F., 2016. Paul Ehrlich (1854-1915) and his contributions to the foundation and birth of translational medicine. J. Innate Immun. 8 (2), 111–120.

Verma, D., Gulati, N., Kaul, S., Mukherjee, S., Nagaich, U., 2018. Protein based nanostructures for drug delivery. Int. J. Pharm. 2018, 9285854.
Vivero-Escoto, J.L., Slowing, I.I., Wu, C.-W., Lin, V.S.Y., 2009. Photoinduced intracellular controlled release drug delivery in human cells by gold-capped mesoporous silica Nanosphere. J. Am. Chem. 131 (10), 3462–3463.
Wang, J., Yang, H., 2018. Superelastic and pH-responsive degradable dendrimer Cryogels prepared by Cryo-aza-Michael addition reaction. Sci. Rep. 8 (1), 7155.
Wang, L., Shi, J., Liu, R., Liu, Y., Zhang, J., Yu, X., Gao, J., Zhang, C., Zhang, Z., 2014a. Photodynamic effect of functionalized single-walled carbon nanotubes: a potential sensitizer for photodynamic therapy. Nanoscale 6 (9), 4642–4651.
Wang, Z., Niu, G., Chen, X., 2014b. Polymeric materials for Theranostic applications. Pharm. Res. 31 (6), 1358–1376.
Wang, H., Huang, Q., Chang, H., Xiao, J., Cheng, Y., 2016. Stimuli-responsive dendrimers in drug delivery. Biomater. Sci. 4 (3), 375–390.
Williams, M.J., Corr, S.A., 2013. Chapter 2—Magnetic nanoparticles for targeted Cancer diagnosis and therapy. In: Summers, H. (Ed.), Frontiers of Nanoscience. Elsevier, pp. 29–63.
Wörner, C., Mülhaupt, R., 1993. Polynitrile- and polyamine-functional poly(trimethylene imine) dendrimers. Angew. Chem. Int. Ed. 32 (9), 1306–1308.
Yan, L., Zhao, F., Li, S., Hu, Z., Zhao, Y., 2011. Low-toxic and safe nanomaterials by surface-chemical design, carbon nanotubes, fullerenes, metallofullerenes, and graphenes. Nanoscale 3 (2), 362–382.
Yang, K., Feng, L., Shi, X., Liu, Z., 2013. Nano-graphene in biomedicine: theranostic applications. Chem. Soc. Rev. 42 (2), 530–547.
Yang, K., Feng, L., Liu, Z., 2016. Stimuli responsive drug delivery systems based on nano-graphene for cancer therapy. Adv. Drug Deliv. Rev. 105, 228–241.
Yigit, M.V., Moore, A., Medarova, Z., 2012. Magnetic nanoparticles for Cancer diagnosis and therapy. Pharm. Res. 29 (5), 1180–1188.
Yokoyama, M., Satoh, A., Sakurai, Y., Okano, T., Matsumura, Y., Kakizoe, T., Kataoka, K., 1998. Incorporation of water-insoluble anticancer drug into polymeric micelles and control of their particle size. J. Control. Release 55 (2), 219–229.
Yoo, D., Lee, J.-H., Shin, T.-H., Cheon, J., 2011. Theranostic magnetic nanoparticles. Acc. Chem. Res. 44 (10), 863–874.
Zhang, C., Pan, D., Luo, K., She, W., Guo, C., Yang, Y., Gu, Z., 2014a. Peptide dendrimer–doxorubicin conjugate-based nanoparticles as an enzyme-responsive drug delivery system for Cancer therapy. Adv. Healthc. Mater. 3 (8), 1299–1308.
Zhang, J., Ye, Y., Chen, Y., Pregot, C., Li, T., Balasubramaniam, S., Hobart, D.B., Zhang, Y., Wi, S., Davis, R.M., Madsen, L.A., Morris, J.R., LaConte, S.M., Yee, G.T., Dorn, H.C., 2014b. Gd3N@C84(OH)x: a new egg-shaped Metallofullerene magnetic resonance imaging contrast agent. J. Am. Chem. 136 (6), 2630–2636.
Zhang, C., Pan, D., Li, J., Hu, J., Bains, A., Guys, N., Zhu, H., Li, X., Luo, K., Gong, Q., Gu, Z., 2017. Enzyme-responsive peptide dendrimer-gemcitabine conjugate as a controlled-release drug delivery vehicle with enhanced antitumor efficacy. Acta Biomater. 55, 153–162.
Zhang, J., Jiang, C., Figueiró Longo, J.P., Azevedo, R.B., Zhang, H., Muehlmann, L.A., 2018. An updated overview on the development of new photosensitizers for anticancer photodynamic therapy. Acta Pharm. Sin. B 8 (2), 137–146.
Zhao, W., Zhuang, S., Qi, X.-R., 2011. Comparative study of the in vitro and in vivo characteristics of cationic and neutral liposomes. Int. J. Nanomedicine 6, 3087–3098.
Zhou, Y., Quan, G., Wu, Q., Zhang, X., Niu, B., Wu, B., Huang, Y., Pan, X., Wu, C., 2018. Mesoporous silica nanoparticles for drug and gene delivery. Acta Pharm. Sin. B 8 (2), 165–177.
Zolnik, B.S., González-Fernández, A., Sadrieh, N., Dobrovolskaia, M.A., 2010. Nanoparticles and the immune system. Endocrinology 151 (2), 458–465.

CHAPTER 3

Nanobiomaterials in hard tissue repair

Poulomi Sengupta
Department of Chemistry, School of Science, Indrashil University, Rajpur, Gujarat, India

3.1 Introduction

Since the dawn of civilization, human beings have faced various challenges for survival. The majority of the challenges originated for better food, shelter, and health. Prehistoric men, having a developed brain, tried several innovative ideas to satiate their ever-growing demands for living longer and better. Since then, billions of years have passed, and the zeal for a better living continued. It drove the human race to develop better therapeutics and useful materials to earn a flexible and painless living. "Biomaterials" are one of those discoveries, which have helped the human race to earn a physically comfortable life.

Biomaterials are foreign objects used inside (sometimes outside) the human body. The origin of the material is not necessarily biological. The prefix "bio" comes for its location of use, which is inside a biological species (Black, 1982; Ratner et al., 2004). They are used mainly for three purposes: (1) to support in the recovery from an ailment; (2) to improve functionality (movement); and (3) to correct an abnormality (look better). For a long time, the use of biomaterials is common for such applications. For example, to fix a broken bone, traditionally a wooden plank is used, but the discovery or the first use was never formally reported. In ancient times, Egyptians used horse-hair to close open wounds. The probable reasons for selecting this material were as follows: (1) horse-hair is biocompatible (nontoxic to the human body); (2) it is biodegradable; and (3) it is readily available. It is surprising to learn that even in the modern age, the biomaterials we use are based on these three key points. Later, seashells were reported to fill in the gap of a lost tooth. This was more for aesthetic purposes than for any practical reason. Ancient (even modern) Indians used gold plating on an existing

Nanotechnology in Medicine and Biology
https://doi.org/10.1016/B978-0-12-819469-0.00005-8

tooth both for strengthening and for showing off their wealth. All these are examples of ancient biomaterials.

With time, like every other field, the field of biomaterials also progressed; and instead of horse-hair and conch shell, many more objects were being used inside/outside the human body. After the Civil War, in the United States, several soldiers were left without their limbs. As a result, they tried different external materials to have control in day-to-day life. The materials were mainly metallic and wooden. Artificial limbs not only enhanced their flexibility, but also assisted in boosting their confidence and they looked "normal" as any other individual. Fig. 3.1A indicates a comic character Captain Hook from the famous "Peter Pan" series using a hook hand after losing his real hand. However, until this time, the material was metallic or wooden.

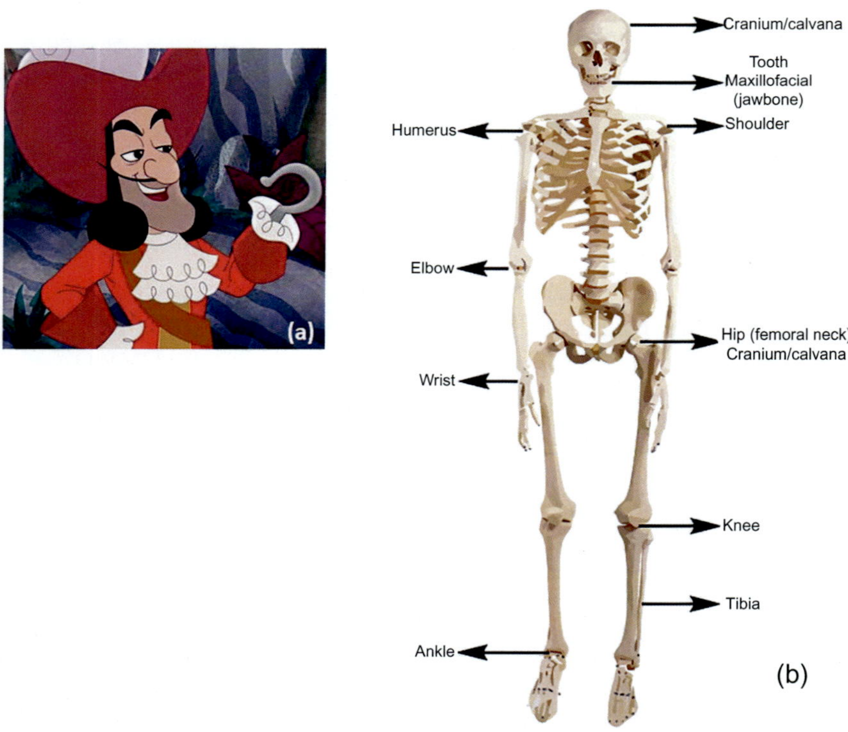

Fig. 3.1 (A) Captain Hook, a character from Peter Pan uses a "Hook hand." (B) Different locations in the human body for hard tissue engineering. ((A) Screenshot from Jake and the Never Land Pirates Television series. Screenshot from Captain Hook videos. Disney Junior, Disney Series. https://jakeandtheneverlandpirates.fandom.com/wiki/Captain_Hook# (Accessed 9 November 2020). Copyright 1953 Disney Junior.)

The next (20th) century witnessed a revolution in polymer synthesis. With the discovery of different man-made polymers, material science took a large leap forward. Polymers have different surface textures, porosity, surface area, flexibility, and functional groups available which can be used for different purposes inside the human body as illustrated in Fig. 3.1B. During a similar time, the characterization techniques [e.g., X-ray crystallography, XRD (X-ray diffraction), XPS (X-ray photoelectron spectroscopy), ICP-MS (inductively coupled plasma mass spectrometry), and ICP-AES (inductively coupled plasma atomic emission spectroscopy)] have also tremendously progressed. This made the characterization of man-made materials smoother. In 1948, plastic contact lenses were developed using poly(methyl methacrylate) (PMMA). In 1949, it was successfully implanted in humans. During 1956, McKee and Watson Farrar pioneered the "total hip" with an acetabular cup. Later during 1968–72, the first total knee replacement surgery was performed which has become quite a regular affair in today's senior citizens. Later, the natural scientific intellect combined various materials of different origin, which resulted in the discovery of composites of various strength and durability. The later years saw many more important discoveries in the field of biomaterials; for example, the replacement of the heart valve, heart implants, the discovery of the lab-grown functional kidney, and the lab-grown brain. For the past 40 years, nanotechnology knocked the doors of material science. Hence, a bunch of completely new/ improved materials poured in which were excellent tissue replacement materials. The field of tissue engineering accumulated many attractive problems and nanotechnology had acquired an immense amount of potential. However, in this chapter, we will limit ourselves to the "hard tissue engineering" part. Hard tissue engineering is equally interesting as well as challenging as regular tissue engineering, but it focuses more on hard tissue, which includes bone fixation and bone replacements as point out in Fig. 3.1B, rather than replacing organs (like the heart, brain, and kidney). Hence, perhaps the level of complicacy is a little lower, but it has very wide challenges and innumerable applications. Here, in this chapter, we will focus on certain aspects of biomaterials used specifically for hard tissue engineering, especially the type and function. A brief discussion about guided bone regeneration is also included.

3.2 Biomaterials in hard tissue engineering

As discussed in the introductory part, traditionally, several materials of natural origin have been used for hard tissue engineering; for example, metals, wood, and conch. During the 20th century, with the tremendous advancements in polymer science and material science, scientists and medical practitioners started thinking about bio-mimicking a lost organ using the foreign material placed inside a live tissue. This was quite a revolutionary thought, as it was unprecedented. For that purpose, physical similarity (including shape size), surface texture, superficial rigidity, elasticity, biodegradability, bioresorbability, and nonbiodegradability were some of the important criteria. With fast advancements in fields like chemistry and material science, materials like calcium phosphates, hydroxyapatite, graphene, graphene-oxide, different polymers (highly contributing to biodegradability, malleability, etc.), bare metals, are considered to be of high importance (Zhang et al., 2018). Some materials used in hard tissue engineering are listed in Table 3.1. Scaffolds made out of these materials were expected to function as an excellent extracellular matrix (ECM), which must "replace" an existing hard tissue inside the human body. Cells binding to the three-dimensional scaffolds and proliferating is a key important step for the success of one scaffold in vivo. To direct the binding of cells onto the scaffolds, biomolecules can be immobilized to the scaffold structure to enhance cell-material interactions. The schematic is represented in Fig. 3.2.

Table 3.1 Materials used in hard tissue engineering.

No.	Type of material	Examples
1	Carbon and polyester composites	Carbon nanomaterials Titanium-reinforced PLGA (poly lactic-*co*-glycolic acid)
2	Crystalline ceramics	Hydroxyapatite Calcium metaphosphate Tricalcium phosphate
3	Amorphous glasses	Bioglass Silica
4	Composites	Hydroxyapatite/poly(ε-caprolactone), chitosan and and/or collagen Poly(lactic acid)/tricalcium phosphate, silica, and/or ceramic Titanium/calcium phosphate, poly(vinyl alcohol), and/or boron
5	Metals	Alumina Stainless steel Titanium

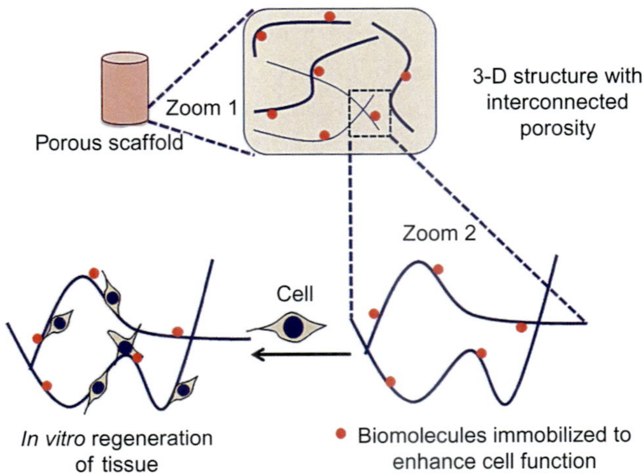

Fig. 3.2 Schematic representation of a solid scaffold containing biological molecules and it is in vitro application in the regeneration of tissues.

3.2.1 Problems in biomaterials

Although by this time (the late 1970s), it was possible to develop superficial mimics with proper size, shape, biodegradability, and bioresorbability similar to the missing organ/tissue inside the human body, proper integration with the existing tissue was a serious challenge. At the beginning of the journey, the market for hard tissue engineering did not grow significantly, mainly because of two reasons: (1) Engineered tissues miserably failed mainly because of in vivo dislocations, which led to multiple repetitive corrective interventions. (2) Apart from that, there were chances of immunological rejection (Williams, 2019).

3.2.2 Why nanobiomaterials are a potential solution?

Nanomaterials, due to their proper size, shape, and surface properties have brought a revolution to the field of hard tissue engineering. By adjusting different reaction parameters and conditions, it has been possible to play around the strength, hardness, softness, porosity, malleability, etc. All of these properties help in the manufacturing of scaffolds, constructs, meshes, and matrices wherever necessary and aid in the proper positioning and anchorage of the foreign materials inside the human body. Also, it was possible to change the surface composition by chemical treatment, which enhanced proper attachment with existing tissues, apart from overcoming immune rejection. We can briefly list the advantages introduced by nanotechnology:

(i) Formation of a porous material having interconnected pores that allowed easy passage of nutrients, cells, drug, etc. Nanotechnology can be exploited to construct surfaces that resemble the ECM by making nanofibers, nanostructured scaffolds, nanotopographical surfaces, which ultimately help in "biomimicking" an existing tissue.

(ii) High porosity leads to lower weight in the replacement tissue and higher surface-to-volume ratio: This higher surface area provides more of a chance for new cells to adhere and make a strong foundation. The nanotechnology-based technique can help in creating smaller particle sizes and higher surface area.

(iii) Surface charge and surface functionality generation: With the help of plasma treatment it is possible to create a charge on the surface of scaffolds which helps in cellular adhesion followed by proliferation to create an active tissue with time. The surface charge and functionality can encourage ECM formation which is ultimately useful in the replacement of hard tissue.

So, existing materials were re-engineered and morphological changes in nanodimensions were introduced. Some of those were successful in in vitro experiments and are listed in Table 3.2.

Table 3.2 Nanobiomaterials used in hard tissue engineering.

S. No.	Materials	Applications
1	Hydroxyapatite	Artificial bone Bone regeneration therapy Dental tissue regeneration
2	Metal nanoparticles	Tissue and cartilage regeneration therapy Dental tissue regeneration
3	Carbon nanostructures	Nanocomposite in regeneration, nanoscale sensors Cartilage regeneration therapy Joint replacement therapy
4	Nanocomposite films	Fiber strengthening in regenerative therapy
5	Porous scaffolds	Bone reformation and bone implants Tooth regeneration
6	Nanohybrid membrane	Bone regeneration therapy Periodontal regeneration Endodontic regeneration

3.3 Nanobiomaterials in tissue engineering

3.3.1 Polymeric nanobiomaterials

Polymers, due to their controlled synthetic procedures, can have various chemical and physical properties which enable their successful use as "scaffolds" in solid tissue replacement. Apart from that, there are natural polymers (mostly animal proteins and carbohydrates like silk, collagen, chitosan, etc.), which due to their strength and biocompatibility can be used for hard tissue replacements. Using nanotechnology, it is possible to procure porous, fiber-like structures from the polymers. Here, we plan to discuss the polymers used for hard tissue engineering in two segments.

3.3.1.1 Polymers of natural origin

Certain naturally extracted protein-based polymers, for example, silk, wool, collagen, gelatin can be molded in a scaffold (singly or in unison with a synthetic polymer) with high mechanical strength so that it can act as a hard tissue replacement (Ha et al., 2013). Some carbohydrate-based natural polymers like chitin, chitosan, polysaccharides, cellulose, starch, and alginate can also be molded into scaffolds of definite shape, size, and porosity (Sell et al., 2010). The biggest advantage of naturally occurring polymers is their biocompatibility and immune-acceptance, which replaces a damaged hard tissue smoothly. These naturally occurring polymers can be extracted in different molecular weights, electrospun to create several nanosized features (porous scaffolds or fibers) that can be used for replacing hard tissues. Most importantly, polymers like collagen and elastins are found to carry the -RGD-(-Arginine-Glycine-Aspartic acid-) sequence, which recognizes cellular receptors. So, cellular attachment is vastly improved which can successfully lead to a firm replacement.

3.3.1.2 Synthetic polymers

Synthetic polymer-based hard tissue replacements gained popularity after polymer synthesis was under control. Synthetic polymers have several advantages, which place them very high in the field of hard tissue engineering. These can be tuned to degrade over an optimal period (in vivo). Regarding the challenges posed by the smooth translation of polymeric scaffolds, Williams (2019) mentioned that the rate at which a polymeric scaffolds degrade, affects the cellular adhesion process.

Hence, control over one (polymer degradability) will directly affect the other (cellular adhesion). With advanced synthetic chemistry skills, it is possible to achieve fine control in biodegradation. Apart from that, by controlling the nature of the linker, substituent, and molecular weight, different physical properties (melting point, softness, rigidity, and rheological properties) can be attributed toward the final product. Moreover, by the application of different tools (solvent casting, gas foaming, particulate leaching, electrospinning, fluid-deposition molding, and extrusion) porosity, crystallinity, the surface-to-volume ratio, and surface roughness can be fine-tuned which directly contributes to the fate of the polymeric scaffold after implantation (Quirk et al., 2004). Functional groups present in the side chains can also impart hydrophilic or hydrophobic properties which decides the extent to which the scaffolds can be comfortable in vivo. They can be easily produced industrially hence cheaper. Nanopatterning also greatly contributes toward the attachment of bone cells. For example, Xi Chen et al. in 2013 *ACS Nano* showed that by combining polymers PCL [poly(ε-caprolactone)] and PAA [poly(acrylic acid)], mineralization of calcium is possible on nanofibers (Chen et al., 2013, Fig. 3.3).

The most common polymer for constructing a three-dimensional scaffold used in hard tissue engineering is high-density polyethylene (HDPE). These, owing to their rigidity and pore formation capability (as a scaffold), are commercially used in hard tissue replacements. HDPE, being hydrophobic, has challenges to integrate with the existing tissue, but there are surface modification techniques available for the safe alteration of the surface behavior. Polyhydroxy esters, including poly(vinyl alcohol) (PVA), poly(lactic acid) (PLA), poly(glycolic acid) (PGA), PLGA, poly-L-lactic acid (PLLA), polyethylene oxide (PEO), and PCL are examples of some synthetic polymers widely tested for hard tissue engineering. To enhance mechanical properties and cellular adhesion and proliferation, the incorporation of nanoparticles (e.g., apatite component, carbon nanostructures, and metal nanoparticles) has been extensively investigated.

3.3.2 Ceramic nanobiomaterials

3.3.2.1 Bioceramics

In the quest of finding the perfect material for hard tissue engineering, several materials have been developed by thorough research. Among those, bioceramics are popular choices as they have very similar chemical and crystallographic properties with those of bones. Moreover, they are bioactive, biocompatible, and able to form good complexes with bones. Porcelain was the first bioceramic used as a tooth crown in the 18th century. Calcium

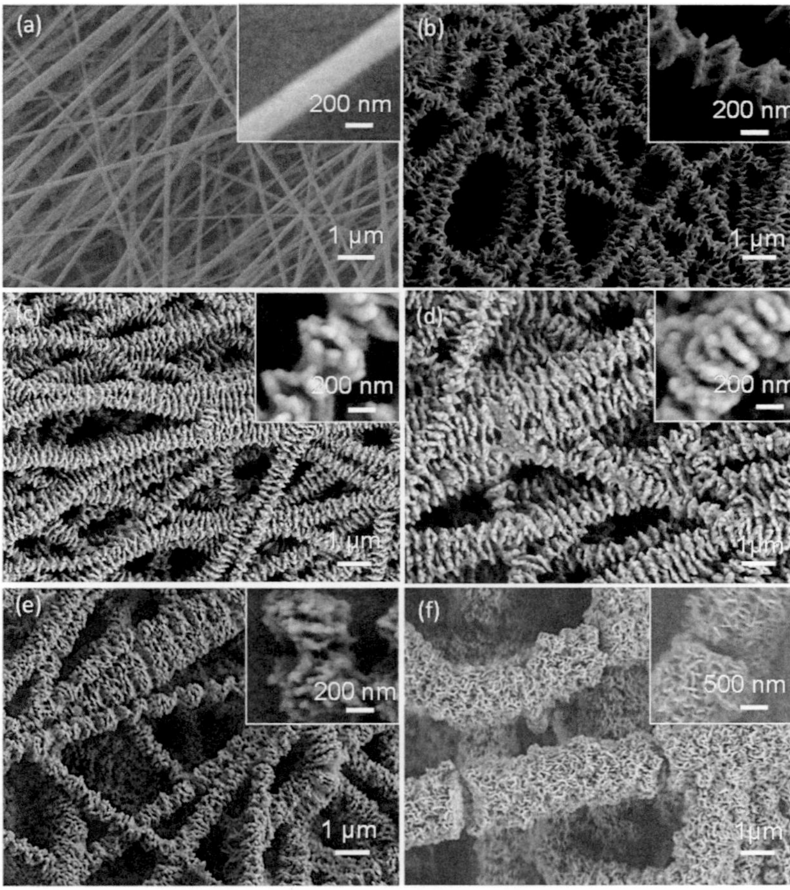

Fig. 3.3 SEM image of (A) PCL nanofiber, (B) PCL-PAA block nanofibers, (C–F) Mineralization at different time point. (From Chen, X., Wang, W., Cheng, S., Dong, B., Li, C.Y., 2013. Mimicking bone nanostructure by combining block copolymer self-assembly and 1D crystal nucleation. ACS Nano 7(9), 8251–8257. Copyright © 2013 American Chemical Society.)

phosphate ceramics are very basic among these, but they are inherently stiff (and hence) degrading. They need to be mixed with another biodegradable polymer to develop a better composition. HA (hydroxyapatite) $Ca_{10}(PO_4)_6(OH)_2$ (Freed et al., 1994), β-TCP (β-tricalcium phosphate), and BCP (biphasic calcium phosphate) are a few examples. But these basic units have been modified with higher porosity, nanopatterning keeping in mind the basic need for bone tissue engineering: that is osteoinnductivity, osteoconductivity, and osseointegration. By generating porosity, it is possible to control the degradation rate of the implant material (LeGeros, 2002; Fisher et al., 2001). Synthetic hydroxyapatite is shown to encourage osteoconduction and can be incorporated into bone without showing any immune rejection (Klein et al., 1983; Ducheyne and Qiu, 1999). Reduction in the grain size of ceramics (< 60 nm) has successfully shown the enhancement in the attachment of more osteoblasts (Webster et al., 1999). Studies showed increased calcium deposition of osteoblasts when the grain size was under 100 nm (Webster et al., 2001) and the nano-sized materials were more active compared with the micro-sized ones. Guo and colleagues fabricated 54%–81% porous calcium-deficient porous HA and by in vitro and in vivo studies, proved the porous HA has osteogenic outcomes (Guo et al., 2009). Placing mesenchymal stem cells (MSCs) on nanosized HA and β-TCP resulted in a 1.3 times enhancement in bone formation. Calcium phosphate is another basic and simple ceramic very useful for supporting bone tissue engineering. But due to its brittle nature, its use as a scaffold is restricted. Rather it has been found as a coating material covering metallic and polymeric meshes (Wolke et al., 1994; Feddes et al., 2004) ultimately leading to better osteogenecity.

3.3.2.2 Bioglass: Bioactive ceramic materials

Bioglasses also fall into this category of materials (ceramics) and work very efficiently (mainly due to their high mechanical strength) when they are built into three-dimensional porous nanostructures (LeGeros, 2002). The main ingredients for the bioglass ceramic are Ca and P. These increase the effectiveness of the bioglasses as they are present in bones as well (Hench, 1998, 2006). Some other precursors like MgO or CaF_2, and Na_2O or K_2O, can also be added to bioglasses. Even Al_2O_3 and B_2O_3 can also replace SiO_2 in bioglasses, which increase the hydrophilicity in the scaffolds leading to a better integration with the existing active tissues (DeAza et al., 2007). These form strong chemical interactions with existing bone and form an apatite layer when it comes close to the body fluid (Hench, 1991). Products like Bioglass 45S5, 58S, 70S30C, S53P4, BCT bioactive glass, and bioactive glass sol-gel derived foam scaffolds are successfully marketed for tooth- and bone-related tissue engineering (Fig. 3.4).

3.3.3 Metallic nanobiomaterials

Although polymers and ceramics are found to be excellent materials for solid tissue engineering purposes, replacing a bone needs very high mechanical strength in which a polymer (synthetic or artificial) was unable to provide. Ceramics and bioglasses could provide mechanical strength but

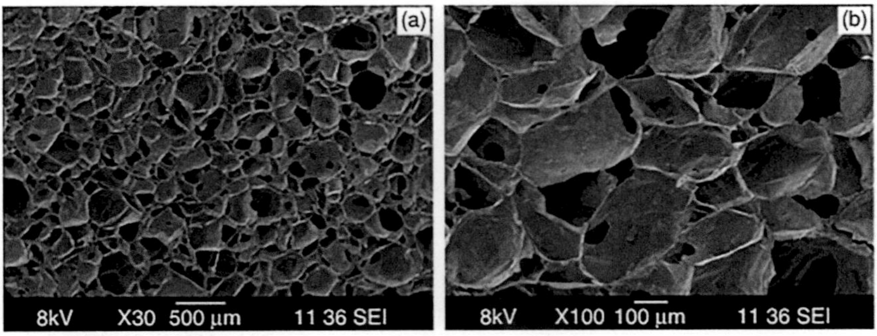

Fig. 3.4 SEM (scanning electron microscopy) images of a bioglass chitosan scaffolds. (From Erol, M., Boccaccini, A.R., 2011. Nanoscaled bioactive glass particles and nanofibres. in: Bioactive Glasses Materials, Properties and Applications. Woodhead Publishing Limited, pp. 129–161. Copyright © 2011 Woodhead Publishing Limited.)

they were brittle in certain cases. So, recently there is a fast-growing interest in the use of biodegradable metals. Metals like magnesium, due to its inherent strength and ductility, are key for building scaffolds used for hard tissue engineering applications. Metallic magnesium, and as an alloy with rare earth elements (Di Mario et al., 2004; Peeters et al., 2005; Witte et al., 2005; Hanzi et al., 2009), Ca-Mg alloys (Zhang and Yang, 2008; Li et al., 2008), pure iron (Peuster et al., 2001; Peuster et al., 2006), and their alloys are well-researched in the field of hard tissue engineering. Magnesium has a density close to natural bones (1.8–2 g/cm^3) and degrades in vivo through electrochemical processes. Magnesium can be made into porous scaffolds by nanotechnological ways, which encourage new bone formation (Xu et al., 2007). Apart from that, Witte et al. (2007) observed fast degradation in porous magnesium under in vivo circumstances. Nano-indenting and pore formation has helped magnesium metals to increase surface area and anchor better with the existing tissues. An example of porous magnesium scaffold with different topologies has been represented in Fig. 3.5(A-H).

Apart from magnesium, iron (Fe) and its alloy are well researched in hard tissue engineering. Fe foam, when coated by calcium-phosphate, has been found to encourage the accommodation and proliferation of MSCs. Titanium (along with a TiO_2 layer on the surface) has been commercialized as a hard tissue replacement scaffold. Porous Nitinol (nickel-titanium alloy) has a shape memory effect and portrays high biocompatibility and plasticity. They have a Young's modulus and compressibility identical to bones, hence, they are largely used in vivo, and in the treatment of scoliosis (Tarnita et al., 2009).

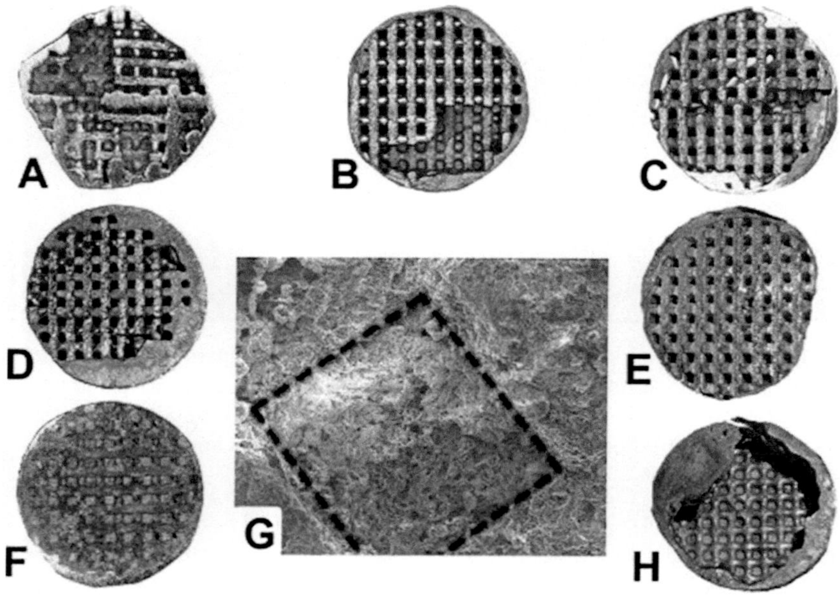

Fig. 3.5 Schematic representation of a magnesium scaffold (produced by salt leaching). (From Kirkland, N.T., Kolbeinsson, I., Woodfield, T., Dias, G.J., Staiger, M.P., 2011. Synthesis and properties of topologically ordered porous magnesium. Mater. Sci. Eng. B 176, 1666– 1672.)

3.3.4 Nanobiomaterials from carbon

The main goal of replacing a damaged hard tissue is to build up mechanical strength in the affected organ. As a result, carbon-originated nanoparticles due to their high mechanical strength and durability are very well researched in the field of tissue engineering. Different carbon analogs like graphene, carbon nanotubes, fullerenes, and nanofibers (Dresselhaus et al., 2001) have been thoroughly examined. Carbon is satisfactorily biocompatible and already used in clinical applications like artificial heart valves. Carbon nanomaterials having true nanometric features (< 100 nm), express exceptional mechanical, thermal, optical, and electrical properties (Harrison and Atala, 2007). Additionally, the carbon nanoparticles can be assembled to a three-dimensional structure. These advantages work in unison in building three-dimensional shapes and functions. Moreover, the surface chemistry of the carbon nanoparticles is under control, so it is possible to functionalize those with molecules of interest to promote cellular adhesion. As a result, carbon nanoparticles are coming up as the next-generation material to repair and regenerate hard tissues (Veetil and Ye, 2009; Haniu et al., 2012). New opportunities in the field of carbon-based nanoparticles have encouraged the use of carbon-based nanocomposites.

Carbon nanotubes (CNTs) (both single-walled and multiwalled) possess a honeycomb-like structure that encourages the ingress of newly formed tissue and provides very strong mechanical support. Moreover, because of the mesh-like structure, carbon nanotubes conduct electricity pulses; this property has successfully attracted many innovative devices including composites, sensors, and nanoscale electronic devices (Saito et al., 1998; Lee et al., 2000). Multiwalled carbon nanotubes (MWNTs) were found to grow mouse fibroblast cells. These tubes can be easily modified by chemical means to corresponding acid, carbonyl groups, etc., which can further be used for the functionalization with required biomolecules. These carbon networks can be used as a biocompatible mesh for restoring and reinforcing damaged tissues. The electrical conductivity of nanotubes also contributes to cellular growth. Osteoblast proliferation on PLLA/MWNT (multiwalled nanotube) nanocomposites under alternating current stimulation was investigated (Supronowicz et al., 2002). SWNT (single-walled nanotubes) or MWNTs have proven to be nontoxic and can even help cells proliferate (Shi et al., 2008). The sidewalls of carboxylic functionalized SWNTs exhibited a nucleation surface to induce the formation of a biomimetic apatite coating (Armentano et al., 2008).

Nanodiamonds are also important in terms of tissue engineering. They are made by detonation and dispersed into single particles to increase the surface area of the composites. Nanodiamonds are functionalized and blended with different polymers (PLLA) to increase in strain to failure and fracture energy. Both of these points are important for bone tissue engineering (Zhang et al., 2012). Growth and proliferation of these hybrid nanocomposites are also faster.

3.3.5 Nanobiomaterial composites

Composites are biomaterials where more than one class of material is employed in the scaffolds. Bone tissue is a combination of both hard and soft materials. Nowadays, different types of materials are combined and used in artificial joints and bone implants. This is to combine several contributions from different scaffolds, which stimulate specific responses at the molecular level. The main reasons behind the concept of composite materials are as follows:

1. Reinforce the structural integrity of the scaffolds by changing the mechanical properties of the materials when a component of different origin (inorganic) is added to the bulk materials (organic polymeric).
2. The polymer itself intensifies its bioactivity with the inorganic materials.
3. The inorganic material can help in decreasing the erosion of the bulk polymer.

Common material combinations are synthetic polymers with bioceramic and synthetic/natural polymers with metals. HA-collagen nanocomposite systems have gained popularity in the recent literature (Liao et al., 2004). HA is found to degrade slower and be highly osteoconductive. However, it is not osteoinductive. To overcome this drawback, HA can be made into a composite with collagen, which carries osteoinductive growth factors and osteogenic potential cells. Depending on these experimental results, the nano HA-collagen-osteoblast system was developed along with PLA (Liao et al., 2004). These constructs support cellular adhesion, proliferation, migration, integration in the segmental defect (in vivo), and new bone formation.

Osteoblast adhesion on nanoscale ceramics improved significantly in composition with PLGA (Liu et al., 2005). Up to three times more osteoblasts adhered to PLGA when it contained nanophase in comparison with conventional titania having the same weight ratio and porosity (Smith and Webster, 2005). Nanoscale carbon fibers witnessed significantly greater in vitro osteoblast function and mineral deposition (Elias et al., 2002; Price and Webster, 2004). The osteoblasts and deposited minerals evenly oriented themselves on carbon nanofibers placed on the surface (Khang and Webster, 2006).

Other than encouraging results in osteoblast orientation and enhanced attachments, nanoscale materials have been found to portray enhanced strength that can truly mimic bone. Recently, carbon nanotubes, and alumoxane nanoparticles have been examined as reinforcing fillers for biodegradable polymers (Shi et al., 2005). The size, shape, orientation, and dispersion of the fillers dictate the extent of performance in the case of composites (Horch et al., 2004).

Apart from these, there are several examples of improved nanocomposites tried in the field of hard tissue engineering (Fig. 3.6). Silk fibroin portrayed excellent mechanical strength and biodegradability while combined with silica-based bioglass (Mieszawska et al., 2010). PLGA microspheres have been combined with calcium phosphate cement to serve as porogens that accelerate degradation and bone growth (Renno et al., 2013). Yu et al.

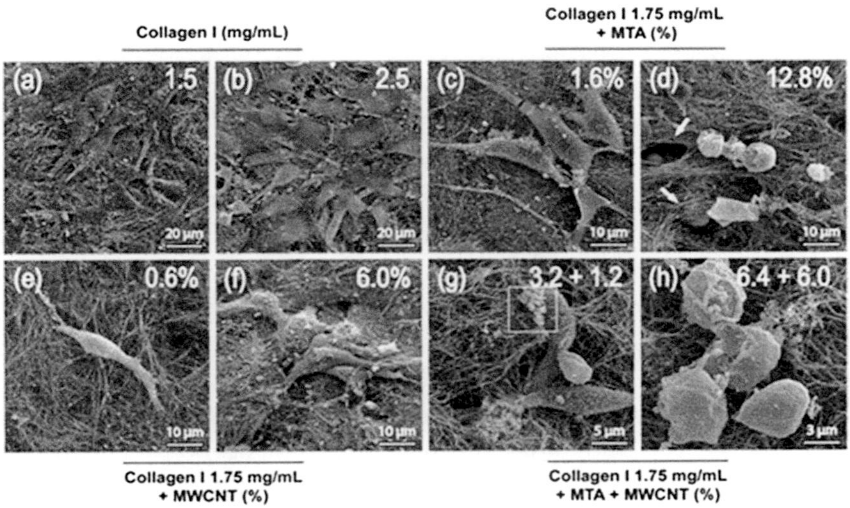

Fig. 3.6 Scanning electron microscopy of MC3T3-E1 cells grown on different biocomposites. (A, B) Collagen I. (C–H) Collagen mixed with MTA (mineral trioxide aggregate) and MWNT (multiwalled nanotube) in different quantities. (From Thalita, M., et al., 2016. A novel 3D bone-mimetic scaffold composed of collagen/MTA/MWCNT modulates cell migration and osteogenesis. Life Sci. 162, 115–124. Copyright © 2016 Elsevier B.V.)

fabricated macrochanneled CaP (calcium phosphate) scaffolds that maintain three-dimensional integrity in scaffolds which collagen hydrogels inside the pores to ensure cell distribution and retention (Yu et al., 2012).

3.4 Role of stem cells

Bone tissue is a combination of both mineral and organic matrix with cellular components. The organic matrix is composed of collagen and calcium phosphates (like hydroxyapatite). It has osteoblasts, osteoclasts, and osteocytes as cell components. For bone reconstruction, different material properties like hardness, porous nature are important. For cellular attachment, cell growth and differentiation nanoscaffolds, various nanomatrices have been used. The basic components most popularly used in this regard are nano-HA (Sato et al., 2005), collagen, electro-spun silk (Jin et al., 2004), anodized titanium, and nanostructured titanium surfaces (Yao et al., 2008). Although the problem of a proper scaffold was in control, there was always a risk involving the use of primary osteoblasts due to the following reasons:

(i) The restricted availability and inherent donor site morbidity of the material.

(ii) The limited proliferative capability of the tissue.
(iii) The patient age-dependent behavior.
(iv) The greater risk of dedifferentiating during in vitro culture.

To avoid these problems, stem cells may be a better choice because of their large proliferative capacity and their ability to differentiate into various cell types. Although the nanofeatures present in the scaffolds are very important, for the efficiency of a scaffold to properly produce hard tissues, the role of stem cells is of utmost importance. Among different types of stem cells somatic stem cells (that naturally exist in human bodies), embryonic stem (ES) cells (that are derived from culturing embryos or fertilized eggs), and induced pluripotent stem (iPS) cells (that are artificially produced) have all been well researched. Among these three types of stem cells, somatic stem cells have been most utilized in medical treatments. Somatic stem cells are better accepted because those originate from the human body. There are several types of somatic stem cells, such as neural stem cells, mesenchymal stem cells, and hematopoietic stem cells. Mesenchymal stem cells can differentiate into various tissues and organs such as bone, cartilage, and fat cells (Arvidson et al., 2011). Mesenchymal stem cells (MSCs) from various sources are found to differentiate into osteoblasts on different nanofibers. Natural (collagen or silk fibroin Jang et al., 2009), synthetic degradable polymers (PLA, PCL, PLGA; Hu et al., 2008, 2009), a mixture of synthetic and natural polymers also showed the desired differentiation of MSCs. Bone marrow derived MSCs exhibited promising results in terms of differentiation on nano-HA, PLGA, and nano-HA-PLGA composites (Lock and Liu, 2011). CNTs on the other hand portray dramatically enhanced effects in selective cellular differentiation into osteoblast like cells (Mooney et al., 2008).

Growth factors are proteins that encourage cells to differentiate and proliferate. Both BMP-2 (bone morphogenic protein 2) and BMP-7 exhibit important roles in the differentiation and proliferation of osteocytes. Growth factors such as the fibroblast growth factor (FGF), transforming growth factor (TGF)-β, insulin-like growth factor 1 (IGF)-1, and platelet-derived growth factor (PDGF) do not exhibit an ectopic osteoinductive capacity, they do have osteogenic properties (Solheim, 1998). The scaffolds are chemically modified with these growth factors and implanted in the necessary locations. Growth factors encourage the formation of bones to fill up the void created by mishap.

Different materials have been tried for the purpose of bone regeneration. They can broadly be classified into mainly two subcategories: biodegradable and nonbiodegradable (Fig. 3.7). Collagen (Zhao et al., 2009), poly-L-lactic

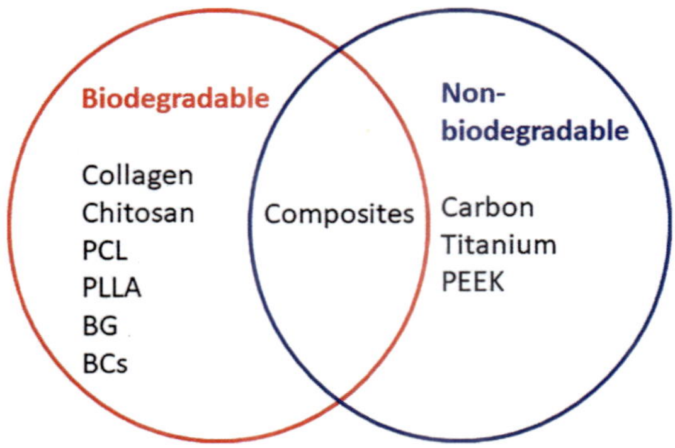

Fig. 3.7 Scaffolds for regeneration contain biodegradable, nonbiodegradable as well as composite scaffolds. Some examples from each category are included. *BC*, bioresorbable ceramics; *BG*, bioglass; *PEEK*, polyether ether ketone.

glycolic acid (Chang et al., 2007), resorbable bioactive glass (BG) (Fernandes et al., 2018), and bioresorbable ceramics (BCs) including β-tricalcium phosphate (TCP) (Han and Dai, 2013) are used as biodegradable materials, while metals (e.g., titanium) (Li et al., 2007; Takizawa et al., 2018), carbon (Aoki et al., 2009), and polyetheretherketone (PEEK) (Nakahara et al., 2010) are used as nonbiodegradable materials. Advantages of biodegradable scaffolds lie in the osseous replacement that degrade at the same time as bone regeneration, providing a more biomimetic regeneration with less risk of infection and foreign body reactions; however, when used for filling large bone defects, residual bone defects may remain. Nonbiodegradable scaffolds do not replace bone and can serve as a spacer or bone substitute to fill bone defects and transmit load (Fig. 3.6).

3.5 Conclusion and future perspectives

Hard tissue engineering is a field in infancy. There is a lot of hope regarding this field. Worldwide many groups are working on the development of new functional hard body replacements. This field will soon highlight exciting new areas of stem cell biology with the understanding of intrinsic bone regeneration in health and disease. Most importantly, biomaterial and nanomaterials are like two sides of a coin, which gives many hands to tune the properties. The increased surface area, surface roughness, micropatterning, etc. can immensely help the field to develop more bio-similar products. Especially inventions like "biocomposites" and "nanocomposites" can assemble beneficial properties from several materials at once. Still there are active challenges like immune rejection, which requires more interdisciplinary knowledge. So, there is a lot of scope for future work and this field will no doubt keep us inspired and enthusiastic about new developments.

References

Aoki, K., Usui, Y., Narita, N., Ogiwara, N., Iashigaki, N., Nakamura, K., Kato, H., Sano, K., Ogiwara, N., Kametani, K., Kim, C., Taruta, S., Kim, Y.A., Endo, M., Saito, N., 2009. A thin carbon-fiber web as a scaffold for bone-tissue regeneration. Small 5, 1540–1546.

Armentano, I., Alvarez-Pérez, M., Carmona-Rodríguez, A.B., Gutiérrez-Ospina, I., Kenny, J.M., Arzate, H., 2008. Analysis of the biomineralization process on SWNT-COOH and F-SWNT films. Mater. Sci. Eng. C 28, 1522–1529.

Arvidson, K., Abdallah, B.M., Applegate, L.A., Baldini, N., Cenni, E., Gomez-Barrena, E., Granchi, D., Kassem, M., Konttinen, Y.T., Mustafa, K., Pioletti, D.P., Sillat, T., Finne-Wistrand, A., 2011. Bone regeneration and stem cells. J. Cell. Mol. Med. 15, 718–746.

Black, J., 1982. The education of the biomaterialist: report of a survey. J. Biomed. Mater. Res. 16 (2), 159–167.

Chang, P.C., Liu, B.Y., Liu, C.M., Chou, H.H., Ho, M.H., Liu, H.C., Wang, D.M., Hou, L.T., 2007. Bone tissue engineering with novel rhBMP2-PLLA composite scaffolds. J. Biomed. Mater. Res. A 81A, 771–780.

Chen, X., Wang, W., Cheng, S., Dong, B., Li, C.Y., 2013. Mimicking bone nanostructure by combining block copolymer self-assembly and 1D crystal nucleation. ACS Nano 7 (9), 8251–8257.

DeAza, P.N., De Aza, A.H., Pena, P., Aza, S.D., 2007. Bioactive glasses and glass-ceramics. Bol. Soc. Esp. Cerám. Vidr. 46, 45–55.

Di Mario, C., Griffiths, H., Goktekin, O., Peeters, N., Verbist, J., Bosiers, M., Deloose, K., Heublein, B., Rohde, R., Kasese, V., Ilsley, C., Erbel, R., 2004. Drug-eluting bioabsorbable magnesium stent. J. Interv. Cardiol. 17 (6), 391–395.

Dresselhaus, M.S., Dresselhaus, G., Eklund, P.C., 2001. Science of Fullerenes and Carbon Nanotubes. Academic Press, San Diego.

Ducheyne, P., Qiu, Q., 1999. Bioactive ceramics: the effect of surface reactivity on bone formation and bone cell function. Biomaterials 20, 2287–2303.

Elias, K.L., Price, R.L., Webster, T.J., 2002. Enhanced functions of osteoblasts on carbon nanofiber compacts. Biomaterials 23, 3279–3287.

Feddes, B., Wolke, J.G., Vredenberg, A.M., Jansen, J.A., 2004. Initial deposition of calcium phosphate ceramic on polyethylene and polydimethylsiloxane by rf magnetron sputtering deposition: the interface chemistry. Biomaterials 24, 633–639.

Fernandes, H.R., Gaddam, A., Rebelo, A., Brazete, D., Stan, G.E., Ferreira, J.M.F., 2018. Bioactive glasses and glass-ceramics for healthcare applications in bone regeneration and tissue engineering. Materials 11, 2530–2584.

Fisher, J.P., Holland, T.A., Dean, D., Engel, P.S., Mikos, A.G., 2001. Synthesis and properties of photocross-linked poly(propylene fumarate) scaffolds. J. Biomater. Sci. Polym. Ed. (12), 673–687.

Freed, L.E., Novakovic, G.V., Biron, R.J., Eagles, D.B., Lesnoy, D.C., Barlow, S.K., 1994. Biodegradable polymer scaffolds for tissue engineering. Biotechnology 12, 689–693.

Guo, H., Su, J., Wei, J., Kong, H., Liu, C., 2009. Biocompatibility and osteogenicity of degradable Ca-deficient hydroxyapatite scaffolds from calcium phosphate cement for bone tissue engineering. Acta Biomater. 5, 268–278.

Ha, T.L.B., Quan, T.M., Vu, D.N., Si, D.M., 2013. Naturally derived biomaterials: preparation and application. In: Andrades, J.A. (Ed.), Regenerative Medicine and Tissue Engineering. InTech (Chapter 11).

Han, D., Dai, K., 2013. Prefabrication of a vascularized bone graft with beta tricalcium phosphate using an in vivo bioreactor. Artif. Organs 37, 884–893.

Haniu, H., Saito, N., Matsuda, Y., Tsukahara, T., Usui, Y., Narita, N., Hara, K., Aoki, K., Shimizu, M., Ogihara, N., Takanashi, Okamoto, S.M., Kobayashi, S., Ishigaki, N., Nakamura, K., Kato, H., 2012. Basic potential of carbon nanotubes in tissue engineering applications. J. Nanomater., 343747.

Hanzi, A.C., Dalla Tore, A.S., Sologubenko, A.S., Uggowitzer, P.J., 2009. Design strategy for microalloyed ultra-ductile magnesium alloys for medical applications. Mater. Sci. Forum 89 (6), 75–82.

Harrison, B.S., Atala, A., 2007. Carbon nanotube applications for tissue engineering. Biomaterials 28, 344.

Hench, L.L., 1991. Bioceramics: from concept to clinic. J. Am. Ceram. Soc. 74, 1487–1510.

Hench, L.L., 1998. Bioceramic. J. Am. Ceram. Soc. 81, 1705–1728.

Hench, L.L., 2006. The story of Bioglass®. J. Mater. Sci. Mater. Med. 17, 967–978.

Horch, R.A., Shahid, N.A., Mistry, S., et al., 2004. Nanoreinforcement of poly(propylene fumarate)-based networks with surface modified alumoxane nanoparticles for bone tissue engineering. Biomacromolecules 5, 1990–1998.

Hu, J., Liu, X., Ma, P.X., 2008. Induction of osteoblast differentiation phenotype on poly (l-lactic acid) nanofibrous matrix. Biomaterials 29, 3815–3821.

Hu, J., Feng, K., Liu, X., Ma, P.X., 2009. Chondrogenic and osteogenic differentiations of human bone marrow-derived mesenchymal stem cells on a nanofibrous scaffold with designed pore network. Biomaterials 30, 5061–5067.

Jang, J.H., Castano, O., Kim, H.W., 2009. Electrospun materials as potential platforms for bone tissue engineering. Adv. Drug Deliv. Rev. 61, 1065–1083.

Jin, H.J., Chen, J., Karageorgiou, V., Altman, G.H., Kaplan, D.L., 2004. Human bone marrow stromal cell responses on electrospun silk fibroin mats. Biomaterials 25, 1039–1047.

Khang, D., Webster, T.J., 2006. Selective adhesion and mineral deposition by osteoblasts on carbon nanofiber patterns. Int. J. Nanomedicine 1, 65–72.

Klein, C.P., Driessen, A.A., de Groot, K., van den Hooff, A., 1983. Biodegradation behavior of various calcium-phosphate materials in bone tissue. J. Biomed. Mater. Res. 17, 769–784.

Lee, C.J., Park, J., Kang, S.Y., Lee, J.H., 2000. Growth and field electron emission of vertically aligned multiwalled carbon nanotubes. Chem. Phys. Lett. 326, 175–180.

LeGeros, R.Z., 2002. Properties of osteoconductive biomaterials: calcium phosphates. Clin. Orthop. Relat. Res. 395, 81–98.

Li, J.P., Habibovic, P., van den Doel, M., Wilson, C.E., de Wijn, J.R., van Blitterswijk, C.A., de Groot, K., 2007. Bone ingrowth in porous titanium implants produced by 3D fiber deposition. Biomaterials 28, 2810–2820.

Li, Z., Gu, X., Lou, S., Zheng, Y., 2008. The development of binary Mg–Ca alloys for use as biodegradable materials within bone. Biomaterials 29 (10), 1329–1344.

Liao, S.S., et al., 2004. Osteoblasts adherence and migration through three-dimensional porous mineralized collagen based composite: nHAC/PLA. J. Bioact. Compat. Polym. 19, 117–130.

Liu, H., Slamovich, E.B., Webster, T.J., 2005. Increased osteoblast functions on nanophasetitania dispersed in poly-lactic-co-glycolic acid composites. Nanotechnology 16, S601–S608.

Lock, J., Liu, H., 2011. Nanomaterials enhance osteogenic differentiation of human mesenchymal stem cells similar to a short peptide of BMP-7. Int. J. Nanomedicine 6, 2769–2777.

Mieszawska, A.J., Fourligas, N., Georgakoudi, I., Ouhib, N.M., Belton, D.J., Perry, C.C., Kaplan, D.L., 2010. Osteoinductive silk–silica composite biomaterials for bone regeneration. Biomaterials 31, 8902–8910.

Mooney, E., Dockery, P., Greiser, U., Murphy, M., Barron, V., 2008. Carbon nanotubes and mesenchymal stem cells, biocompatibility, proliferation and differentiation. Nano Lett. 8, 2137–2143.

Nakahara, H., Misawa, H., Yoshida, A., Hayashi, T., Tanaka, M., Furumatsu, T., Tanaka, N., Kobayashi, N., Ozaki, T., 2010. Bone repair using a hybrid scaffold of self-assembling peptide PuraMatrix and polyetheretherketone cage in rats. Cell Transplant. 19, 791–797.

Peeters, P., Bosiers, M., Verbist, J., Deloose, K., Heublein, B., 2005. Preliminary results after application of absorbable metal stents in patients with critical limb ischemia. J. Endovasc. Ther. 12 (1), 1–5.

Peuster, M., Wohlsein, P., Brügmann, M., et al., 2001. A novel approach to temporary stenting: degradable cardiovascular stents produced from corrodible metal—results 6–18 months after implantation into New Zealand white rabbits. Heart 86 (5), 563–569.

Peuster, M., Hesse, C., Schloo, T., Fink, C., Beerbaum, P., von Schnakenburg, C., 2006. Long-term biocompatibility of a corrodible peripheral iron stent in the porcine descending aorta. Biomaterials 27 (28), 4955–4962.

Price, R.L., Webster, T.J., 2004. Increased osteoblast viability in the presence of smaller nano-dimensioned carbon fibers. Nanotechnology 15, 892–900.

Quirk, R.A., France, R.M., Shakesheff, K.M., Howdle, S.M., 2004. Supercritical fluid technologies and tissue engineering scaffolds. Curr. Opin. Solid State Mater. Sci. 8, 313–821.

Ratner, B.D., Hoffman, A.S., Schoen, F.J., Lemons, J.E., 2004. Biomaterials Science: An Introduction to Materials in Medicine, second ed. Academic Press.

Renno, A.C.M., Van De Watering, F.C.J., Nejadnik, M.R., Crovace, M.C., Zanotto, E.D., Wolke, J.G.C., Jansen, J.A., Van Den Beucken, J., 2013. Incorporation of bioactive glass in calcium phosphate cement, in vivo evaluation. Acta Biomater. 9, 5728–5739.

Saito, R., Dresselhaus, G., Dresselhaus, M.S., 1998. Physical Properties of Carbon Nanotubes. Imperial College Press, London.

Sato, M., Slamovich, E.B., Webster, T.J., 2005. Enhanced osteoblast adhesion on hydrothermally treated hydroxyapatite/titania/poly(lactide-co-glycolide) sol-gel titanium coatings. Biomaterials 26, 1349–1357.

Sell, S.A., Wolfe, P.S., Garg, K., McCool, J.M., Rodriguez, I.A., Bowlin, G.L., 2010. The use of natural polymers in tissue engineering: a focus on electrospun extracellular matrix analogues. Polymers 2, 522–553.

Shi, X., Hudson, J.L., Spicer, P.P., 2005. Rheological behavior and mechanical characterization of injectable poly(propylene fumarate)/single-walled carbon nanotube composites for bone tissue engineering. Nanotechnology 16, S531–S538.

Shi, X., Sitharaman, B., Pham, Q.P., Spicer, P.P., Hudson, J.L., Wilson, L.J., Tour, J.M., Raphael, R.M., Mikos, A.G., 2008. *In vitro* cytotoxicity of single-walled carbon nanotube/biodegradable polymer nanocomposites. J. Biomed. Mater. Res. A 86A, 813–823.

Smith, T.A., Webster, T.J., 2005. Increased osteoblast function on PLGA composites containing nanophase titania. J. Biomed. Mater. Res. 74A, 677–686.

Solheim, E., 1998. Growth factors in bone. Int. Orthop. 22, 410–416.

Supronowicz, P.R., Ajayan, P.M., Ullmann, K.R., Arulanandam, B.P., Metzger, D.W., Bizios, R., 2002. Novel current-conducting composite substrates for exposing osteoblasts to alternating current stimulation. J. Biomed. Mater. Res. 59, 490–506.

Takizawa, T., Nakayama, N., Haniu, H., Aoki, K., Okamoto, M., Nomura, H., Tanaka, M., Sobajima, A., Yoshida, K., Kamanaka, T., et al., 2018. Titanium fiber plates for bone tissue repair. Adv. Mater. 30, 1703608.

Tarnita, D., Tarnita, D., Bîzdoaca, N., Mîndrila, I., Vasilescu, M., 2009. Properties and medical applications of shape memory alloys. Rom. J. Morphol. Embryol. 50, 15–21.

Veetil, J.V., Ye, K., 2009. Tailored carbon nanotubes for tissue engineering applications. Biotechnol. Prog. 25, 709–721.

Webster, T.J., Ergun, C., Doremus, R.H., Siegel, R.W., Bizios, R., 1999. Osteoblast adhesion on nanophase ceramics. Biomaterials 20 (11), 1221–1227.
Webster, T.J., Ergun, C., Doremus, R.H., Siegel, R.W., Bizios, R., 2001. Enhanced osteoclast-like cell functions on nanophase ceramics. Biomaterials 22, 1327–1333.
Williams, D.F., 2019. Challenges with the development of biomaterials for sustainable tissue engineering. Front. Bioeng. Biotechnol. 7, 127.
Witte, F., Kaese, V., Haferkamp, H., Switzer, E., Meyer-Lindenberg, A., Wirth, C.J., Windhagen, H., 2005. In vivo corrosion of four magnesium alloys and the associated bone response. Biomaterials 26 (17), 3557–3563.
Witte, F., Ulrich, H., Rudert, M., Willbold, E., 2007. Biodegradable magnesium scaffolds: part I: appropriate inflammatory response. J. Biomed. Mater. Res. A 81 (3), 748–756.
Wolke, J.G.C., vanDijk, K., Schaeken, H.G., de Groot, K., Jansen, J.A., 1994. Study of the surface characteristics of magnetron-sputter calcium phosphate coatings. J. Biomed. Mater. Res. 28 (12), 1477–1484.
Xu, L., Yu, G., Zhang, E., Pan, F., Yang, K., 2007. In vivo corrosion behavior of Mg–Mn–Zn alloy for bone implant application. J. Biomed. Mater. Res. A 83 (3), 703–711.
Yao, C., Slamovich, E.B., Webster, T.J., 2008. Enhanced osteoblast functions on anodized titanium with nanotube-like structures. J. Biomed. Mater. Res. A 85, 157–166.
Yu, H.S., Jin, G.Z., Won, J., Wall, E.I., Kim, H.W., 2012. Macrochanneled bioactive ceramic scaffolds in combination with collagen hydrogel: a new tool for bone tissue engineering. J. Biomed Mater. Res. A 100A, 2431–2440.
Zhang, E., Yang, L., 2008. Microstructure, mechanical properties and bio-corrosion properties of Mg–Zn–Mn–Ca alloy for biomedical application. Mater. Sci. Eng. A 497 (1–2), 111–118.
Zhang, Q., Mochalin, V.N., Neitzel, I., Hazeli, K., Niu, J., Kontsos, A., Zhou, J.G., Lelkes, P., Gogotsi, I.Y., 2012. Mechanical properties and biomineralization of multifunctional nanodiamond-PLLA composites for bone tissue engineering. Biomaterials 33, 5067–5075.
Zhang, K., Wang, S., Zhou, C., Cheng, L., Gao, X., Xie, X., Sun, J., Wang, H., Weir, M.D., Reynolds, M.A., Zhang, N., Bai, Y., Hockin, H., Xu, K., 2018. Advanced smart biomaterials and constructs for hard tissue engineering and regeneration. Bone Res. 6, 31.
Zhao, J., Shinkai, M., Takezawa, T., Ohba, S., Chung, U., Nagamune, T., 2009. Bone regeneration using collagen type I vitrigel with bone morphogenetic protein-2. J. Biosci. Bioeng. 107, 318–323.

CHAPTER 4

Application of nanobiomaterials in soft tissue engineering

Dhara Jajal[a] and Sejal Shah[b]
[a]Charotar University of Science and Technology, Changa, Gujarat, India
[b]Department of Microbiology, School of Science, RK University, Rajkot, India

4.1 Introduction

In the past few decades, tissue engineering (TE) has gained a lot of attention from researchers of various scientific disciplines like biology, engineering, material science, and medicine. This is because the technology has the tremendous potential to regenerate, restore, or repair the injured or lost human tissue and even organs. Tissue and organ damage or loss of their functionality is one of the most prevalent health challenges of all the time that can occur due to several factors, for example, diseased conditions, trauma, congenital defects, and ageing. As many tissues/organs have limited self-repairing capacity most of the time transplantation remains to be the available cure for such tissue/organ damage. However, a lack of donor sources, damage occurred to donors, and graft rejection are some of the significant challenges faced in existing clinical transplantation (Luo et al., 2019).

In the present scenario, TE has become the cutting edge branch of regenerative medicine and has the potential to reconstruct a wide range of tissue like bone, skin, ligaments, and blood vessels. The key elements required for the TE include cells, scaffold, and growth factors that are usually referred to as the "tissue engineering triad" (Kumar et al., 2018). Selecting the biomaterials and designing of the scaffold are crucial parameters in determining the success of tissue regeneration. Scaffold supports the tissue and promotes tissue repair or the regeneration process. Nanotechnology has several advantages in fabricating scaffold structures that has driven much attention nowadays in developing newer scaffolds made up of nanomaterials that can mimic the native tissue more efficiently. In this context, nanomaterials are thought to be ideal in scaffold generation as they can improve cell adhesion, proliferation, and stem cell differentiation compared

Nanotechnology in Medicine and Biology
https://doi.org/10.1016/B978-0-12-819469-0.00006-X

with other microscopic biomaterials. The types of nanomaterials used for TE include nanofibers, nanotubes, nanocomposite, nanoparticles, and many more which are selected depending on the tissue to be engineered (Lin et al., 2014). Biologically derived nanoparticles might have a role in tissue enggineering (Ghosh et al., 2021; Shah and Ghosh, 2020).

4.2 Tissue engineering

TE is the interdisciplinary approach aimed to achieve successful strategies dedicated to human tissue reconstruction, repair, and restoration of their normal functions in conditions where their self-repairing capacity is affected by disease or injury. TE mainly involves the combination of life sciences and engineering principles. TE implicates different approaches that can be divided into three broader spectra: (i) the injured tissue at a specific site can be repaired by injection or transplantation of isolated cells; (ii) the targeted site can be healed with tissue inducing materials such as peptide, polysaccharides, or growth materials, and (iii) the three-dimensional (3D) scaffold can be prepared to grow tissue in a biomimic environment. Among all, the TE approach using 3D scaffolds have been very much in demand because of its potential to fabricate a whole tissue or organ with all the essential biomimetic properties of the original tissue or organ (Zhu et al., 2014). For the recovery of the damaged tissue, these scaffold constructs either implanted at the injury site directly or they can be cultured in vitro to develop into the specific tissue that can be transplanted later. The scaffold is vital for tissue generation as it principally acts as an artificial extracellular matrix when specialized cells or stem cells are cultured on it. Further, numerous growth factors and mechanical or biophysical stimuli are added on to the cell-seeded scaffold that induces cell proliferation and differentiation, ultimately leading to the tissue formation of interest. Such crucial interplay of cells, growth signals, and scaffold leads to tissue regeneration, which is commonly known as the TE triad (Kumar et al., 2018). Fig. 4.1 represents the illustration of each component of the TE triad with the key steps involved in the TE process.

TE empowers the synthesis of the almost all human tissues including soft and hard tissues. Hard tissues are bone, dental, and craniofacial tissues. Human soft tissues are largely described as a group of tissues needed to connect and support other tissues and to protect the organs by surrounding them. They are mostly multifaceted, preliminarily comprised of fibrous biomolecules

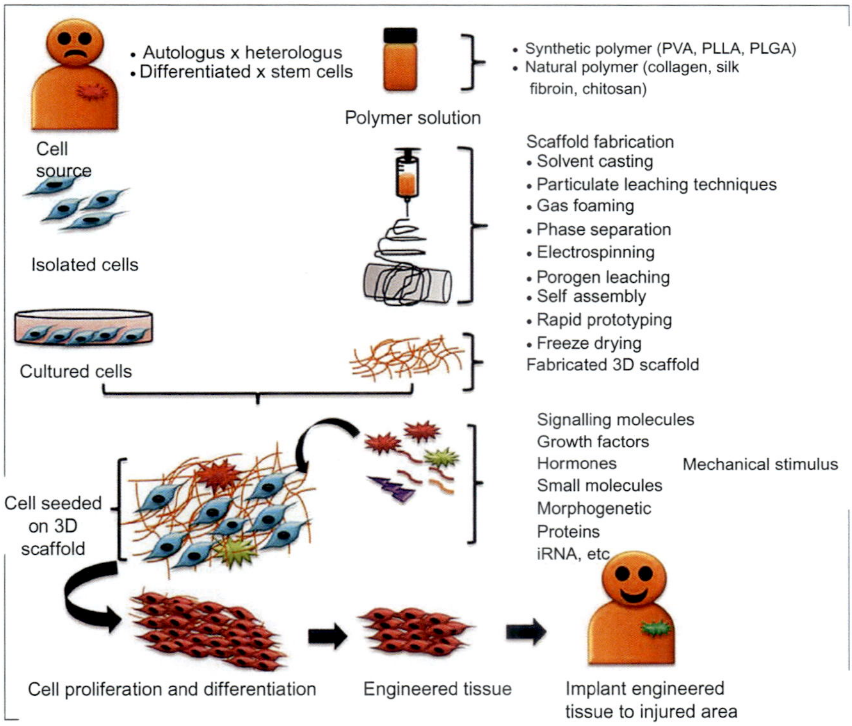

Fig. 4.1 ***Tissue engineering triad consists of the scaffold as a 3D support, cells and external signals.*** (Reproduced with permission from Kumar, V., Naqvi, S. Gopinath, P., 2018. Applications of nanofibers in tissue engineering. In: Application of Nanomaterials. Woodhead Publishing. p. 179–203. Copyright © 2018 Elsevier Ltd.)

and composite structures. Soft TE aims to restore or reconstruct such soft tissues that include cartilage, ligaments, nerves, blood vessels, and skin.

4.2.1 Nanotechnology in scaffold designing

The scaffold is 3D synthetic frameworks composed of biocompatible materials assisting the de novo synthesis of tissues or organs. 3D architectures of the scaffold should be interconnected and highly porous to allow diffusion of nutrients and cell infiltration into the 3D matrix. Moreover, such morphology of the scaffold permits cells to eliminate the waste products from the scaffold. Gradually, a scaffold should be degraded upon transplantation, and the resultant products should have the ability to be removed from the 3D scaffold and exit the body without causing any toxicity to other tissues or organs (Kumar et al., 2019). It is known that the scaffold is the most essential in TE; performing many key functions that include the following:

(i) promotes cell adhesion by interacting with chemical groups and ligands presented by scaffold materials and extracellular matrix (ECM) deposition; (ii) allows the adequate transport of nutrients, gases, and growth or signaling factors required for the cell viability, growth, and differentiation; (iii) degrades in a controlled manner at the rate which matches to the regeneration rate of tissue being formed; and (iv) creates the least inflammation (Langer and Tirrell, 2004). A vast range of biomaterials, synthetic and natural, are extensively used in the synthesis of scaffolds in such a way that they perform desired functions necessary for tissue generation. Scaffold biomaterials should be very specific, having certain essential characteristics for the successful TE summarized in Fig. 4.2. Till date, various biomaterials that can be classified as polymers, metals, or composites depending on their chemical nature are explored in TE.

Nanotechnology offers a great potential in designing and fabricating nanoscopic scaffolds using similar biomaterials as previously used but with an improved ability to mimic the native tissue. Hence, modern approaches in regenerative medicine envisage the amalgamation of nanotechnology in developing novel nanobiomaterials with superior regeneration potential. Looking into soft human tissues, cells are embedded in the ECM that mainly consists of interconnected nanofibers along with various small organic compounds. The ECM provides mechanical support to the resident cells and directs distinct functions of cells. Additionally, the ECM has an essential function in regulating the storage of the growth and signaling factors as well as in secreting these biological factors (Hudita et al., 2019).

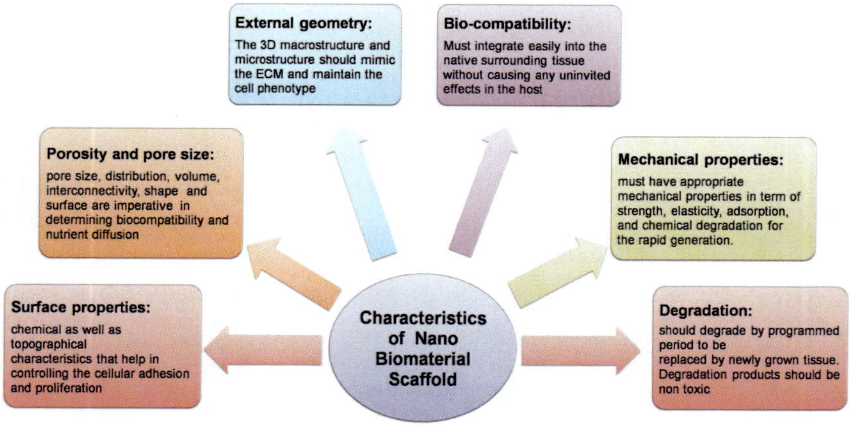

Fig. 4.2 ***The characteristics determining an ideal biomaterial scaffold for tissue engineering.*** ECM, extracellular matrix; 3D, three-dimensional.

The current advancements in nanotechnology have enabled the development of a nanoscaled biomimetic environment with specific biochemical, mechanical, and electrical properties that is homologous to the ECM. Furthermore, the interplay between tissue cells and biomimetic nanopatterns drives dynamic changes in the ECM and stimulates stem cell differentiation (Kim et al., 2012). Thereby, nowadays, de novo tissues are being engineered by employing these nanobiomaterials for improved cell adhesion, proliferation, and differentiation. As discussed, designing of the microenvironment in a scaffold modulates the phenotype and decides the cell fate that has triggered growing innovations in scaffold fabrication.

4.2.2 Nanobiomaterials in soft tissue regeneration

The advancement of nanotechnology has triggered growing innovations in nanoscopic scaffold fabrication. Biomimetic nanomaterials are produced by several methods that principally include electrospinning, phase-separation, and molecular self-assembly. Further, the surface modification of the scaffold or biomaterial allows performing certain functions required for tissue generation. The techniques like blending and coating of nanoscaffolds, chemical leaching, wet chemical methods, and plasma treatment are used for surface modification (Chen et al., 2013). Among all, electrospinning has grasped a huge attention in fabricating nanofibrous scaffolds as it provides high porosity and facility to adjust pore size distribution, enhancing cell functionality (Nemati et al., 2019). Soft tissues, in general, have interwoven fibrous ECM structures at the nanoscale due to which nanofibrous scaffolds are mainly implemented in their regeneration. Moreover, scaffolds are made up of nanofibers and provide high surface area and porosity, as well as impart similarity to the physical features of the natural ECM making them promising for engineering soft tissues.

Numerous synthetic and natural polymers are implemented in fabricating scaffolds, where the selection of the polymer depends on the tissue that needs to be synthesized. Natural polymers commonly utilized in TE include collagen, chitosan, fibrin, gelatin, alginate, hyaluronic acid, and cellulose. They can be resident polymers of the tissue's own inherent bioactivity, possess surface ligands required for cell interactions and offer superior cell proliferation and differentiation compared with synthetic polymers. Conversely, synthetic polymers serve more flexibility in fabrication, processing, and surface modification and are more economical than natural polymers (Nemati et al., 2019). Some of the widely utilized synthetic polymers are poly-ε-caprolactone (PCL), polylactic acid (PLA), poly(L-lactic acid)

(PLLA), polyglycolic acid (PGA), poly[lactic-*co*-poly(glycolic acid)] (PLGA), poly(L-lactic acid)-*co*-poly(ε-caprolactone) (PLLA-PCL), and polyurethane (PU). Researchers construct hybrid scaffolds with better physical and biological properties to exploit the benefits of both natural and synthetic polymers. Some of the different nanofibrous scaffolds employed for reconstructing cartilage, neural, and vascular tissues are summarized in Table 4.1.

Furthermore, various other nanomaterials like carbon nanotubes (CNTs), nanowires, or nanoparticles (NPs) can be reinforced into the structured scaffold to modulate the scaffold property for improved performance. Such nanocomposites facilitate enhancement and the emergence of the new functional characteristic of the scaffold ultimately resulting in superior tissue regeneration (Hudita et al., 2019). In this chapter, we describe the regeneration of soft tissues, that is, cartilage, tendons and ligaments, neural, and cardiovascular tissues using the different nanoscopic scaffolds.

4.3 Nanobiomaterials in cartilage tissue engineering

4.3.1 Cartilage tissue

Cartilage is a flexible connective tissue that provides support to the adjacent tissues, acts as a structural scaffold or absorbs shocks during physical activities. Several areas of the human body such as joints, ribs, nose, ear, trachea, and intervertebral discs, have cartilage tissue (Oseni et al., 2011). Cartilage is avascular and nutrients can be only transported through diffusion making cell growth and tissue regeneration limited in the existing hypoxic environment leading to a restrictive self-regenerative capacity. Cartilage can be injured in several ways including a recurrent stress in the joint that can cause irreversible damage that ultimately requires joint replacement. The increased prevalence of tracheal and nasal cancers has augmented the frequent cases of radical resection as a part of its critical treatment. Further, congenital disorders about the malformation of the ear and nose, and accidental trauma involve cartilage damage (Chiu and Waldman, 2016; Oseni et al., 2011).

Human cartilage is classified into three types differing by structure, elasticity, and strength: hyaline or articular cartilage, fibrocartilage, and elastic cartilage (Holban et al., 2016; Oseni et al., 2011). The cartilage tissue composition includes specialized cells (chondrocytes) embedded in an extracellular matrix (ECM) consisting a network of collagen, elastin, glycoproteins, and proteoglycans—the constituents and their proportions vary for different cartilage (Chiu and Waldman, 2016).

Table 4.1 Nanofibrous scaffold studied for soft tissue engineering applications.

Materials	In vitro/in vivo model	Cells	Potential application
Self-assembled nanofiber			
Peptide amphiphile (PA) containing collagen (PA-collagen)	In vitro	Granule cells and Purkinje cell	Neural TE
RADA16 (Ac-ADARADARADARADA-COHN$_2$)	In vitro	Neural stem cells	Neural TE
RAD16-I peptide	Adult rats	Rat Schwann cells and embryonic NPCs	Neural TE
KLD-12 peptide (AcN-KLDLKLDLKLDL-CNH$_2$)	In vitro	Bovine chondrocytes	Cartilage TE
Peptide amphiphile (PA) combining with TGF	Omentum of Rats	Human mesenchymal stem cells	Cartilage TE
Phase separation nanofiber			
Chitosan/poly(ε-caprolactone) blend	In vitro	Bovine chondrocyte	Cartilage TE
Poly-L-lactide	In vitro	Human aortic smooth muscle cells	Vascular TE
Electrospinning nanofiber			
Poly(L-lactic acid)	In vitro	Neural stem cells	Neural TE
Poly(ε-caprolactone)	In vitro	Human mesenchymal stem cell	Cartilage TE
Poly(L-lactic-*co*-ε-caprolactone) (75:25)	In vitro	Smooth muscle cell	Vascular TE
Gelatin-modified PET nanofibers	In vitro	Endothelial cells	Vascular TE
Poly(ε-caprolactone)-collagen	Rabbit aorta-iliac bypass model	Vascular cells	Vascular TE

TE, tissue engineering.

Reproduced with permission from Chen, H., Truckenmüller, R., Van Blitterswijk, C., Moroni, L., 2013. Fabrication of nanofibrous scaffolds for tissue engineering applications. In: BT-Nanomaterials in Tissue Engineering. Woodhead Publishing Series in Biomaterials. Woodhead Publishing. p. 158–183.

Articular cartilage is zonally structured into four central compartments, viz., superficial (10%–20%), middle (40%–60%), deep (30%), and calcified (5%). Human adult articular cartilage is a glass-like (hyaline) complex tissue containing the ECM exclusively produced by its distinct cell type, chondrocytes. Although a plethora of molecular components make up the ECM of cartilage, it is composed mainly of type II collagen and cartilage-specific proteoglycan, aggrecan (Fig. 4.3). The number of chondrocytes and the amount of ECM components, that is, collagen, proteoglycans, and water vary from superficial to deep layers and occur in abundance close to the calcified zone (Holban et al., 2016). Collagen II fibrils (account for up to 60% of dry cartilage weight) confer the tissue with high tensile strength. In contrast, the aggrecan proteoglycans (which comprise ~35% of dry cartilage weight) allow the tissue to sustain high compressive loads. Numerous glycosaminoglycan (GAG) side chains, precisely chondroitin sulfate and keratan sulfate polysaccharides are covalently linked with aggrecan. Several aggrecan monomers are attached to a typical long hyaluronan polysaccharide chain (Fig. 4.3). The high negative charge densities imparted by chondroitin sulfate and keratan sulfate build an osmotic potential that moves water into the cartilage from the adjacent tissues and synovial fluid of the joint cavity, thereby, making water content of articular cartilage up to 80% that has a critical role in its load-bearing function (Fuentes-Mera et al., 2017).

Fibrocartilage is located in the intervertebral discs, costochondral joints, sacroiliac joints, pubic symphysis, and meniscus. It integrates with the dense fibrous connective tissue of tendons and ligaments. It is a more rigid form of cartilage and unlike the other types of cartilage characterized by an abundance of both collagen I and II fibers harboring scattered chondrocytes within the matrix. The collagen fibers may have specific orientations depending on the site of fibrocartilage, as an example, the annulus fibrous (of the intervertebral disc) and meniscus possess longitudinal and circumferential fibers (Chiu and Waldman, 2016; Holban et al., 2016).

Elastic cartilage provides support, flexibility, and helps to define and maintain the shape in the various human body parts, for example, the pinna and Eustachian tube of the ear. Although histologically similar to hyaline cartilage, it contains elastic fibers lying in a solid matrix consisting mainly of collagen II and aggregating proteoglycans (Chiu and Waldman, 2016). The flexibility to withstand repeated bending is due to these elastic fibers present in the tissue. Like most hyaline cartilages, the elastic cartilage is surrounded by the perichondrium. In contrast, it does not generally ossify or calcify (Kim et al., 2011).

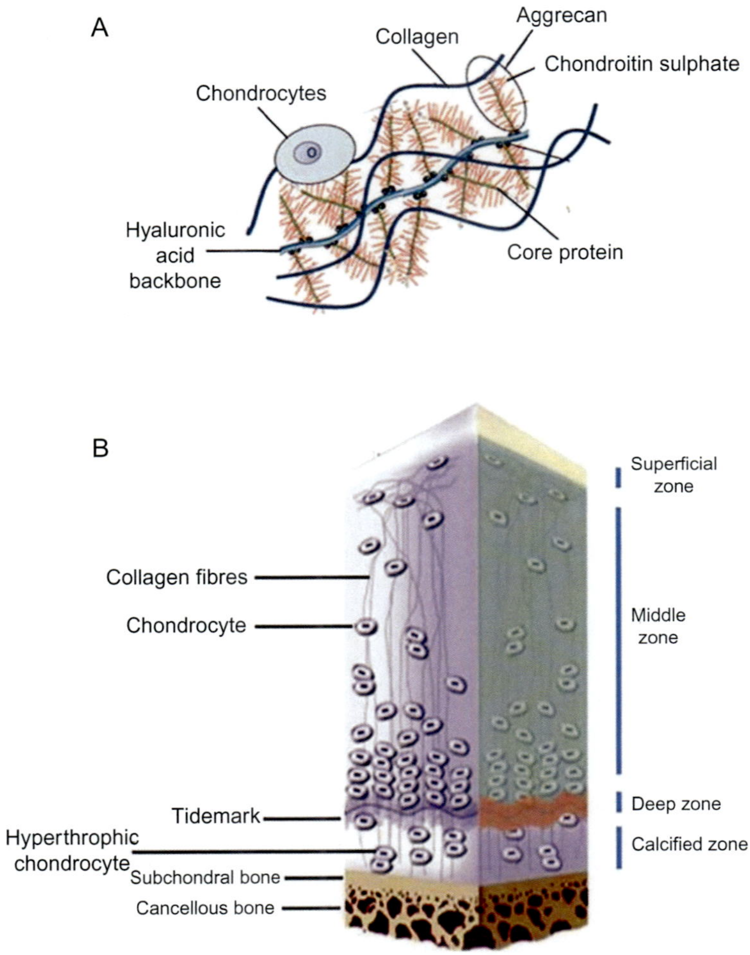

Fig. 4.3 ***Components of ECM and 3D structure of the articular cartilage.*** (A) Molecular assembly of extracellular matrix proteins. (B) 3D organization of normal articular cartilage. (Reproduced with permission from Fuentes-Mera, L., Camacho, A., Moncada-Saucedo, N.K. and Peña-Martínez, V., 2017. Current applications of mesenchymal stem cells for cartilage tissue engineering. In: Mesenchymal Stem Cells-Isolation, Characterization and Applications. IntechOpen. p. 149–184. Copyright © 2017.)

4.3.2 Rationale for cartilage tissue engineering

Articular cartilage impairment is the most frequently experienced among all cartilage damage. Long-term stresses and road accidents can cause permanent damage in the joints, leading to the development of osteoarthritis. The destruction of the matrix organization and increased permeability that occurs during osteoarthritis leads to the high water content in cartilage resulting in diminished stiffness and load-bearing capacity. On injury to the tissue, usually, inflammation occurs that depends on the intrinsic vascularization of the tissue. The injured cartilage has limited self-repairing capacity due to a lack of direct blood supply. Thus cartilage regeneration relies on articular chondrocytes and their metabolism, including the synthesis of ECM molecules. As chondrocyte progenitor cells found in blood and marrow cannot propagate to the damaged region, they are not able to restore the tissue. Moreover, fibrocartilaginous repair leads to scar formation which is associated with an increased risk for the gradual development of secondary osteoarthritis (Holban et al., 2016). It is known that like hyaline cartilage, fibrocartilage also lacks an innate capacity to self-repair after disease or injury. Though researchers have put significant effort to engineer distinct fibrocartilage tissues, the development of functionality equivalent to fibrocartilage remains obscure (MacBarb et al., 2013).

The malformation in the structure of the nose and ear are found in congenital disorders. In the case of the ear, both acquired and congenital disabilities can cause external ear deformities. Additionally, accidental fractures may lead to significant damage to the ear and nose cartilage, whereas nasal fractures are half of all facial fractures. These malformations may also require cartilage reconstruction. Tracheal defects resulting from trauma, inflammation or illness and due to congenital or benign stenosis need tracheal reformation. In general, malignancy incidences of the ear, nose, and trachea are rising and that often requires resection followed by replacement or reconstruction (Chiu and Waldman, 2016).

The treatment modalities for the cartilage lesions are majorly aimed to either manage the symptoms of the disease or to repair or replace the damaged tissue. Tissue regeneration involves the formation of analogous new tissue with the native articular cartilage, whereas repair leads to tissues with inferior properties. Symptoms like swelling, stiffness of the joints and pain can be managed by reducing body weight loss and changing lifestyle through physical exercise. Various anti-inflammatory, nonsteroidal drugs, and other pharmacological agents, as well as injection of a hyaluronic acid solution into the joint, are used to manage the symptoms. However, when these noninvasive approaches are no longer adequate, several surgical procedures are available to be applied to treat the disease or cartilage damage. At this point, replacement of the damaged joint with prosthesis remains the standard gold treatment as it is quite successful in reducing pain and improving quality of life. However, it requires revised surgery because of previous implant failure caused by infection, fatigue failure, or implant loosening, making it nonfavorable for younger patients (Mahendran and St-Pierre, 2019). As a result, the development of tissue- and cell-based interventions is increasing.

Till date, many strategies have been studied to restore the integrity of cartilage. The choice of the most appropriate therapeutic modality depends on the multiple factors; for example, in treating articular cartilage injuries factors like location, the patient's age, depth, history, associated injuries, knee stability, meniscal injuries, and limb mechanical axis, need to be considered. None of the mentioned interventions have been found to be ultimately successful. Depending on the type of the therapeutic method, it possesses drawbacks like excessive trauma of the bone, thermal necrosis, low quality of the repaired tissue, and multiple surgeries. Encouraging results have been observed for osteochondral allografts or/and autograft transplantation. However, the treatment is not so frequently used due to poor amalgamation of the grafts, disease transmission, donor site morbidity, and limited treatable defect sizes (Holban et al., 2016). The researchers have combined different approaches or successfully modified them to overcome the shortcomings; nonetheless, they remain to be warranted extensively. Presently, cartilage TE is the most popular and rapidly evolving approach as the developed technologies have shown potential to regenerate cartilage tissues with similar complexity of the native tissue.

4.3.3 Cartilage tissue engineering

Researchers are investigating several cell types and various biomaterials to form desired 3D scaffolds, and multiple signaling molecules to offer new and better insights into the repair of cartilage damage. Chondrocytes are specialized cells resident to cartilage because of which they are commonly used in engineering the cartilaginous tissues. The chondrocytes can be isolated from different zones of the articular cartilage where most commonly full depth chondrocytes have been used for transplantation as well as in vitro TE. They are obtained from the low weight-bearing autologous or allogenic cartilage tissue (Fuentes-Mera et al., 2017). Nowadays, the use of stem cells has been growing for cartilage TE because they possess a high proliferative capacity and multilineage differentiation potential. Mesenchymal stem cells (MSCs), a precursor of chondrocytes, have shown higher proliferation rates compared with chondrocytes and possess a vast differentiation potential leading to effective chondrogenesis. Bone marrow-derived MSCs undergo chondrogenic differentiation by applying appropriate conditions, even showing elevated osteochondral differentiation when implanted in vivo (Chiu and

Waldman, 2016). MSCs achieve the cartilage formation by producing various ECM macromolecules including fibronectin, collagen(s), proteoglycans, and GAGs, as well as a wide range of cytokines and growth factors. Moreover, they are easily accessible from several tissues, such as bone marrow, adipose tissue, and synovial membrane (Somoza et al., 2014). The other approach uses co-culturing of the multiple cell types to impersonate the structural organization of the original cartilage tissue (Chiu and Waldman, 2016).

Successful chondrogenesis and proliferation of the chondrocytes require growth factors such as TGF-β1, fibroblast growth factor 2 (FGF-2), and platelet-derived growth factor-BB (PDGF-BB). In the case of MSCs, chemokines and growth factors induce its differentiation into chondrocytes, maintain the chondrocyte morphology, and allow for the formation of the cartilage matrix. Such growth factor and signaling molecules include transforming growth factor-β (TGF-β), fibroblast growth factor (FGF), hedgehog, bone morphogenic protein (BMP), insulin-like growth factor (IGF), and wingless/Int (Wnt). The application of TGF-β members, BMP-2 and IGF-1 in producing cartilage tissue constructs have been shown to improve their compressive and tensile properties. Further, these growth factors help in expressing various ECM proteins like collagen, GAGs and other proteoglycans aiding tissue formation (Chiu and Waldman, 2016; Fuentes-Mera et al., 2017).

The scaffolds can be built using natural (e.g., collagen) or synthetic materials and tailored as either monophasic (comprising chondral phase) or multiphasic (imitating the osteochondral unit). Hitherto, engineered cartilage tissues have not achieved mechanical properties and biochemical composition precisely the same as the native tissue (Chiu and Waldman, 2016). Hence, current developments in cartilage TE are focused on yielding engineered tissues that have improved structure and functionality.

4.3.4 Nanobiomaterials in cartilage tissue engineering

A plethora of studies have been conducted on scaffold formation using various types of nanobiomaterials to ultimately enhance the functionality of the constructed cartilage tissues. The researchers have used different methods for generating nanoscale components, where electrospinning and 3D fiber deposition have shown improved quality of the nanostructured scaffolds. The use of nanobiomaterials has allowed for the fabrication of the mechanical environment via reinforcement and at the same time, their characteristic conductivity encourages the electrical stimulation of the tissue and cells.

They further incorporate nanoscale dimensions into the scaffold structure that is believed to enhance the cell-cell communication as well as cell interactions with the scaffold, improving the functional performance of the engineered cartilage tissue. It is suggested that topology of the scaffold, as well as the pattern and spacing of the adhesive ligands modulates cell transduction (Mahendran and St-Pierre, 2019). Thereby, the nanoscale features may affect cell behavior and interactions leading to better production of the ECM proteins, ultimately forming the tissue construct imitating the native cartilage tissue.

4.3.4.1 Nanofibers in cartilage tissue engineering

Synthetic and natural nanofibrous matrices are largely utilized for cartilage regeneration. The synthetic polymers, such as PCL, PGA, and PLGA, as well as natural polymers like gelatin, collagen, and chitosan, can be easily fabricated to form nanofibrous or nanoporous structures. Electrospinning technique predominates in the synthesis of nanoscopic scaffolds for cartilage TE (Chiu and Waldman, 2016).

Li et al. (2005) created 3D scaffolds from a synthetic biodegradable polymer, PCL that had resembled collagen fibrils of the cartilage tissue. The nanofibers had a diameter of 700 nm, were distributed uniformly and randomly oriented in the scaffold. In vitro, the scaffold supported the multilineage differentiation of bone marrow-derived human mesenchymal stem cells and the resultant tissue successfully expressed the genes related to chondrogenesis (i.e., aggrecan, collagen type II, X, and other cartilage-specific ECM proteins) in the TGF-β1 containing chondrogenic medium. In their previous study, fetal bovine chondrocytes were seeded on the same PCL nanoscaffold that supported the chondrocytic phenotype and in turn cartilage formation (Fig. 4.4A and B). In another in vivo study, electrospun, chitosan-coated/uncoated PCL (fibers of 400 nm in diameter) scaffolds were implanted under the periosteum in rabbits and their results were comparable with that of Li et al. (2005) (Chiu and Waldman, 2016). They found better cartilage formation at the longer duration of implantation in the uncoated scaffolds. The periosteal cells migrated in the transplanted nanoscaffold in vivo, and as it had produced engineered cartilage in vitro, it was thought to be responsible for the same in vivo. Thus the scaffold structure and composition and the culture medium played a significant role in determining the functionality of the tissue cells. The results of the previous research incorporating the scaffold made up of nanoscopic PCL fibers showed a vast potential to be explored further in cartilage TE.

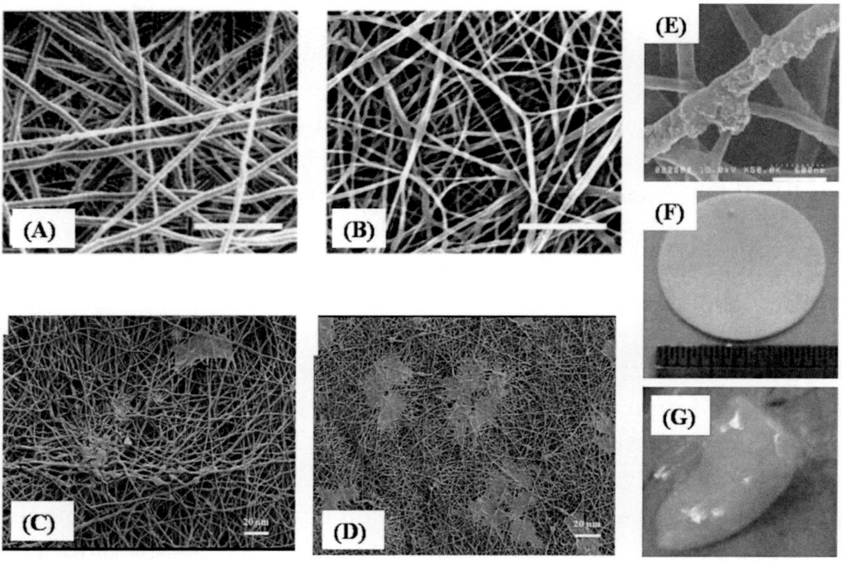

Fig. 4.4 ***Nanoscaffolds used in cartilage tissue engineering: (A, B) Electrospun nanofibrous polycaprolactone scaffolds.*** (A) Scanning electron microscopy image of polycaprolactone scaffolds with fibers 500–900 nm in diameter, (B) Nanofibrous scaffold incubated in cell culture medium for 21 days. Fibers and pores are maintained having no significant structural degradation. (C, D) SEM images of the chondrocyte attached to the electrospun scaffold of poly(3-hydroxybutyrate-*co*-3-hydroxy valerate) (PB). (C) PB scaffold and (D) PB scaffold reinforced with 1% graphene oxide enhances chondrocyte proliferation and ECM production. (E–G) Electrospun nanofibrous poly(L-lactic acid) (PLLA) membranes modified by treatment with oxygen plasma and subsequent covalent grafting of cationized gelatin molecules. (E) SEM image of nanofibrous membrane. (F) Bulk appearance of nanofibrous membrane before implantation into rabbits. (G) Bulk appearance of the tissue constructs 4 weeks after implantation into rabbits. ((A, B) Reproduced with permission from Li, W.J., Tuli, R., Okafor, C., Derfoul, A., Danielson, K.G., Hall, D.J., Tuan, R.S., 2005. A three-dimensional nanofibrous scaffold for cartilage tissue engineering using human mesenchymal stem cells. Biomaterials 26(6), 599–609. Copyright © 2005 Elsevier Ltd. (C, D) Reproduced with permission from More, N., Srivastava, A., Kapusetti, G., 2020. Graphene oxide reinforcement enhances piezoelectric and mechanical properties of poly (3-hydroxybutyrate-co-3-hydroxy valerate) based Nanofibrous scaffolds for improved proliferation of chondrocytes and ECM production. ACS Appl. Biol. Mater. 3(10), 6823–6835. Copyright © 2020 American Chemical Society. (E–G) Reproduced with permission from Chen, J.P., Su, C.H., 2011. Surface modification of electrospun PLLA nanofibers by plasma treatment and cationized gelatin immobilization for cartilage tissue engineering. Acta Biomater. 7(1), 234–243. Copyright © 2011 Elsevier Ltd.)

Turner et al. (2014) created a scaffold of electrospun nanoscale polycarbonate urethane fibers and grown bovine annulus fibrosus cells on them to study their cellular and molecular behavior modulated by tensile forces. The tension was applied either during the entire culture duration (monotonic condition) or removed after 24 h (relaxed). The cells cultured in the relaxed condition showed higher proliferation, more collagen synthesis and increased *TGFβ-1* gene expression. In contrast, the cells were more aligned on the monotonic strained scaffolds that led to a greater scaffold elastic modulus. Thereby, to engineer the annulus fibrosus may require determination of the optimal elastic modulus and applied tensile forces to mimic the native tissue in a better manner. Chen and Su (2011) modified the surface of the electrospun nanoscopic PLLA fiber membranes by oxygen plasma that introduced carboxylate groups on the surface on which they added cationic gelatin molecules. In vitro, when rabbit articular chondrocytes were cultured, it enhanced their viability, proliferation and differentiation on the modified membranes as compared to the unmodified membranes. SEM analysis showed better cell infiltration while maintaining cell morphology. Moreover, the modified membrane enhanced chondrogenic properties of the cells as increased production of GAGs, collagen and aggrecan were observed and also successfully formed the cartilage tissue in vivo after 28 days of implantation (Fig. 4.4E–G).

Apart from electrospinning, the thermal phase separation method was applied to synthesize a semicrystalline iblock copolymer, poly(β-caprolactone)-*block*-poly(L-lactide) (PCL-*b*-PLLA) nanofibrous scaffold (He et al., 2009). The homogenous solution of PCL-*b*-PLLA/tetrahydrofuran was quenched to −20°C or below and subsequently gelled for 2 h as PCL and PLLA microcrystals were present. The structured nanoscaffold possessed increased specific surface area and protein adsorption than the solid-walled scaffold. The cartilage cells seeded on this new nanoscaffold demonstrated spherical chondrocyte-like phenotype and more significant amounts of cartilaginous ECM protein (collagen II and aggrecan) secretion. The other study designed peptide amphiphiles via nanofibers self-assembly having a binding property for TGF-β 1 and evaluated the chondrogenic effect of human MSCs cultured on the scaffold. The results in a rabbit model highlighted the cartilage synthesis forming complete articular cartilage even in the presence/absence of an exogenous growth factor (Profire and Constantin, 2019). A similar type of study reported a nanostructured hydrogel scaffold containing a self-assembled peptide (KLD-12, Lys-Leu-Asp) and encapsulated chondrocytes within the synthesized hydrogel.

The resultant scaffold showed successful cartilage regeneration by promoting chondrocyte-specific phenotype and synthesis of the cartilaginous ECM (Holban et al., 2016).

4.3.4.2 Nanocomposites in cartilage tissue engineering

Besides using nanoscaled polymers for scaffold generation, nanocomposites have been extensively studied to create more relevant scaffolds in terms of functionality matching to the native cartilage tissue. Since graphene has favorable properties to support cellular growth and differentiation, it is widely used to form cartilage tissue scaffolds. One such hybrid scaffold is made up of chondroitin sulfate methacryloyl, poly(ethylene glycol) methyl ether-ε-caprolactone acryloylchloride, and graphene oxide (GO) that was evaluated in vitro as well as in vivo after culturing chondrocytes over the scaffold. In comparison with the pure scaffold, this novel scaffold exhibited significantly improved biocompatibility and cell proliferation, in turn, aiding better cartilage regeneration (Profire and Constantin, 2019). The most recent study, optimally reinforced GO in the poly(3-hydroxybutyrate-*co*-3-hydroxy valerate) (PB) based nanofibrous scaffold enhanced the piezoelectric property of the scaffold, resulting in vitro in the improved proliferation of chondrocyte and ECM production (Fig. 4.4C and D). The other studies reported piezoelectric PB reinforced with barium titanate, a 3D PVDF-TrFE scaffold and an electrospun PVDF scaffold that significantly induced chondrogenesis with a better ability to repair or regenerate cartilage tissue. This is because piezoelectricity allows the tissue to respond to the mechanical stimuli and generate electrical cues to support remodeling of the cartilage (More et al., 2020).

Also, many researchers have suggested hydrogels as the potential candidate for creating cartilage scaffolds due to their increased resemblance to the native ECM. Newer hydrogels were constructed by embedding cellulose nanocrystals in different concentrations to upgrade the features required for cartilage rebuilding. These hydrogels showed the potential to be used in articular cartilage regeneration because of their cartilage-like features such as a porous surface (allowing cellular filtration), significant mechanical characteristics, and proper water absorption (Profire and Constantin, 2019). The other study reinforced nanohydroxyapatite into poly(vinyl alcohol) (PVA) composite gels by a freeze/thaw technique. Varying the nanohydroxyapatite content, PVA concentration and freeze/thaw cycle times of the synthesized scaffold could lead to modified mechanical properties of the hydrogel. Besides, one can incorporate metallic nanoparticles, such as gold, into polymers to fabricate polymer-metal nanoparticle composites, for instance, gold nanoparticles were added to hydrogels made of porcine collagen II. These nanoparticles of the hydrogels encouraged cartilage cell growth and expression of the cartilage-specific proteins due to certain favorable properties (optical, electronic, and biological properties) of the gold (Chiu and Waldman, 2016).

4.4 Nanobiomaterials in tendon/ligament tissue engineering

4.4.1 Tendon/ligament tissue

Tendons and ligaments are components of the musculoskeletal system, made up of collagen fibers. They play a pivotal role in aiding joint stability and facilitating mobility via transferring forces within the musculoskeletal system. Both tendons and ligaments are connective tissues that mainly distinguished in terms of what they connect. Tendons connect muscle to bone or other structures while ligaments attach bone to bone, the former being responsible for the movements of bone or structure. In contrast, the latter holds the bone and provides stability (Lake et al., 2020). Primarily, both tissues consist of similar constituents including collagen, proteoglycans (aggrecan, versican, decorin, and biglycan), elastic fibers, glycoproteins, other minor proteins, and water. These tissues are highly hydrated as they contain 65%–75% water. On the other hand, type I collagen is the major component of the tissues representing 70%–80% of the dry weight of the tissue (Rumian et al., 2007). The amount and distribution of collagen and different cross-linking between collagen molecules affect the mechanical properties of the tissues. Moreover, the quantity and location of the proteoglycans, as well as glycoproteins and minor collagens, are also thought to vary according to functional demands and loading environments (Lake et al., 2020). Further, the cellular component of the tendon and ligament commonly include fibroblasts, while progenitor cells, chondrocyte-like cells are found in some regions and inflammatory cells during tendinopathy conditions. These tissues possess reduced cell density and limited vascularization which may contribute to the limited healing and regenerative potential (Yang et al., 2013).

4.4.2 Rationale for tendon/ligament tissue engineering

Tendons and ligaments become frequently injured or damaged because of the high mechanical demands placed on them. Besides, trauma, accidents, tumor resection, and atrophy are further responsible for the injury of these tissues. Tendons and ligaments possess reduced cell density and limited vascularization, which may contribute to the limited healing and regenerative potential (Mogoşanu et al., 2016). The available treatment methods are not capable of providing the optimal mechanical strength. Similarly, auto/allografts have limited applications in treating conditions due to tissue rejection and disease transmission. In this scenario, TE seems an ideal approach to restore the injured tendon/ligament tissue. Like cartilage TE, the scaffold for creating tendon/ligament tissues must meet the physiological needs of the resident tissue and permit the cellular response for better healing and regeneration.

4.4.3 Nanobiomaterials in tendon/ligament tissue engineering

Tendons and ligaments are fibrous tissues due to which natural or synthetic polymers are most commonly used to construct fibrous scaffolds for their regeneration. Such scaffolds can generate uniaxial alignment and possess highly porous structures aiding cell filtration and hence they mimic the anisotropy of the native tissue. Many studies have utilized natural fibers such as collagen, chitosan, and silk for tendon and ligament rebuilding. However, more beneficial properties of the synthetic polymers such as spinnability, excellent mechanical integrity, and cost-effectiveness make them better candidates for TE of tendons/ligaments. Besides, several previous studies have shown that nanofibers of PCL, PLGA, PGA, PLLA, etc. are promising candidates for making scaffolds to regenerate tendons as they allow for cell adhesion, proliferation, and differentiation (Mogoşanu et al., 2016; Nemati et al., 2019).

In vitro studies have successfully synthesized PGA, PLLA, and polylactic-*co*-glycolic acid 82:18 (PLAGA) scaffolds to show their potential applications in tendon/LTE. Another study employed electrospun PLGA nanofiber to construct a biodegradable nano-microfibrous scaffold that encouraged cell growth, differentiation, and function making them promising for tendon/LTE reconstruction (Mogoşanu et al., 2016). Recent work by Perikamana et al. (2018) suggested an aligned polydopamine-coated PLLA nanofiber scaffold with immobilized platelet-derived growth factor-BB in a gradient for tendon regeneration. The scaffold showed the ability for promoting stem cell proliferation and tenogenic differentiation. At day 14, the researchers found significantly increased expression of tenomodulin, a protein required for tenocyte proliferation and tendon maturation, in the aligned scaffold compared with random nanofiber scaffolds. The earlier study employed a 3D multilayered hybrid scaffold containing PCL-poly (ethylene glycol) nanofibers into a porous chitosan matrix. The study demonstrated more in-depth cell filtration and more cell viability in the 3D aligned nanofiber-embedded scaffold (3D-AL) compared with 3D random (3D-RD) and porous control scaffolds (Jiang et al., 2015). There are other studies available indicating improved cell infiltration, tenogenic differentiation, and collagen formation in the aligned multilayer nanofiber scaffold and the scaffold containing growth factors like bFGF (Nemati et al., 2019; Griffin and Kalaskar, 2016). An in vivo study by Liu et al. (2013) constructed bFGF-loaded dextran glass nanoparticles on PLLA fibers and found evidence of tendon healing in the rat model. The healing was because of the release of bFGFs from the designed scaffold for the extended duration.

The tendon-bone insertion site is the complex tissue that needs strong materials in combination with mineralized and unmineralized tissues possessing varied strength and stiffness owing to its distinct composition from the tendon tissues. Kolluru et al. (2013) designed hydroxyapatite-reinforced PLGA nanofibrous scaffold that provided the enhanced surface mineralization and hardening behavior required for the tendon-bone interface site. The other approach to recapitulate this distinct tissue is to manage the mineral deposition of the scaffold. Few investigations have been carried out for controlling the mineralization along the nanofibers that in turn showed good cell attachment.

4.5 Nanobiomaterials in neural tissue engineering

4.5.1 Neural tissue engineering

Injured tissue in the central nervous system (CNS) and its repair is a big challenge and very complicated for researchers as well as for neurosurgeons. Neural TE (NTE) is the best and alternative approach to repair damaged tissue. Neural scaffolds with nanofibrous structures that mimic the natural extracellular matrix (ECM) have been found to be the best potential tool for NTE. Researchers have explored two main fabrication methods for nerve tissue regeneration: electrospinning and self-assembly. The electrospinning method generates fibers ranging from micrometer to nanometer, which can be introduced at the injured site by implantation, whereas self-assembled fibers with tens of nanometers that can be directly injected into the CNS system at the injured site are of great value. Both the fibrous scaffolds would have a significant role in the enhancement in neurite extension and axon regrowth. Hence, nanofibrous scaffolds have been proven as a functional tool for neural tissue regeneration (Cao et al., 2009).

Neural scaffolds and constructs should be ideally designed in such a way that it should have less toxicity, a proper structure support and axon extension for tissue regeneration. The cytotoxicity of the biodegradable components can be controlled by many different ways such as altering molecular weight, fabrication process, chain branching, and/or crosslinking degree. Nowadays, synthetic polymers with electrical conductivity are the better option for neural tissue repair such as polypyrrole (PPy) and polyaniline (PANI). Due to the superconductivity and cytocompatibility of PPy, it has been widely studied and used as a synthetic biopolymer. In vivo and in vitro studies have proven its efficacy as an excellent biopolymer for nerve tissue regeneration (Lee et al., 2009).

The CNS, central nervous system, transmits signals across the human body and coordinates such signals thoroughly. The limitation of the nervous system is that it cannot repair itself after injury. Hence, it ends up in memory loss, sensory loss, neuropathic pains resulting in tissue damage. To repair the tissue, many therapeutic approaches have been attempted, for nerve tissue regrowth. The most approachable technique is nerve TE that involves a nanoscaffold or microscaffold to facilitate tissue regeneration (Chen et al., 2013).

Advanced neural hopeful strategies offer an idealized substitute for nerve repair and regeneration and entails in vitro repair with a scaffold using surgical implantation at the injured site. Nano biomaterials developed using nanobiotechnology include grains, particles, fibers or other constituent components with basic smaller substructural units less than 100 nm in size. Initially, human ECMs have inbuilt into them microarchitecture and nanoarchitecture. Hence, nanobiomaterial-derived scaffolds which mimic the natural architecture with physiochemical properties are high in demand nowadays and can be a promising advanced approach.

Neural cell arrangement in the human body is found within a 3D ECM with a nanoinfrastructure or microinfrastructure. It is now clear that 3D nanoscaffolds with biomimetic features have the potential solution for improving severe clinical conditions for the whole nervous system especially the brain, spinal cord, and neurodegenerative afflictions. Till date, a number of nanotechniques have been introduced for neural tissue regeneration, here, we have discussed several nanobiomaterials for NTE for nervous tissue repair using a different type of biomimetic nanoscaffolds (Cao et al., 2009).

4.5.2 Nanobiomaterials for neural regeneration

The human system can easily recognize the foreign body and elicit an immune response or rejection. Nanoscale objects can rapidly be identified by antibodies and rejected, whereas larger objects may elicit an inflammatory response around them. To ensure the biocompatibility of any biomaterial, it should have the ability for corrosion resistance as the internal environment composition varies in terms of pH as well as it must have a low thermal conductivity to prevent thermal shock. The patient's health, age, immunological disorders, and tissue permeability also affect the biocompatibility of bio nanomaterials. Based on the nature of the biomaterials, whether it is a metal, ceramic, or polymer, can be classified into different applications in the medical field.

Nanobiomaterials have been widely used to impair injured nerve tissue by improving axon outgrowth and accelerating the connection between artificial tissue and targeted tissue to be repaired. Carbon nanotubes (CNTs) and carbon nanofibers (CNFs) have been proven as wonderful nanobiomaterials to date. Due to their exceptional mechanical properties, excellent electrical conductivity, and unique surface chemical properties, CNTc have been well studied for NTE (Seidlits et al., 2008). Previous studies have reported its potential, especially patterned CNTs, for neural tissue growth without the purifying and functionalizing process (Fig. 4.5).

CNFs have the same properties as CNTs, with a comparable lower cost for the same function as well they can be quickly produced. CNTs and CNFs, both having the same size as neurites in the nanometer range, can be useful to control neural functions and activity, which biomimic the neural tissue environment at pertinent injury sites. The main key factor to emphasize CNFs and CNTs for TE is their nm size especially for neural tissue regeneration. Earlier studies have reported that neuron cells grown on multi-walled carbon nanotubes (MWCNTs), show a threefold increase number of neurite branches and a twofold increase in neurite branch length, when it was coated with 4-hydroxynonenal (Hu et al., 2004). A further study reported an increasing number of growth cones and neurite branches with positively charged MWCNT-EN (ethylenediamine) compared with negatively charged MWCNT-COOH. Another study with single-wall CNTs from the same research group demonstrated an increase in length and number of branches for neurites when single-wall CNTs, grafted with PEI (polyethyleneimine) as a copolymer (SWCNTPEI) were used (Hu et al., 2005). A study with modified MWCNTs by amino group accelerated neurite

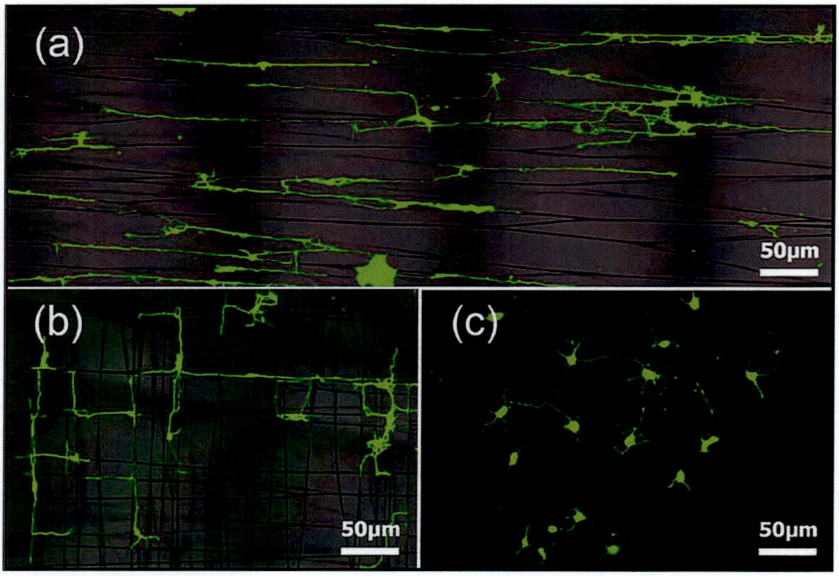

Fig. 4.5 ***Confocal microscopy images of neurons (green) cultured for 5 days on: (A) parallel-aligned carbon nanotube (black lines) substrates, (B) crosslinked carbon nanotubes (black lines) substrates, and (C) a polystyrene substrate.*** (Reproduced with permission from Fan, L., Feng, C., Zhao, W., Qian, L., Wang, Y., Li, Y., 2012. Directional neurite outgrowth on superaligned carbon nanotube yarn patterned substrate. Nano Lett. 12(7), 3668–3673. Copyright © 2012 American Chemical Society.)

outgrowth in terms of both ways at dorsal root ganglion (DRG) neurons and rat pheochromocytoma cells (PC12) by upregulating the level of the active extracellular signal-regulated kinase. CNTs can improve or enhance neurite growth and branching by any number of ways, whether chemical functionalization or using a copolymer. Hence, CNTs have proven well as a neural scaffold material. One more study investigated single-wall CNT polymer thin film membranes for the differentiation, adhesion, and viability of neurons, it was further studied that the viability of neurons can be extended for up to 10 days and, can induce cell differential as well. Studies have reported that SWCNTs have higher electrical conductivity, and hence can stimulate neurons to repair nerve tissue. CNTs can enhance the neuronal circuit network as they have good electrical conductivity, mostly needed for a successful neural transplant (Gheith et al., 2006).

Carbon nanofibers are the second alternative, which have the same function as CNTs; it also can induce neural growth and neurite extension just like CNTs. A team of scientists has developed a CNF electrode using a thin film of polypyrrole, which are polymers and have properties of electronic conductivity (Nguyen-Vu et al., 2006). The study further proved stem cell differentiation and glial scar tissue formation using CNFs when injected in vivo into the rat brain. The research has proven the role of CNF in delivering stem cells to an injured brain where stem cells have differentiated into neurons to repair damaged neural tissue. CNTs and CNFs have the ability to generate a good cell-implant interface, which has merits over various others nanomaterials to repair neural injuries.

Moreover, graphene, which has suitable electronic conductive properties, has shown its potential for neural regeneration. Graphene neither possesses neurotoxicity nor biocompatibility alteration, which makes it unique, and very easy to deposit on nonconducting and flexible biopolymer surfaces. Apart from that, a graphene-coated surface has shown increased growth in neurite number and length compared with others (Zhu et al., 2014).

4.5.3 Nanostructured polymers as neural tissue engineering scaffolds

There are two types of biomaterials that exist for neural scaffold fabrication, natural biomaterials, and synthetic biomaterial. Each has their merits and demerits for neural regeneration. Natural biomaterials are like proteins, peptides, or polysaccharides, which biomimic the tissue or organ environment, but the process of extraction and purification alter its properties, which is not advisable for the transplant. On the other hand, synthetic biomaterials have a higher degree of modulation capacity due to their flexible structure and properties, but not able to mimic the natural environment and lack the biocompatibility. Collagen has proved itself one of the best natural rich biomaterials that mimics the ECM used as a 3D scaffold, having pertinent advantages such as biodegradability, biocompatibility, cell proliferation, and differentiation capacity, it can cross-talk with native tissue, which makes it a unique biomaterial. The central lacuna for collagen usage as a biomaterial is its mechanical strength to withstand physical forces undamaged after implantation (Yu et al., 2011). Another natural biomaterial which has same specification invoking a minimal inflammatory response is silk fibroin which consists of the recurrent amino acid sequence (Gly-Ser-Gly-Ala-Gly-Ala) widely used for TE. Several polysaccharides and their derivatives are already reported as a natural biomaterial. Chitosan, a cationic polysaccharide polymer composed of d-glucosamine and *N*-acetyld-glucosamine subunits, have the potential for neural stem cell differentiation and proliferation with less toxicity to fibroblasts and neuroblasts. Moreover, several other polysaccharides, such as alginate, hyaluronic acid, cellulose, and dextran also have shown outstanding performance in neural tissue regeneration when used alone or in combination with others.

Synthetic polymer biomaterials such as aliphatic polyesters mainly poly-L-lactic acid (PLLA), PCL, PGA, PLGA, and poly(organo) phosphazenes, widely used for their unique specifications such as mechanical strength, biocompatibility, biodegradability, and surface chemistry are well known for neural regeneration. Manipulated PCL nanofibrous scaffolds with topical plasma treatment induce Schwann cell adhesion and proliferation. PCL can be easily degraded using surface hydrolysis of ester linkages and it can be manipulated with copolymerizing it with other polymers. PLLA scaffolds have shown promising nerve cell differentiation and proliferation in terms of fiber dimension and alignment; nanofibers have shown tremendous growth in neurite branches and length compared with microfibers. PGLA-based polymers have shown wonderful regrowth of axons along with nanofibers without provoking an immune response. PGLA degradation can comparatively be manipulated by setting the ratio of PGA/PLA. Polyamides and polyurethanes have not been used much for neural scaffolds, due to issues of biodegradability. Degradation of such synthetic polymers increases the toxicity of the degraded components, crystallize tissue, and can have high tissue activity, which all need to be resolved. Toxicity and degradation rates are the prime factors for not using such biopolymers or synthetic materials for tissue regeneration, which limits its usage and application for neural tissue regeneration. Despite such advanced polymers and techniques, in vivo complications can arise due to such said factors (Zhu et al., 2014).

4.6 Nanobiomaterials in cardiovascular tissue engineering

4.6.1 Cardiac tissue engineering

The main aim of cardiac TE (CTE) is the replacing and regeneration of injured myocardial tissue with natural or synthetic contractile heart tissue made up of biopolymers or biomaterials. Bio nanomaterials used for CTE must be biocompatible and biodegradable and should biomimic the cardiac ECM properties. 3D polymeric scaffolds prepared for the CTE especially for function enhancement and maturation of the tissue is very much in demand nowadays. Some of the natural polymers, such as alginate, chitosan, and heparin, are being used for CTE. Alginate scaffolds with gold nanowires prepared and used as a 3D cardiac patches where alginate was used as a natural polymer has improved electrical communication among adjacent cardiac cells. Alginate scaffolds with magnetic properties have shown the promotion of vessel-like organization in vitro of aortic endothelial cells; electrically conductive chitosan/carbon scaffolds with electro conductive properties implanted with neonatal rat heart cells; and CTE achieved by peptide alginate complexes, along with intact ECM proteins, through the cross-talk of integrin receptors on the cell surface and mediation of cell adhesion and signaling (Mogoşanu et al., 2016). Alginate scaffolds using heparin-binding peptide G (HBP), resulted in promoting cardiac tissue regeneration. Magnetic alginate scaffolds are being used for the promotion of in vitro vessels like the organization of aortic endothelial cells (ECs). A study with the chitosan/carbon scaffold has shown electro conductive properties successfully implanted with neonatal rat heart cells (Maity, 2018).

Synthetic polymers designed with a structural similarity to the ECM, such as electrospun poly(methyl glutarimide) nanofibers, have shown cell differentiation and proliferation into contractile tissue filaments with structure similarities to the ECM, promoting cardiac cell alignment, and proliferation into contractile tissue filaments. One more study reported that hydrogels with electroconductive properties infused with homogeneously dispersed gold nanoparticles elevated expression of connexin 43 at the level of neonatal rat CMs. A hydrogel containing poly(2-hydroxyethylmethacrylate-co-methacrylic acid) was found as a potent functional template for proangiogenic scaffolds and were able to enhance vascularization and integration of human embryonic stem cell (hESC)-derived CMs (Mogoşanu et al., 2016).

4.6.2 Vascular tissue engineering

Blood vessels play a very important role in the transportation of gases to and from the heart as well as for the exchange of chemicals and water between the tissue and blood (Chen et al., 2013). Vascular TE (VTE) is mainly used to create blood vessels with artificial surrogates, which are non-immunogenic and must have suitable mechanical and biological properties without any susceptibility to thrombosis. Various nanomaterials have been designed during recent decades, especially for arterial regeneration and vascular cell seeding. Biodegradable scaffolds were prepared for tissue-engineered vascular grafts (TEVGs), which can be grown and remodeled from native vessels extracted from coronary artery bypass if it is nonimmunogenic and nonthrombogenic in nature. Angiogenesis promotion and vascular network formation can be managed by biocompatible and biodegradable scaffold platforms. A study reported novel TEVGs having biocompatibility and biodegradability properties with a synthetic gel-based scaffold (Mogoşanu et al., 2016).

Natural polymers, such as alginate and collagen, have shown tremendous efficacy for VTE as they have a role in improved angiogenesis by controlling VEGF delivery from injectable alginate hydrogels in an ischemic murine model. A complex vascular phenomena, angiogenesis, thrombosis, and cardiovascular physiopathology, have been studied using a 3D tissue type I collagen hydrogel scaffold using in vitro studies. Certain synthetic or semisynthetic polymers such as PCL, type I collagen, and methacrylate gelatin (GelMA) are being made and used for the fabrication of scaffolds for successful vascular tissue regeneration. Novel cell seeding techniques have been developed using alginate hydrogel scaffolds with adipose-derived stem cells that differentiate into rat endothelial progenitor cells. PCL type I collagen scaffolds in vascular reconstruction have shown biochemical stability in a rabbit model. Moreover, it has shown potential for blood vessel engineering. Apart of this, GelMA hydrogels have shown a remarkable effectiveness for the elongation of fibroblasts, myoblasts, ECs, and cardiac stem cells (Mogoşanu et al., 2016).

Specific synthetic polymers with biocompatibility and biodegradability properties have demonstrated tremendous applications for VTE, such as EC outgrowth proliferation isolated from blood using PLLA scaffolds. Further, Using an electrospinning technique, a copolymer nanoscaffold made up of poly(L-lactic acid)-*co*-poly(ε-caprolactone) (PLLA-PCL) at a ratio of 75 to 25, respectively (75:25), demonstrated similarity in terms of mechanical strength to the human coronary artery, which supported smooth muscle cell proliferation (Mogoşanu et al., 2016).

Nanofibers with gelatin used for blood vessel engineering have also shown improvement for the proliferation of ECs. One more synthetic polymer that has shown the potential for blood vessel engineering is PET, used as tissue-engineered vascular grafts made up of decellularized matrices. Angiogenesis for ocular disease model can be promoted using poly-(D,L-lactide-*co*-glycolide) microspheres with recombinant human vascular endothelial growth factors. A hydrogel prepared with poly(*N*-isopropylacrylamide-*co*-propylacrylic acid-*co*-butyl acrylate) (p[NIPAAm-*co*-PAA-*co*-BA]) with fibroblast growth factor (bFGF) has shown increased angiogenesis in ischemic hind limbs. There are merits of natural and synthetic nanomaterials to repair the VTE. However, there are certain limitations for smaller diameter vessel engineering due to the increased incidence of thrombosis and graft rejection as well as infection (Mogoşanu et al., 2016).

ForVTE, a nanofibrous scaffold was prepared from biodegradable poly(L-lactic-*co*-ε-caprolactone) (PLLA-CL) (75:25), which resembled the natural ECM having same mechanical properties which support smooth muscle cell adhesion and proliferation. A PET nanofibrous scaffold was prepared to overcome graft rejection by surface modification with gelatin because only the surface was covered by epithelial cells following a degenerative state. They observed that the gelatin-modified surface with PET nanofibers supported the proliferation of endothelial cells and maintained the cell phenotype. One more study with PCL-collagen scaffolds for vascular regeneration in a rabbit aortal-iliac bypass model showed enough mechanical for cell growth and other physiological conditions (Chen et al., 2013).

4.7 Conclusions and future perspectives

There is a strong demand for TE in medicine today due to unavailability of organ or graft rejection during organ transplantation. Important progress has been shown during the past decade in nanomedicine and nanotechnology (Turakhia et al., 2018; Turakhia et al., 2019; Turakhia et al., 2020; Prasen and Sejal, 2020). Here, we have discussed the nanobiomaterials used to design scaffolds for regenerating different soft tissues such as cartilage, neural, tendons, ligaments, and cardiovascular tissues. Nanopolymers are predominately used for scaffold synthesis where both natural and synthetic polymers have certain merits and demerits. Natural polymers have excellent biocompatibility and aid superior cell proliferation and differentiation compared with synthetic polymers. On the other hand, synthetic polymers can be easily fabricated to achieve desired scaffold characteristics and more economical. The selection of the nanobiomaterial is largely dependent on the tissue being synthesized.

Researchers have optimized scaffold designs for the regeneration of soft tissues. However, there is a lacuna in the application of TE for different diseases which has revealed numerous major challenges. There is a need for in vivo studies for better understanding the application of TE. Further studies are also required to overcome the neovascularization of the synthetic tissue scaffold. This is the era of 3D/4D bioprinting, due to the complexity of the organ and various biological processes between the organs; the current strategy shows the limitations. A 2D model of tissue cannot mimic the environment in the human body, for that 3D and 4D models have to be prepared and validate the results using TE (Profire and Constantin, 2019). As personalized TE and regenerative medicine (TERM) have shown significant potential toward disease treatment, studies need to be performed toward better personalized strategy which decreases the time and cost as well. Patients have to wait longer for their personalized tissue or organ as it's a laborious process taking much time, and involve tedious steps, such as scaffold designing, cell isolation, seeding, or proliferation. Moreover, there are chances of inflammation and immunogenic responses. Although nanobiomaterials used in the TE represent a big revolution, studies are still needed to be performed for its toxicity, biodegradability, and anti-inflammatory response as well as interactions between materials and cells. Hence, bench to bedside applications ofTE has faced some challenges as discussed, and need to be addressed in the near future.

References

Cao, H., Liu, T., Chew, S.Y., 2009. The application of nanofibrous scaffolds in neural tissue engineering. Adv. Drug Deliv. Rev. 61 (12), 1055–1064.

Chen, J.P., Su, C.H., 2011. Surface modification of electrospun PLLA nanofibers by plasma treatment and cationized gelatin immobilization for cartilage tissue engineering. Acta Biomater. 7 (1), 234–243.

Chen, H., Truckenmüller, R., Van Blitterswijk, C., Moroni, L., 2013. Fabrication of nanofibrous scaffolds for tissue engineering applications. In: BT-Nanomaterials in Tissue Engineering. Woodhead Publishing Series in Biomaterials. Woodhead Publishing, pp. 158–183.

Chiu, L., Waldman, S., 2016. Nanomaterials for Cartilage Tissue Engineering. IAPC Publishing, Zagreb, Croatia, pp. 417–451.

Fuentes-Mera, L., Camacho, A., Moncada-Saucedo, N.K., Peña-Martínez, V., 2017. Current applications of mesenchymal stem cells for cartilage tissue engineering. In: Mesenchymal Stem Cells-Isolation, Characterization and Applications. IntechOpen, pp. 149–184.

Gheith, M.K., Pappas, T.C., Liopo, A.V., Sinani, V.A., Shim, B.S., Motamedi, M., Wicksted, J.P., Kotov, N.A., 2006. Stimulation of neural cells by lateral currents in conductive layer-by-layer films of single-walled carbon nanotubes. Adv. Mater. 18 (22), 2975–2979.

Ghosh, Sougata, Shah, Sejal, Webster, Thomas, 2021. Recent trends in fungal biosynthesis of nanoparticles. ungi Bio-Prospects in Sustainable Agriculture, Environment and Nanotechnology 3 (Volume 3: Fungal metabolites and Nano-technology), 403–452. https://doi.org/10.1016/B978-0-12-821734-4.00018-6.

Griffin, M., Kalaskar, D., 2016. Applications of Nanomaterials in Mechano-Sensitive Tissues. IAPC-OBC Publishing, pp. 385–416.

He, L., Liu, B., Xipeng, G., Xie, G., Liao, S., Quan, D., Cai, D., Lu, J., Ramakrishna, S., 2009. Microstructure and properties of nano-fibrous PCL-b-PLLA scaffolds for cartilage tissue engineering. Eur. Cell. Mater. 18, 63–74.

Holban, A.M., Andronescu, E., Curutiu, C., Ditu, L.M., Chifiriuc, M.C., Lazar, V., 2016. Bioactive nanomaterials for cartilage and muscle regeneration. In: Nanobiomaterials in Soft Tissue Engineering. William Andrew Publishing, pp. 261–297.

Hu, H., Ni, Y., Montana, V., Haddon, R.C., Parpura, V., 2004. Chemically functionalized carbon nanotubes as substrates for neuronal growth. Nano Lett. 4 (3), 507–511.

Hu, H., Ni, Y., Mandal, S.K., Montana, V., Zhao, B., Haddon, R.C., Parpura, V., 2005. Polyethyleneimine functionalized single-walled carbon nanotubes as a substrate for neuronal growth. J. Phys. Chem. B 109 (10), 4285–4289.

Hudita, A., Galateanu, B., Costache, M., 2019. Nanobiomaterials for tissue engineering. Materials for Biomedical Engineering. In: Nanobiomaterials in Tissue Engineering. Elsevier, Amsterdam, pp. 1–21.
Jiang, W., Li, L., Zhang, D., Huang, S., Jing, Z., Wu, Y., Zhao, Z., Zhao, L., Zhou, S., 2015. Incorporation of aligned PCL–PEG nanofibers into porous chitosan scaffolds improved the orientation of collagen fibers in regenerated periodontium. Acta Biomater. 25, 240–252.
Kim, S.Y., Hong, D.K., Im, M., Lee, Y., Lee, J.H., Seo, Y.J., 2011. A case of auricular ossification. Ann. Dermatol. 23 (Suppl 2), S261–S263.
Kim, D.H., Provenzano, P.P., Smith, C.L., Levchenko, A., 2012. Matrix nanotopography as a regulator of cell function. J. Cell Biol. 197 (3), 351–360.
Kolluru, P.V., Lipner, J., Liu, W., Xia, Y., Thomopoulos, S., Genin, G.M., Chasiotis, I., 2013. Strong and tough mineralized PLGA nanofibers for tendon-to-bone scaffolds. Acta Biomater. 9 (12), 9442–9450.
Kumar, V., Naqvi, S., Gopinath, P., 2018. Applications of nanofibers in tissue engineering. In: Application of Nanomaterials. Woodhead Publishing, pp. 179–203.
Kumar, M., Brar, A., Vivekanand, V., Pareek, N., 2019. Possibilities and perspectives of chitosan scaffolds and composites for tissue engineering. In: Materials for Biomedical Engineering. Elsevier, Amsterdam, pp. 167–203.
Lake, S.P., Liu, Q., Xing, M., Iannucci, L.E., Wang, Z., Zhao, C., 2020. Tendon and ligament tissue engineering. In: Principles of Tissue Engineering. Academic Press, pp. 989–1005.
Langer, R., Tirrell, D.A., 2004. Designing materials for biology and medicine. Nature 428 (6982), 487–492.
Lee, J.Y., Bashur, C.A., Goldstein, A.S., Schmidt, C.E., 2009. Polypyrrole-coated electrospun PLGA nanofibers for neural tissue applications. Biomaterials 30 (26), 4325–4335.
Li, W.J., Tuli, R., Okafor, C., Derfoul, A., Danielson, K.G., Hall, D.J., Tuan, R.S., 2005. A three-dimensional nanofibrous scaffold for cartilage tissue engineering using human mesenchymal stem cells. Biomaterials 26 (6), 599–609.
Lin, P.C., Lin, S., Wang, P.C., Sridhar, R., 2014. Techniques for physicochemical characterization of nanomaterials. Biotechnol. Adv. 32 (4), 711–726.
Liu, S., Qin, M., Hu, C., Wu, F., Cui, W., Jin, T., Fan, C., 2013. Tendon healing and anti-adhesion properties of electrospun fibrous membranes containing bFGF loaded nanoparticles. Biomaterials 34 (19), 4690–4701.
Luo, H., Cha, R., Li, J., Hao, W., Zhang, Y., Zhou, F., 2019. Advances in tissue engineering of nanocellulose-based scaffolds: a review. Carbohydr. Polym. 224, 115–144.
MacBarb, R.F., Makris, E.A., Hu, J.C., Athanasiou, K.A., 2013. A chondroitinase-ABC and TGF-β1 treatment regimen for enhancing the mechanical properties of tissue-engineered fibrocartilage. Acta Biomater. 9 (1), 4626–4634.
Mahendran, J., St-Pierre, J.P., 2019. Nanomaterials applications in cartilage tissue engineering. In: Nanoengineering Materials for Biomedical Uses. Springer, Cham, pp. 81–105.
Maity, S., 2018. Use of nanostructured materials in soft tissue engineering. In: Nanobiomaterials. Woodhead Publishing, pp. 465–480.
Mogoşanu, G.D., Grumezescu, A.M., Mogoantă, L., Bejenaru, L.E., Bejenaru, C., 2016. Applications of nanobiopolymers for soft tissue engineering. In: Nanobiomaterials in Soft Tissue Engineering. William Andrew Publishing, pp. 83–109.
More, N., Srivastava, A., Kapusetti, G., 2020. Graphene oxide reinforcement enhances piezoelectric and mechanical properties of poly (3-hydroxybutyrate-co-3-hydroxy valerate) based Nanofibrous scaffolds for improved proliferation of chondrocytes and ECM production. ACS Appl. Biol. Mater. 3 (10), 6823–6835.
Nemati, S., Kim, S.J., Shin, Y.M., Shin, H., 2019. Current progress in application of polymeric nanofibers to tissue engineering. Nano Converg. 6 (1), 1–16.
Nguyen-Vu, T.B., Chen, H., Cassell, A.M., Andrews, R., Meyyappan, M., Li, J., 2006. Vertically aligned carbon nanofiber arrays: an advance toward electrical–neural interfaces. Small 2 (1), 89–94.

Oseni, A.O., Crowley, C., Boland, M.Z., Butler, P.E., Seifalian, A.M., 2011. Cartilage tissue engineering: the application of nanomaterials and stem cell technology. In: Tissue Engineering for Tissue and Organ Regeneration. IntechOpen, pp. 233–266.
Perikamana, S.K.M., Lee, J., Ahmad, T., Kim, E.M., Byun, H., Lee, S., Shin, H., 2018. Harnessing biochemical and structural cues for tenogenic differentiation of adipose derived stem cells (ADSCs) and development of an in vitro tissue interface mimicking tendon-bone insertion graft. Biomaterials 165, 79–93.
Prasen, V., Sejal, S., 2020. Nanocarbons-Mediated water purification: an application towards wastewater treatment. In: Environmental Nanotechnology for Water Purification. Scrivener Publishing LLC, pp. 57–99.
Profire, L., Constantin, S.M., 2019. Nanomaterials in tissue engineering. In: Polymeric Nanomaterials in Nanotherapeutics. Elsevier, pp. 421–436.
Rumian, A.P., Wallace, A.L., Birch, H.L., 2007. Tendons and ligaments are anatomically distinct but overlap in molecular and morphological features—a comparative study in an ovine model. J. Orthop. Res. 25 (4), 458–464.
Seidlits, S.K., Lee, J.Y., Schmidt, C.E., 2008. Nanostructured scaffolds for neural applications. Nanomedicine 3, 183–199.
Shah, S., Ghosh, S., 2020. Medicinal prospects of marine flora and fauna for drug discovery. In: Marine Niche: Applications in Pharmaceutical Sciences. Springer, pp. 321–345. https://doi.org/10.1007/978-981-15-5017-1_18.
Somoza, R.A., Welter, J.F., Correa, D., Caplan, A.I., 2014. Chondrogenic differentiation of mesenchymal stem cells: challenges and unfulfilled expectations. Tissue Eng. Part B Rev. 20 (6), 596–608.
Turakhia, B., Turakhia, P., Shah, S., 2018. Green synthesis of zero valent iron nanoparticles from Spinaciaoleracea (spinach) and its application in waste water treatment. J. Adv. Res. Appl. Sci. 5 (1), 46–51.
Turakhia, B., Chikkala, S., Shah, S., 2019. Novelty of bioengineered iron nanoparticles in nanocoated surgical cotton: a green chemistry. Adv. Pharm. Sci. 2019.
Turakhia, B., Divakara, M.B., Santosh, M.S., Shah, S., 2020. Green synthesis of copper oxide nanoparticles: a promising approach in the development of antibacterial textiles. J. Coat. Technol. Res. 17 (2), 531–540.
Turner, K.G., Ahmed, N., Santerre, J.P., Kandel, R.A., 2014. Modulation of annulus fibrosus cell alignment and function on oriented nanofibrous polyurethane scaffolds under tension. Spine J. 14 (3), 424–434.
Yang, G., Rothrauff, B.B., Tuan, R.S., 2013. Tendon and ligament regeneration and repair: clinical relevance and developmental paradigm. Birth Defects Res. C Embryo Today 99 (3), 203–222.
Yu, W., Zhao, W., Zhu, C., Zhang, X., Ye, D., Zhang, W., Zhou, Y., Jiang, X., Zhang, Z., 2011. Sciatic nerve regeneration in rats by a promising electrospun collagen/poly (ε-caprolactone) nerve conduit with tailored degradation rate. BMC Neurosci. 12 (1), 1–14.
Zhu, W., O'Brien, C., O'Brien, J.R., Zhang, L.G., 2014. 3D nano/microfabrication techniques and nanobiomaterials for neural tissue regeneration. Nanomedicine 9 (6), 859–875.

CHAPTER 5

Nanobiomaterials for wound healing

Amarjitsing Rajput[a,b], Roshan Keshari[a], Runali Patil[a,c], and Rinti Banerjee[a]
[a]Nanomedicine Laboratory, Department of Biosciences and Bioengineering, Indian Institute of Technology Bombay, Powai, Mumbai, Maharashtra, India
[b]Department of Pharmaceutics, Poona College of Pharmacy, Bharti Vidyapeeth Deemed University, Erandwane, Pune, Maharashtra, India
[c]IIT Bombay-Monash Research Academy, Indian Institute of Technology Bombay, Powai, Mumbai, Maharashtra, India

5.1 Introduction

With a uniquely regenerative property, the skin is a protective barrier for the internal outline of the body. Cuts and various wounds are potential threats to the skin, and they can be turned into significant risks if not healed or treated it properly. Disruption in the integrity of the skin epithelium is termed as a wound. These disruptions can be covered to the dermis, causing more profound injury and also exceeding subcutaneous fat, muscles, and even covering bone (Enoch and Price, 2004). Wounds are classified as chronic and acute broadly based on the healing period and severity. Obesity and diabetes are major risk factors world-wide for chronic wounds (Homaeigohar and Boccaccini, 2020). More than 8.2 million people suffer with or without infections and show a significant prevalence of injury. Averagely, 180,000 deaths occur every year due to burn and burn-related wounds (WHO, 2020a). Management of severe burn wounds and diabetic wounds like foot ulcers are very challenging owing to the complexities associated with it.

5.1.1 Types of wounds

Wounds are majorly classified as acute and chronic wounds depending on their severity and healing duration. At the same time, diabetic wounds and burn wounds can be counted as a separate class of wounds due to their complex management and treatment. Complications associated with wound management in diabetic patients are regulated by several factors like shrunk

Nanotechnology in Medicine and Biology
https://doi.org/10.1016/B978-0-12-819469-0.00004-6

growth factor production and compromised angiogenesis with reduced cell migration including unrestrained expression of factors like metalloproteinases (MMPs) (Lee et al., 2019). Burn wounds majorly involve tissue destruction because of the transfer of heat/energy, and sources can be flame, hot liquids or objects, alkaline chemicals, and electrical objects (Jeschke et al., 2020). Depending on the depth of injury, burn injuries can be classified as superficial which is restricted to the epidermis, while partial-thickness involves deep scarring with pain and requires a week to a month for recovery, and full-thickness which is associated with a prolonged treatment, severe pain, and skin grafting needed for improvement (Saghazadeh et al., 2018).

Acute wounds mostly heal by the routine cascade of inflammation with tissue formation as well as remodeling time. Accidental and surgical wounds can be counted as severe wounds. These wounds can heal within a few days with the routine wound healing process of the body. At the same time, wounds that cannot heal within 90 days can be termed as chronic wounds concomitant with comorbid pathological conditions like diabetes and obesity impairing wound healing. Venous leg ulcers due to variable or insufficient blood flow in veins and increased blood pressure and vascular permeability, thermal burns, and diabetic foot ulcers causing peripheral neuropathy leading to decreased foot sensation, are commonly found in chronic wounds (Ghosh and Clark, 2007).

5.1.2 Biological cascade of wound healing

Various growth factors wound healing mediators, kinins like chemokines, formed blood elements, and cytokines, and cells like parenchymal cells contribute to the progression of wound healing. The wound healing process involves phases: homeostasis and inflammation, proliferation where granulation tissue formation takes place, and matrix remodeling with scar formation.

5.1.2.1 Hemostasis and inflammation

At the site of blood vessel tissue injury, vessel closure which also acts as plugs formed by fibrin aggregation clogs wound tissue discontinuity promoting homeostasis. This is an instantaneous response to injury. These clots also act as a matrix for wound repair. Cells like neutrophils and platelets contribute to the process of homeostasis. Activated platelets which bind to collagen exposed at the injury site are a vital factor to stimulate growth factors (TGF-α,β) and blood leukocytes. Various factors like thrombospondin, fibronectin, sphingosine-1-phosphate, and von Willebrand factor are responsible for the advanced stimulation of platelets. Inflammation lasts for 3–4 days after injury incidence and the body's immediate response to the injury or the wound. A pool of leukocytes is characteristic of the inflammation phase. Inflammation occurs mainly due to the release of histamine and other amines from granules filled with these mediators by mast cells. Fluid retention at the injured site causes swelling, and also recruitment of neutrophils to remove foreign bodies, and matrix debris are other signs of inflammation, which can be seen in the wound healing process after 24–48 h. Specialized cell adhesion molecules expressed on endothelial cells additionally attract neutrophils. In later stages, stimulated lymphocytes and monocytes differentiate into macrophages. Macrophages and additionally phagocytes remain and matrix debris, pathogens, and also produce growth factors like cytokines, platelet-derived growth factor (PDGF), and tumor necrosis factor α and β which contribute to inflammation at the site of the wound or injury (Ghosh and Clark, 2007; Homaeigohar and Boccaccini, 2020; Saghazadeh et al., 2018). The role of macrophages is controlled by stimulated monocyte chemoattractants.

5.1.2.2 Proliferation

The proliferation phase starts with a reduction in the number of inflammatory cells at the wound site, and the proliferation of fibroblasts takes place. The proliferation phase continues until the wound heals completely. Angiogenesis is a crucial portion of this phase, followed by re-epithelization. Proliferation involves the migration of fibroblasts, synthesis of collagen, angiogenesis, the formation of tissue granulation, and epithelialization. Fibroblast migration is responsible for the production of fibronectin (a protein matrix), collagen, and hyaluronan. This new extracellular matrix is a key factor for wound repair (Ghosh and Clark, 2007; Enoch and Price, 2004).

Later, fibroblast migration is responsible for the synthesis of collagen. Exposed collagen at the wound site stimulates platelet aggregation and the initiation of a growth factor cascade and also involves the formation of the fresh extracellular matrix. As epidermal cells start migrating at the wound site, the requirement for blood supply for micronutrition, marks the initiation of angiogenesis. Proangiogenic factors like fibroblast growth factor 2 (FGF-2), vascular endothelial growth factor (VEGF), and PDGF play a pivotal role in angiogenesis. These factors attract macrophages and granulocytes for the initiation of angiogenesis. The microvascular network of baby capillaries develops thoroughly into granulation tissues. Endothelial progenitor cells are also one of the critical factors for revascularization pooled during the response to injury (Ghosh and Clark, 2007; Wang et al., 2019; Homaeigohar and Boccaccini, 2020).

Granulation tissue formation is the next process in wound healing. Pinkish granular appearance indicates a capillary loop on the wounded portion. This tissue consists of a newly formed extracellular matrix with collagen, fibroblasts, and a capillary network. These granular tissues allow for the beginning of the process of re-epithelialization. Keratinocytes migrate at wound site beds. The recruitment of keratinocytes is a result of activated growth factors like epidermal growth factor and keratinocyte growth factor, stimulated by inflammatory cytokines (Demidova-Rice et al., 2012).

The next epithelialization process that starts is termed as "epiboly" in which a monolayer of epidermis covers the exposed wound area. The leap-frog fashion of cell movements observed in the extracellular matrix containing fibronectin, fibrinogen, tenascin as well as vitronectin with type I collagen. Cell generation can happen in the case of a large loss of epidermis. The stratified epithelium is re-established by this re-epithelialization process. Moist wounds accelerate the rate of epithelialization. This also improves dermal integrity (Enoch and Price, 2004).

5.1.2.3 Matrix remodeling and scar formation

The granulation phase leads to matrix remodeling. Tensile strength of the wound covering increases with mature collagen strips and bundles. This contraction of connective tissue is the result of responses of TGF-AED-A fibronectin tenascin C and, tissue tension, to differentiated fibroblasts. After about 21 days, the collagen making-braking cycle continues with the extracellular matrix. Collagen degradation takes place by matrix metalloproteinases (MMPs), which is a matrix remodeling enzyme that also supports the healing cascade. With the progression of remodeling, the role of MMPs decreases with increasing activity of tissue inhibitors of metalloproteinases (TIMPs) with TGF-β promoting the accumulation of the matrix. Apoptosis helps to halt the movement of macrophages and fibroblasts cells. Finally, avascular and acellular scars form with halting blood flow and metabolic activities (Demidova-Rice et al., 2012; Enoch and Price, 2004). The normal wound healing process is as shown in Fig. 5.1.

5.1.3 Disease relation in the pathology of wound healing

Disease conditions like diabetes contribute to the altered wound healing process, which causes delays in wound healing or the increasing complexities associated with it, leading to chronic wounds. Neuropathic conditions,

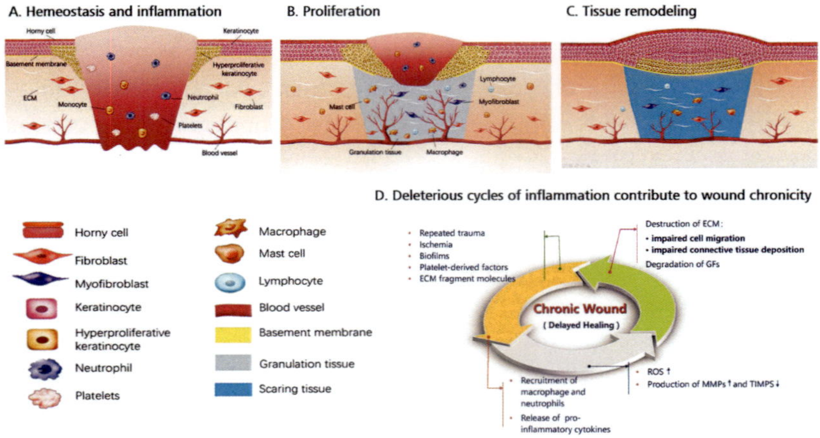

Fig. 5.1 (A–C) Different phases of normal wound healing. Normal wound healing is a complicated biological process, which can be divided into: inflammatory phase (A), proliferation phase (B), and tissue remodeling phase (C). The inflammatory phase occurs shortly after injury, and is characterized by the influx of inflammatory cells. In response to inflammatory cues, neutrophils migrate to the wound first, followed by the monocyte/macrophage lineages, as well as mast cells. As the inflammatory phase subsides, the proliferative phase of tissue repair begins by the migration and hyperproliferation of dermal and epidermal cells within the wound bed. This phase is marked by epithelialization, collagen deposition, angiogenesis, and formation of granulation tissue. The tissue remodeling phase is characterized by matrix remodeling and declined cellularity. During this phase, the wound undergoes contraction, resulting in the formation of a scar with reduced tensile strength. (D) Schematic to show the deleterious cycles of inflammation those contribute to wound chronicity. It is believed that persistent inflammation is a hallmark of chronic nonhealing wounds. Due to repeated tissue injury, microorganisms (e.g., biofilms), and platelet-derived factors stimulate the influx of inflammatory cells and the prolonged release of pro-inflammatory cytokines (e.g., IL-1β and TNFα), leading to elevated levels of ROS and proteases (e.g., MMPs) in the wound bed. Particularly, the protease levels in chronic wounds exceed that of their respective inhibitors. High levels of ROS together with the imbalances between MMPs and TIMPs result in the destruction of ECM components and the degradation of growth factors. The proteolytic destruction of ECM further in turn attracts more inflammatory cells to the wound, and thus, promoting the inflammation into a detrimental vicious cycle and contributing to wound chronicity. *(Reproduced with permission from Kim, H.S., Sun, X., Lee, J.H., Kim, H.W., Fu, X., Leong, K.W., 2019. Advanced drug delivery systems and artificial skin grafts for skin wound healing. Adv. Drug Deliv. Rev. 146, 209–239.)*

ischemia, inherited neutrophil disorders, and edema are some conditions where the risk of chronic wounds can be highlighted. Commonly seen altered physiologies of wound healing in these diseases are chronic infections and thus form microbial biofilms, which may be drug-resistant, prolonging an inflammatory phase, and the incapability of dermal-epidermal cells for epithelialization. Venous hypertension and excess sugar lowers the rate of wound healing (Enoch and Price, 2004). Chronic wounds in diabetes are associated with chronic nerve impairment, bacterial infection, and blood vessel damage, which lead to progressive amputation of appendages (Masood et al., 2019).

Plasma factors and fibrin leaking occurs in venous ulcers due to increases in vein pressure and vascular permeability. Leaked fibrin gets accumulated in the perivascular region, which results in the downregulation of collagen and impaired wound healing processes. It also restricts normal blood vessel function to deprive growth factors related to blood. These complications lead to delayed wound healing in venous ulcers. In the same way, arterial ulcers show an impaired wound healing process, but the occurrence of arterial ulcers is less than venous ulcers. Ischemia is caused due to atherosclerosis and is the main reason for arterial insufficiency of function leading to a delay in wound healing.

Revascularization can help to improve wound healing in arterial ulcers. Pressure ulcers can also cause a chronic wound. Oxygen tension and tissue necrosis in pressure ulcers cause a major alteration in the wound healing process (Demidova-Rice et al., 2012).

5.1.4 Wound management and current treatment

Significant factors that affect wound healing are patient-related factors like diseases like diabetes, immunocompromised conditions, age-related issues, wound-related factors like infection, the extent of the injury, and some local factors like closure period, and homeostasis (WHO, 2020b).

Addressing the control or correction of these chronic wounds not only is focused on removing or relieving etiologic causes, but also aims at metabolic uneasiness, which causes chronicity of the injury. Hence, wound assessment is considered a vital step for wound precision management before the formulation of a treatment plan. This comprises inspection of the wound, patient survey, identification of related clinical data, and past health data of patients. The Bates-Jensen Wound Assessment Tool (BWAT), also known as a pressure sore status tool (PSST) and the Photographic Wound Assessment Tool (PWAT), are some of the mechanisms proposed for wound monitoring and scoring purposes. Wound status can be monitored weekly, and results can be plotted on a continuum of the result status.

Decision-making can be aided by linking clinical actions and assessment findings. TIME, a wound healing based multistep approach, has been used widely for preparing a recipient a wound bed. The TIME framework has been widely accepted for wound treatment and management. TIME involves: T-Tissue, related to foreign components like adherent dressing clothing and bandages, exudates, and biofilms which are all on the wound surface; I-which is the infection treatment involving pharmaceutical management like antiseptics; M-moisture balance to select wound dressings; and E-edge of the wound for observation and assessment (Kim et al., 2019).

Basic steps in the wound and scar treatment involve (i) prevention of infection, thus, protecting from bacterial and contaminants; (ii) removal of debris, dead tissues, and impurities; (iii) appropriate wound drainage; and the (iv) preparation of wound bedding and a suitable wound closure method. Some conventional to modern treatment approaches is nowadays in practice for wounds like a detriment vacuum-assisted closure therapy, platelet-rich plasma treatment, ozonated oil usage, amnion liquid derivative stem cell therapy, use of herbal-Ayurveda-based medicines like *Nigella sativa*, *Hipericum perforatum*, Honey and Propolis and the combination of curcumin with other herbs and oils like Refined Sheep oils and neem oil. The use of antiseptics like povidone-iodine and silver sulfadiazine are also popular. Platelet-rich plasma treatment involves platelet-rich plasma for treatment, taking advantage of platelets being a source of various growth factors involved in the wound healing process.

Vacuum-assisted closure therapy involves exposure of a vacuum at the sore area of the wound at a negative pressure of 125 mmHg for 2 min to remove endemic fluids, debris, and improve perfusion with stimulation of cell proliferation. Amnion liquid derivative stem cell therapy involves amniotic fluid mesenchymal cells that are responsible for pro-inflammatory mediators like hepatocyte growth factor (HGF), vascular endothelial growth factor-A (VEGF-A), and VEGF. Ozonated oil treatment is commonly used to clean the wound and prevent infection due to antimicrobial and antifungal action of ozonated oils (Wang et al., 2019; Canpolat and Alper, 2017). Recently, various biomaterials like polycaprolactone, poly(lactic-*co*-glycolic acid) (PLGA), and poly(ethylene glycol) (PEG) are in consideration for wound dressing materials and nanocarriers for treatment. Also, nanoparticulate drug delivery for wound care and treatment is being explored (Kim et al., 2019; Saghazadeh et al., 2018). The wound healing trend in open wound and open wound treated with antimicrobial dressing is depicted in Fig. 5.2.

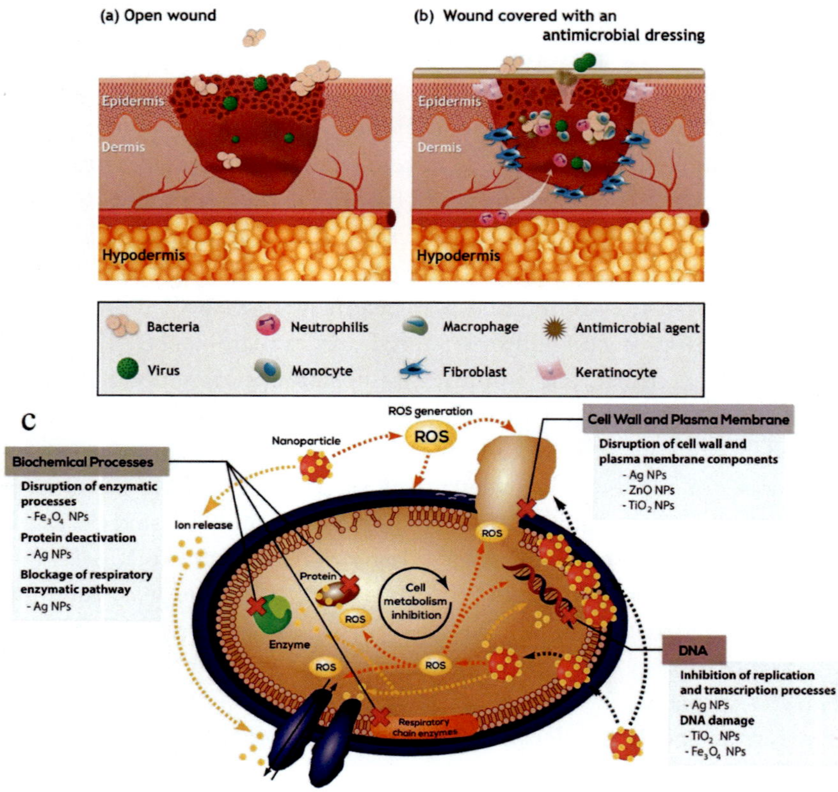

Fig. 5.2 Schematic illustration of the healing trend in: (A) an open wound alone and (B) an open wound treated with an antimicrobial wound dressing. As seen here, the open wound is susceptible to invasion of bacteria, engendering delayed healing due to prolonged inflammation and large release of metalloproteinases, potentially destroying the ECM constituents and hindering the generation of new granulation tissue. In case of applying an antimicrobial dressing, the pathway of pathogens into the wound is blocked and the ones penetrated are efficiently killed. Moreover, provoking the immune system and fibroblast/keratinocyte migration, the healing pace is accelerated. (C) Various mechanisms suggested for the killing function of antibacterial nanoparticles. *(Reproduced with permission from Homaeigohar, S., Boccaccini, A.R., 2020. Antibacterial biohybrid nanofibers for wound dressings. Acta Biomater. 107, 25–49.)*

5.2 Biomaterials for wound healing

5.2.1 Biomaterials from a natural source

5.2.1.1 Protein-based natural polymers

Collagen

Collagen is a versatile material widely used in the medical, dental, and pharmaceutical fields. It is mainly used in wound dressings, burn coverings, bone fillings, and also used as a carrier for collagen-based drug delivery.

Wang et al. developed a new collagen matrix from porcine through decellularization with supercritical carbon dioxide, which is chemically compatible with human skin. An in vitro study was carried out in a porcine skin wound model mimicking human skin, and after 2 or 3 weeks, a reduction in inflammation, complete epithelization, and wound healing was noticed. An in vivo study was carried out in a land-race hybrid male pig, and after 2 or 3 weeks, healing reduction found was found in the group treated with a collagen matrix (Wang et al., 2020).

Mahmoud and Salama prepared norfloxacin collagen/chitosan scaffolds for the treatment of wounds by fusing both high and low viscosity chitosan. An in vivo study was conducted in male albino rats, and after 28 days, it demonstrated that tissue generation was faster compared with an untreated wound. In addition to this, a histopathological study showed an intact epidermal and dermal layer, which was found to be healthy. Finally, all formulated scaffolds released 100% of the drug in 24 h (Mahmoud and Salama, 2016).

Silk fibroin

Silk fibroin is widely used in the biomedical system due to its biocompatibility in nature along with less immunogenicity, partially biodegradability, multifaceted properties, less irritant to the skin with no side effects, and remarkable mechanical properties (Kundu et al., 2013; Zeplin et al., 2014; Rodriguez et al., 2017). Additionally, it has a suitable sustained-release property, muscular flexibility with good air, and moisture permeability. These benefits make silk fibroin a suitable biomaterial for various biological purposes.

Barna et al. determined the healing efficacy of silk fibroin/gelatin (SF/GT) electrospun nanofiber dressings assembled by electrospinning nanotechnology. It was further stuffed with astragaloside IV (AS). In vivo studies were illustrated in female rats divided into four groups and treated with different formulations. The various formulations were a blank control, AS solution, and AS-loaded with SF/GT nanofibers. The prepared formulations were applied to different groups of rats and at the 3rd, 6th, and 9th day of treatment, it was detected that AS-loaded with SF/GT found were more superior and faster in wound healing, promoted angiogenesis and inhibited scar formation by arranging collagen compared with other treatment groups (Barna et al., 2007).

Shefa et al. developed a novel TEMPO-(2,2,6,6-tetramethylpiperidin-1-yl) oxyl-oxidized cellulose nanofiber (TOCN)-silk fibroin scaffold by a freeze-drying method. An in vitro study was analyzed by using L 929 fibroblasts to determine cytotoxicity by using a colorimetric MTT assay. It demonstrates that scaffolds with more silk fibroin support better cell propagation and bonding, and the distribution of natural human keratinocytes. However, an in vivo study carried out using an adult rat model was used to determine wound healing activity. The rats were excised and treated with different percentages of the prepared formulations like a control group, TOCN, TOCN-silk fibroin 2%, and TOCN-silk fibroin 5% and recovery data were recorded on 7th day and 14th day. Results revealed that both the TOCN-silk fibroins (2%) showed rapid wound healing as compared with other groups. Thus it was found to be a superior material in wound healing for clinical applications (Shefa et al., 2017).

5.2.1.2 Polysaccharide-based natural polymers

Hyaluronic acid

Hyaluronic acid (HA) is a natural hydrophilic polysaccharide biologically active material mainly used for tissue engineering and in the drug delivery system (Cho et al., 2003; Lee et al., 2001). It is used to develop high-quality scaffolds, gels (Park et al., 2005; Shu et al., 2004), sponges (Halbleib et al., 2003; Solchaga et al., 2005), films (Liu et al., 2005; Shu et al., 2003), fibers (Milella et al., 2002), and microparticles (Park et al., 2005). It is biocompatible (Ehlers et al., 2001) with the right bacteriostatic properties compared with other matrices such as type 1 collagen and hydroxyapatite (Carlson et al., 2004).

Movahedi et al. developed core-shell structured polyurethane (PU)/starch (ST) and PU/ST (hyaluronic acid) nanofibers using a coaxial electrospinning method. An in vitro study was carried out by using an MTT assay on a mouse fibroblast (L 929) cell lines at an interval of 1, 3, and 7 days. It witnessed that cell proliferation increased from 1 to 7 days along with cell viability more significantly than 80% after 7 days of incubation without any cytotoxicity. An in vivo study was conducted for 14 days by an incision in 18 healthy female Wistar rats. After the incision, wounds were treated with the prepared formulations along with the control group (without scaffolds). After 14 days, the highest wound healing rate was found for the PU/ST (HA) core-shell structure as compared with the PU/ST and control group, and hence it can be used for the treatment of wounds and skin tissue engineering (Movahedi et al., 2020).

Alginate

Alginate is a copolymerized polysaccharide of (1–4) coupled-α-L-guluronic acid and β-D-mannuronic acid monomers along with a polymeric backbone

(George and Abraham, 2006). It is known to be an attractive biomaterial for drug delivery, tissue engineering, and wound healing (Fischer et al., 2017). Although it has attractive properties for biomedical applications, it has two significant drawbacks: deficient in cellular adhesion and in vivo degradation (Sarker et al., 2014).

Bakhsheshi-Rad et al. developed a combination of chitosan-alginate (CS-ALG) nanofiber dressings by an electrospinning method through the incorporating of varying amounts of gentamycin (GN) for antimicrobial infection and wound healing. The addition of gentamycin reduced the diameter of nanofibers along with the enhancement of antibacterial performance. An in vitro study was carried out by using L 929 fibroblast cells, and it reported that the CS-ALG/GN nanofiber with 1%–5% showed exceptional cell adhesion and proliferation compared with the highest concentration (10%) after 3 days. In the same way, an in vivo study was carried out in Balb/C mice with only CS-ALG and CS-ALG/3% GN. It revealed that a lower concentration of gentamycin after 7 days increased the thickness of the dermis, collagen deposition, formation of the new blood vessel, and hair follicles; hence, it can be used for complete skin regeneration (Bakhsheshi-Rad et al., 2020).

Li et al. formulated an in situ injectable curcumin containing nanocomposite hydrogel, along with oxidized alginate and *N,O*-carboxymethyl chitosan and CCS-OA hydrogel as a wound dressing material for wound repair. An in vitro study was conducted in phosphate buffer solution (7.4), which revealed that nano curcumin showed slow or sustained release from the prepared formulation, and its releasing behavior was interpreted using a release kinetic mathematical model. Similarly, an in vivo study was carried out in male adult mice and separated into randomly four groups: a control group, a new CCS-OA hydrogel-treated group, an unmodified curcumin stuffed CCS-OA hydrogel-treated group, and finally a nano curcumin/CCS-OA hydrogel group. Different formulations were tested for 14 days. Better wound closure along with the re-epithelialization of the epidermis and collagen deposition of tissue was observed in the group treated with the nano curcumin/CCS-OA hydrogel (Li et al., 2012).

Chitosan

Chitosan is a high molecular weight and linear polymer. It is obtained from chitin with a composition of biopolymeric polysaccharide of *N*-acetyl-D-glucosamine residues and (1/4)-coupled D-glucosamine (Croisier and Jérôme, 2013). It is biodegradable, bio-adhesive, biocompatible, and widely used in wound dressings and as a formulation of drug delivery carriers (Tan et al., 2009; Zhang and Zhang, 2001; Hu et al., 2013; VandeVord et al., 2002; Dudhani and Kosaraju, 2010; Sarhan et al., 2016). Chitosan is extensively under research in tissue engineering, mostly to target bone, cartilage, and skin (Kim et al., 2008). Due to its versatile use and properties, many FDA-approved chitosan containing products are available in the market (Devlin et al., 2011; Pozza and Millner, 2011; Whang et al., 2005).

Hajji et al. utilized a green method for the production of chitosan-PVA-silver nanoparticles (CS-AgNPs) for antioxidant, antibacterial, and wound healing activities. An in vitro study was carried out using Chinese Hamster Ovary (CHO-K1) cells to determine cytotoxic effects using an MTT assay. It revealed that the cytotoxic effect was dose-dependent (5–200 μg/mL) and no cytotoxicity effect was noticed in this range. However, a complete wound was observed after 12 days of an incision done in an in vivo study performed on male Wistar rats. Another study done by Hajji et al. concluded that chitosan-silver nanoparticles showed higher antioxidant as well as antibacterial activities against both grams-positive (*Staphylococcus aureus*, *Micrococcus luteus*, *Bacillus cereus*) and gram-negative bacteria (*Klebsiella pneumoniae* and *Escherichia coli*) and than the chitosan polymer and silver alone (Hajji et al., 2019).

Abbaszadeh et al. studied the effect of chitosan/selenium nanoparticles for wound healing. An in vivo study performed on male Wistar rats, divided into four groups, that is, the control group (Group 1), methicillin-resistant *S. aureus* (MRSA) (Group 2), MRSA/chitosan (Group 3), and MRSA/chitosan/nanoselenium (Group 4). The in vivo study concluded that on 14 days of treatment, significant differences were found in group 4 and the other groups. Neovascularization and cellular infiltration in group 4 was found to be higher with polymorphonuclear (PMN) cells as well as mononuclear (MNC) cells and more fibroblast cell propagation as compared with other groups. This study proves that the chitosan/selenium nanoparticles are effective for treating wounds (Abbaszadeh et al., 2019).

Starch

Starch is a natural polymeric polysaccharide of homoglucan unit, only constituted by α-D-glucose units (Galliard, 1987; Reis and Cunha, 2001). It is a carbohydrate polysaccharide found in a higher species of plants, tubers, and fruit roots (Naeem et al., 1997). It can be a possible alternative to a synthetic polymer. It is biodegradable, abundantly available, and one of the cheapest biopolymers (Majeed et al., 2014).

Poonguzhali et al. developed symmetric and asymmetric chitosan (C)/PVP(P) films by a salt leaching method containing porous structured nanoparticles for wound dressing and healing. In this preparation, asymmetric chitosan (C)/PVP(P) was coated with stearic acid, whereas symmetric nano starch was kept uncoated. MTT assays were performed to determine cytotoxicity using a NIH3T3 cell line. Cell viability was studied for 1, 3, and 5 days. This study concluded a starch-dependent increment in the cell growth and proliferation of NH3T3 cells. Similarly, an in vivo study was performed using male albino rats by dividing them into three groups: control, CP-S, and CPNS 1%-S and were observed for 7, 14, and 21 days, respectively. From the initial days, the group treated with CPNS 1%-S was found to be superior as compared with the other groups, and complete wound curing and healing were observed around 21 days of treatment (Poonguzhali et al., 2018).

Ahmed et al. prepared hydrogel nanoparticles of starch and PVA in which graphitic carbon nitride (g-C_3N_4) was used as a filler. In this formulation, silver-deposited-titania nanoparticles [Ag@TiO_2 NPs] was used as an antibacterial agent. The prepared hydrogels were prepared by using a solution casting technique at ambient conditions. An in vitro study in distilled, simulated wound fluid, and saline fluid, showed a sustained release behavior of NPs. Additionally, to determine the release profile of the prepared formulation, a mathematical model, the Higuchi model, was used. An in vivo study was performed on female albino mice, dividing them into four groups. The group treated with PVA/Starch/0.14GCN/0.7Ag@TiO_2 NPs showed maximum wound treatment after 7 days (Ahmed et al., 2020).

5.2.2 Biomaterials from synthetic origin

Synthetic biomaterials are majorly used for the reconstruction and regeneration of a variety of tissues, organs as well as in drug delivery. The primary requirements for ideal synthetic biomaterials are biocompatibility, mechanical, chemical, and biological properties. Their use is in tissue engineering for the augmentation of existing tissue, promoting the growth of new tissues, and in organ replacement therapy (Samavedi et al., 2014).

5.2.2.1 Polycaprolactone

It is a semicrystalline biopolymer, widely used for biomedical purposes because of its mechanical properties, in vivo degradation profile, secure processing, and molecular weight-dependent drug release (Mulinti et al., 2018). It offers a thrombogenic potential, and when electrospun into a fiber, it induces hemolysis based on its molecular weight (Horakova et al., 2018; Padalhin et al., 2014). It can also be copolymerized with other lactones like valerolactone (Gunatillake and Adhikari, 2003), or polyesters, to impart additional rigidity, altered hydrolysis, and degradation.

Bakhsheshi-Rad et al. developed nanofibers for wound dressings having antibacterial activity by the electrospinning method. They utilized the antibiotic cephalexin, loaded with polycaprolactone (PCL)-gelatin methacryloyl (GelMA). Its antibacterial efficacy was determined using both gram-positive (*S. aureus*) as well as gram-negative bacteria (*E. coli*). The mechanism of antibacterial efficacy of these nanofibers involved the interaction of the formulation with the cell wall of the bacteria, leading to the rupturing of the bacterial cell membrane causing cell death. An in vivo study in male BALB/c mice with and without antibiotic cephalexin was studied. It showed that the mice treated with only PCL/GelMA had a slightly regenerated epidermal, the formation of new hair follicles, and a sebaceous gland. Still, the group treated with PCL/GelMA-CEX had a thicker epidermis as compared with other groups, the creation of new blood vessels and a reduced inflammatory cell infiltration (Bakhsheshi-Rad et al., 2019).

Hivechi et al. developed a hybrid nanofiber scaffold using a polycaprolactone and gelation (PCL-GEL) electrospinning method. To improve the antibacterial properties, they utilized cellulose nanocrystals and incorporated in PCL-GEL nanofibers. An in vitro study was designed by an MTT assay, cell morphology, and fluorescence staining. It observed that cells could be quickly grown on the scaffold by offering biocompatibility. A further in vivo study was performed on Balb/c mice. Mice were divided into three groups: mice treated with sterile gauze, a PCL/gel scaffold, and CNC incorporated PCL gel scaffolds. After the 7th and 14th days, the mice treated with CNC included a PCL gel scaffold were found to be more effective than the other groups (Hivechi et al., 2020).

5.2.2.2 Poly(lactic-co-glycolic acid)

PLGA is a block copolymerized polymer formed by poly(lactic acid) (PLA) and poly(glycolic acid), widely used in biomedical systems to prepare scaffolds, sutures, and for tissue engineering applications. Because of its excellent cell adhesion and proliferation properties, it is widely used in tissue engineering. It is hemocompatible and biocompatible in nature, and it degrades into a nontoxic metabolic product.

Shefa et al. prepared PLGA-platelet lysates loaded with nanoparticles by using a Pluronic F-127 (thermos-responsive) material. In this formulation, a high amount of lysate was accommodated by using a double emulsion solvent evaporation method. An in vitro study conducted using dermal fibroblast cells and a scratch technique was used to determine the biological activity of the platelet lysate. The scratching of the fibroblast cell resulted in free space generation, and the filling of these open spaces resulted due to the presence of a lysate in the nanoparticles, leading to enhanced repair of the fibroblast cell culture along with cell migration and proliferation. Similarly, an in vivo comparison study of the developed formulation was studied using CD1 mice, in which mice were treated with a control, platelet lysate, PLGA-platelet lysate loaded nanoparticles hydrogel, and platelet lysate hydrogel nanoparticles (PLHN). Mice treated with PLHN showed better recovery compared with other formulations after 10 days (Shefa et al., 2017).

Garcia-Orue et al. developed lipid nanoparticles using *Aloe vera* and PLGA. In this study, in vitro activity was assessed using HaCaT keratinocytes and BalbC/3T3 A31 fibroblasts to determine cytocompatibility and cytotoxicity. For an in vivo study, male dB/db mice were divided into three groups: control, PLGA-*Aloe vera* and PLGA-*Aloe vera* nanoparticles. Fifteen days of treatment revealed that mice treated with PLGA-*Aloe vera* nanoparticles recovered faster than other treatment groups (Garcia-Orue et al., 2019).

5.2.2.3 Poly(vinyl alcohol)

PVA is a biodegradable, water-soluble synthetic polymer with a hydrocarbon backbone that can swell in water and impart strength and stability for various biomedical purposes (Chiellini et al., 2003; Sonker et al., 2017). The branching of PVA increases its mechanical strength along with the improvement in hemocompatibility (Semenova et al., 2016).

Wentao et al. formulated an antibacterial film (PVA@am-ZnO@CuO@Au), which induces disinfection by a reactive oxygen species system. In vitro studies on different bacteria like *E. coli* and *S. aureus* using an irradiating red laser was found to be effective against both. However, an in vivo study in diabetic wounds was demonstrated by comparing results with PVA (control group) and the prepared formulations with and without an irradiating laser. It depicted that after 10 days, the wound treated with PVA@am-ZnO@CuO@Au irradiated at 535 nm was found to be more effective than other treatment groups (Wentao et al., 2019).

Nguyen et al. developed silver nanoparticle gels of different concentrations [like 15, 30, 60 ppm (ppm)] using poly(vinyl alcohol) and chitosan. An in vitro study using gram-positive (*S. aureus*) and gram-negative

(*Pseudomonas aeruginosa*) bacteria demonstrated its usefulness. It was determined using the agar diffusion method and was found to be effective against both of the bacteria. Finally, an in vivo study was carried out using mice and treated with a gel of different concentrations (ppm) along with the marketed product. After 12 days of observation, it was estimated that the group with 60 ppm silver nanoparticles were found to be more effective than the other groups (Nguyen et al., 2019).

5.2.2.4 Poly(lactic acid)

PLA is an aliphatic polyester composed of completely renewable sources such as corn and sugar beets (Drumright et al., 2000). It is biodegradable with a wide range of applications. Despite the full range of its use in the biomedical field, some of its disadvantages have made its applications limited. The bulk erosion of PLA negatively affects the scaffold's integrity, which leads to premature failure by releasing acidic degraded products, causing an inflammatory response (Eglin et al., 2009).

For example, Fang et al. prepared nanofibers consisting of a core and shell made up of two different materials [poly(γ-glutamic acid) (γ-PGA) and PLA, respectively] by a coaxial electrospinning method. An in vitro cytotoxicity study was conducted using an MTT assay with mouse embryonic fibroblast cells (NIH/3T3), which showed good biocompatibility with the prepared core-shell nanofibers. In vivo testing was demonstrated in female Kunming mice, divided into two treated and untreated groups. Results indicated that after 14 days, the mice treated with the core-shell nanofibers were re-epithelialized along with neovascularization and red blood cells to a greater extent compared with the untreated group (Fang et al., 2019).

5.3 Advanced drug delivery systems for wound healing

Several nanocarrier-based drug delivery systems have been studied by various researchers in the case of drug delivery systems for wound healing treatment. These include nanoparticles, polymeric nanoparticles, and lipid-based drug delivery systems. The lipid-based drug delivery systems included solid lipid nanoparticles, nanostructured lipid carriers, and liposomes. Nanocarrier systems act as an important carrier for biologics, which act intracellularly like peptides or nucleic acids. Nano-sized particles provide an additional benefit of the improved penetration of the drug into wound beds as well as increased intracellular uptake of drugs (Kim et al., 2019).

Recent innovation and development in the field of nanotechnology have highlighted several nanocarriers associated with optimal delivery for skin revival. The nanocarrier-based drug delivery systems fasten the wound healing process and also enhance wound healing quality due to following advantages:

(i) They are nontoxic and compatible with the skin.
(ii) They make a wet environment around the skin for acceleration and activation of the wound healing progression.
(iii) A few specific drug delivery systems can enter into the cytoplasmic area beyond the cellular obstacles or enhance the retention of the drug by activating specific transport pathways (Sandhiya et al., 2009).
(iv) Nanocarrier-based drug delivery systems prevent the drug from degradation due to protease enzymes in the wound increasing the therapeutic efficiency of the drug (Losi et al., 2010).
(v) They showed a reduction in the frequency of dosage, which ultimately reduces the cost of the therapy and patient compliance.
(vi) They result in a sustained drug release and maintenance of therapeutic drug concentrations for an extended period (Wang et al., 2019).

Consider the example of nitric oxide, which plays an important role in different pathways such as cellular, inflammatory, angiogenesis, and extracellular matrix deposition and remodeling. Similarly, it exhibits a broad-spectrum of antibacterial properties and also interferes with the synthesis of a biofilm. Hence, many researchers have explored drug delivery systems using high drug loading, controlled release, and reduced cytotoxicity (Hamdan et al., 2017). Similarly, curcumin, is one of the most widely used components of spice turmeric because of its antibiotic and antioxidant properties. It also acts as a stimulating agent for granular tissue production (Krausz et al., 2015).

5.3.1 Nanocarriers for wound healing

5.3.1.1 Inorganic nanoparticles

Nanoparticles are considered as important nanocarrier drug delivery systems for wound healing. The nanoparticles used for wound healing treatment are classified into two types:

1. Nanoparticles which have inherent properties those help in wound closure.
   A. Inorganic
      (a) Metal
      (b) Nonmetal
   B. Organic
      (a) Polymeric
      (b) Nonpolymeric

2. Nanoparticles which act as a carrier for therapeutic agents (Hamdan et al., 2017).

These are described more in the following sections.

Silver nanoparticles

Silver nanoparticles used nowadays may overwhelm problems associated with standard silver compounds. In the case of the silver nanoparticles, smaller particle sizes resulted in more surface area. It is more effective at lower amounts and decreases the toxicities associated with its use. It can change the release of antiinflammatory cytokines to promote faster wound healing without increasing scarring (Hamdan et al., 2017).

Jun et al. studied the wound healing effect and mechanism of silver nanoparticles in healing wounds due to burns using a wound model (chronic). Silver nanoparticles showed a dose-dependent faster healing and enhanced the external appearance of the wound. The study further revealed an increased level of specific markers such as VEGF, IL-6, TGF-β by silver nanoparticles, endorsed wound healing, and reduced inflammation (Tian et al., 2007).

Zulkifli et al. developed hydroxyethyl cellulose-silver nanoparticles into the scaffold to show its antimicrobial capability. Further, studies were conducted using fibroblast cells, and results showed that cells adhered to the surface of scaffolds after co-incubation proving its potential in wound healing and the tissue engineering era due to its high compatibility (Zulkifli et al., 2017).

Chen et al. developed silver-loaded poly(vinyl alcohol), sodium alginate, and carboxymethyl chitosan hydrogel wound dressings. The formulated wound dressing showed antibacterial activity. The developed antibacterial hydrogel was characterized by different wound healing and antibacterial activity properties. The results of the study showed that sodium alginate could reduce to silver nanoparticles, which were small and monodispersed, fulfilling the criteria of an ideal antibacterial material. The silver nanoparticles were uniformly dispersed into the hydrogel with excellent water retention and water absorption capacity. The silver nanoparticle loaded hydrogel showed suitable mechanical properties, antibacterial activities, and biocompatibility. Thus silver nanoparticles loaded in hydrogels are considered a suitable material for wound dressings (Chen et al., 2020).

Shao et al. studied the antibacterial activity of silver nanoparticles charged into chitosan-based membranes. The three chitosan-based membranes were prepared using different concentrations of silver nanoparticles. In vitro silver release and antibacterial properties were studied using a phosphate buffer solution and serum. The antibacterial activity and wound healing efficacy were studied in vivo. The results showed that a higher concentration of silver nanoparticles was required to attain in vivo antibacterial activity. Hence, we conclude that silver nanoparticle loaded chitosan-based membranes can increase the antibacterial activity of biomaterials without changing the wound healing property of the chitosan-based membranes (Shao et al., 2019).

Gold nanoparticles

Gold nanoparticles act as useful drug delivery systems for antimicrobial compounds to enhance wound healing suffering from infections due to its nanosize and large surface area. The large surface area offers more contact area with bacteria resulting in a breakdown of the bacterial membrane and enhanced permeability and respiratory functions (Comune et al., 2017; Chen et al., 2015).

Zepon et al. prepared gold nanoparticles of locust bean gum, κ-carrageenan, land poly(vinyl alcohol), and loaded them into a polymer-based wafer. The wafer-loaded gold nanoparticles were characterized by physicochemical, morphological, mechanical, and swelling properties. Furthermore, antibacterial and in vitro cytotoxicity activities of gold nanoparticles were also studied. Scanning electron microscopy established the wafers' porous structure which was influenced by surface area, mechanical properties, and swelling. These properties were influenced due to the initial amount of silver and the composition of the wafer. Finally, it was concluded that wafers loaded with gold nanoparticles were safe for fibroblast cells acting as a bacterial barrier. Hence, wafer-based gold nanoparticles served as potential materials for wound dressings (Zepon et al., 2020).

Mahmoud et al. formulated various patterns [rod and spheres] and polymer surface-modified (cationic, anionic, and neutral) gold nanoparticles. The formulated nanoparticles were evaluated for different parameters and were finally loaded into the temperature-responsive gel of poloxamer 407. Silver nanoparticle-based hydrogels showed good stability with a slow and sustained release pattern for 48 h using an in vitro study. PEG hydrogel-based gold nanorods (AuNRs) and positively charged poly(allylamine hydrochloride) (PAH) silver nanorods showed outstanding wound healing characteristics in an animal model using topical administration. PEGylated and positively charged silver nanorods-based hydrogels demonstrated increased skin re-epithelization and the impeachment of collagen in the wound post 14 days of treatment compared with the control group. PEG-silver nanorods and PAH-silver nanorods illustrated good in vitro antibacterial potential against *S. aureus* and *P. aeruginosa*. Hence, silver nanorod-based hydrogels served as a potential strategy for wound healing (Mahmoud et al., 2019).

Zinc oxide nanoparticles

Nanoparticles loaded with zinc oxide acting as a suitable antibacterial compound by promoting perforations on the bacterial cell membrane. In addition, zinc oxide nanoparticles loaded in hydrogel-based wound dressings (Hamdan et al., 2017), resulted in increased contact time, advancing keratinocyte migration, and finally enhancing re-epithelization. However, a recent study on microporous zinc oxide nanoparticle based chitosan hydrogel dressings showed their high ability to absorb wound exudates and result in the production of hemostatic blood clots. It also showed antibacterial activity with minimal cytotoxic effects (Shou et al., 2020; Xia et al., 2020).

Kaushik et al. formulated zinc oxide nanoparticles using a wet chemical process. Nanoparticles were defined by XRD, FTIR, and TEM for their structure distribution and particle size. The impact of nanoparticle size on the growth of fibroblast cells (NH3T3) and antimicrobial activity was studied. The growth of fibroblast cells was proportional to zinc oxide nanoparticle size. Calcein-AM fluorescence staining, MTT assay, and F-acting assay demonstrated the development of fibroblast cells with increased biocompatibility. Finally, confocal microscopy and zone of inhibition studies proved the microbial resistance property of zinc oxide nanoparticles (Kaushik et al., 2019).

Arshad et al. developed a thiolated chitosan-alginate bandage loaded with zinc oxide nanoparticles for the cure of surgical site infections. The nanoparticle loaded bandage was characterized by porosity, swelling volume, enzyme degradation (lysozyme), and showed proper wound healing and biodegradation potential. An in vivo study proved it enhanced wound healing and the tissue production activity of developed zinc oxide nanoparticles compared with positive and negative controls. Finally, it was concluded that a thiolated bandage showed an excellent capability to treat surgical site infection, fulfilling the criteria of standard surgical dressings (Arshad et al., 2019).

5.3.1.2 Polymeric nanoparticles

Polymeric nanoparticles are considered a prominent system for drug delivery due to their biocompatibility, biodegradability, injectability, and intracellular potential of delivery. The different physicochemical characteristics of polymer-based nanocarriers can be modified at a molecular stage to increase its drug encapsulation and to modulate its drug release (Chereddy et al., 2014).

Shende et al. prepared and characterized curcumin nanoparticles prepared with the help of polymers (natural, semisynthetic, and synthetic origin) and compared their wound healing activity. Curcumin-based chitosan (natural) and carboxymethyl cellulose (semisynthetic) and PLGA (synthetic) nanoparticles were all prepared using an ionotropic and emulsion solvent evaporation method. In an in vivo wound healing study of chitosan loaded with curcumin, nanoparticles were considered as the promising treatment for wound healing because of its low cost and higher wound healing capability by synergistic action. Finally, the stable noninvasive formulation was developed for wound healing and can be modified into the other drug delivery systems as per requirements (Shende and Gupta, 2020).

5.3.1.3 Lipid-based nanocarrier system

Solid lipid nanoparticles

Solid lipid nanoparticles show a steady drug release because of their condensed structure and ordered molecular confirmation. The drug is encapsulated into a lipid core because of strong interactions (hydrophobic) between the drug and the lipid (Kim et al., 2019).

Arantes et al. developed solid lipid nanoparticles based on retinoic acid (trans) bound with chitosan for healing of diabetic wounds. The prepared solid lipid nanoparticles of all-trans-retinoic acid showed suitable particle sizes (83 ± 6 nm), polydispersity indexes 0.240 ± 0.02, and entrapment efficiencies (98%). A transmission electron microscopy study showed a homogeneous and spherical size structure of the nanoparticles. In addition, an in vivo study showed healing of the wound in diabetic mice treated with retinoic acid-based solid lipid nanoparticles coated with chitosan films compared to a control (chitosan film) without retinoic acid-based solid lipid nanoparticles. All retinoic acid-based solid lipid nanoparticles resulted in decreased leukocyte infiltrates in the wound bed, increased deposition of collagen, and reduced scar tissue. Hence, retinoic acid-based solid lipid nanoparticle-coated chitosan films are a potential treatment for diabetic wound healing (Arantes et al., 2020).

Nanostructured lipid carrier

Nanostructured lipid carriers are next-generation lipid nanoparticles after solid lipid nanoparticles (Naseri et al., 2015). Nanostructured lipid carriers provide higher drug loading by minimizing drug leakage compared with solid lipid nanoparticles because of the existence of an additional component (oil) in its solid lipid structure (Buss et al., 2018).

Ghodrati et al. studied the in vitro antibacterial and acceleratory impact on infected wounds of nanostructured lipid carriers encapsulated with peppermint oil. The prepared nanostructured lipid carrier was characterized for particle diameter, polydispersity index, charge, scanning electron microscopy as well as an in vitro and in vivo wound healing study. During an in vitro study, the antibacterial activity of peppermint oil and peppermint oil loaded nanostructured lipid carriers were studied against *P. aeruginosa, E. coli, S. aureus, Salmonella typhimurium, S. epidermidis, B. anthracis, S. pneumonia*, and *Listeria monocytogenes*. An in vivo study was performed in mice inoculated with *P. aeruginosa* and *S. aureus* by inducing two wounds (5 mm in size). Various parameters were studied, such as wound contraction, histopathological examinations, bacterial count, and molecular analysis. In vivo results revealed that wound deflation rate, collagen deposition, fibroblast intrusion, and re-epithelization were enhanced with mice treated with peppermint oil and peppermint oil loaded nanostructured lipid carriers. Also, results showed a positive impact on FGF-2 and ECF mRNA level expressions. Finally, peppermint oil loaded nanostructured lipid carriers can serve as a useful approach to treat infected wounds by converting them in suitable topical formulations (Ghodrati et al., 2019).

Khezri et al. evaluated the antibacterial and wound healing activity of a *Mentha pulegium* oil loaded nanostructured lipid carrier. The in vitro and in vivo antibacterial property of a nanostructured lipid carrier loaded with *M. pulegium* oil was studied in BALB/c mice. To determine the activity of the nanostructured lipid carrier loaded *M. pulegium* oil on wound healing, bacterial tissue wound contraction, bacterial tissue count, as well as molecular, and histological properties were determined at 3, 7, and 14 days after wound induction. A nanostructured lipid carrier loaded *M. pulegium* oil demonstrated antibacterial properties against *S. epidermidis, S. aureus, L. monocytogenes* and *S. aureus* (gram-positive bacteria) and *P. aeruginosa, E. coli* (gram-negative bacteria) ($P < .01$). A nanostructured lipid carrier loaded *M. pulegium* oil-based gel after being applied topically showed a declining anti-inflammatory activity and an enhancement of the proliferative phase. In addition to this, it also showed enhanced expression of markers such as TGF-β, IL-10, b-FGF, and reduced levels of NF-κB compared with the control group ($P < .05$). Thus the nanostructured lipid carrier loaded *M. pulegium* oil acted as a promising compound for treating an infectious wound (Khezri et al., 2020).

Further, Natarajan et al. formulated pioglitazone loaded nanostructured lipid carrier loaded collagen/chitosan composite scaffolds for diabetic wound healing. The cross-linked scaffold showed low matrix breakdown, optimal porosity, and a controlled release drug profile than a non-crossing-linked scaffold. An in vitro study showed biocompatibility and increased cell growth of a pioglitazone loaded nanostructured lipid carrier-based collagen/chitosan scaffold than a control and nanostructured lipid carrier loaded collagen/chitosan scaffold. The wound healing activity was studied using a streptozotocin-induced diabetic model and showed a higher wound contraction rate for a pioglitazone-loaded nanostructured lipid carrier-based collagen/chitosan scaffold compared with a control, and a nanostructured lipid carrier loaded collagen/chitosan scaffold ($P < .001$). Similarly, the developed formulation indicated a reduction of matrix metalloproteinase 9 levels than the control and nanostructured lipid carrier loaded collagen/chitosan scaffold. Thus the pioglitazone nanostructured lipid carrier-based collagen/chitosan scaffold confirmed its potential to treat diabetic wounds (Natarajan et al., 2019).

Liposomes

Liposomes are lipid bilayer vesicles consisting of phospholipid molecules and are considered as potential drug delivery systems for nanocarriers via a topical route of administration (Chen et al., 2013). Liposomes are suitable nanocarriers for wound healing due to their biodegradability, biocompatibility, safety, and proficiency for encapsulating both hydrophilic (in the aqueous cavity), and lipophilic (in lipid bilayer) drugs (Mitragotri et al., 2014; Değim et al., 2011).

Kumar et al. studied collagen binding to the encapsulation of peptide-tethered vancomycin liposomes in collagen-based scaffolds to treat wound infections. The formulated liposomes were incorporated into a collagen-based hydrogel for treating methicillin-resistant *S. aureus* (MRSA) infections in vitro and in vivo. Collagen mimetic peptide vancomycin nanostructured liposomes bound to a gel to facilitate vancomycin sustained release and increased in vitro antibacterial activity over MRSA than vancomycin-loaded gels or vancomycin liposome loaded gels following bacterial inoculations for 48 h. After that, in vivo studies were conducted in MRSA-infected wounds, and results showed the effectiveness of a developed collagen mimetic peptide vancomycin liposome-based gel up to 9 days than a vancomycin-loaded gel or vancomycin liposome loaded gel (limited to < 2 days). Thus the developed liposome-based gel can be a suitable topical formulation for the prevention of MSRA wound infections (Thapa et al., 2020).

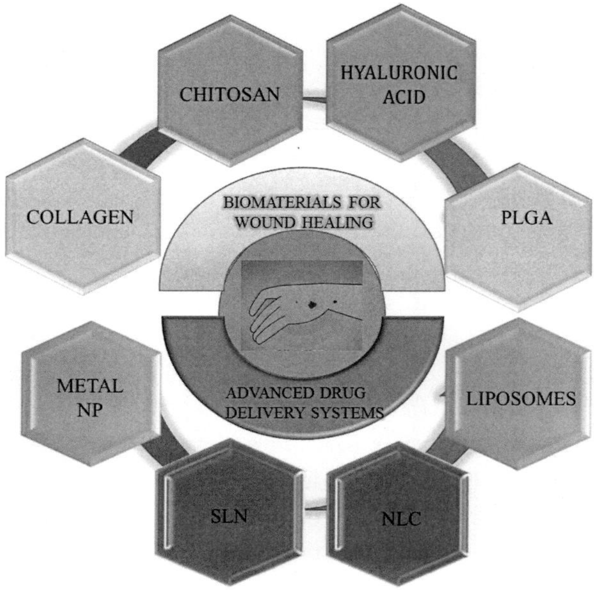

Fig. 5.3 Schematic overview of biomaterials and advanced drug delivery systems for wound healing.

Ferreira et al. developed functionalized nonoven gauze containing piroxicam (an antiinflammatory) loaded liposomes. The mechanism of piroxicam (NSAID antiinflammatory) involves suppression of a constant inflammatory response resulting in improved wound healing. The results proved that the maximum concentration of piroxicam release is attained when gauzes were charged (cationic) with poly(diallyl dimethyl ammonium chloride) (PDDA) with a high level of phospholipid (~ 3000 μM). Finally, the prepared multilamellar vehicles were considered as a suitable carrier due to their biocompatibility and no toxicity to human skin fibroblasts. Hence, functionalized gauzes are regarded as a promising tool to treat chronic wounds (Ferreira et al., 2013).

The schematic overview of biomaterials and advanced drug delivery systems for wound healing is represented in Fig. 5.3.

5.4 Conclusion and future perspectives in wound healing

Compromising various stages like maturation, proliferation, Matrix remodeling and scar formation, inflammation, wound healing is one of the complicated biological cascades involving various biological factors, cells, and processes. Complexity of wounds depends on extent of infection, immunocompromised conditions and various diseased conditions like diabetes. Owing to these complexities in addressing management of wound healing, researchers are focusing on novel biomaterials from natural sources like collagen, hyaluronic acid, alginate, chitosan as well as biomaterials from synthetic origin like polycaprolactone, PLGA. With biomaterials, various nanocarriers like inorganic nanoparticles, organic nanoparticles, lipidic, and polymeric nanoparticles are explored for advance drug delivery wound healing. This review highlights the potential of earlier mentioned advances in wound care and management.

Further advances in wound healing therapy involve the production of split or full-thickness skin alternatives to mimic the natural functioning of the skin. These engineered skin alternatives have managed well, currently using different engineering technologies. Hence, current practices involve the use of different skin substitutes as an auxiliary and advancement of the quality of life. The researchers are exploring various advances and ingenious techniques for wound healing and skin regeneration. The recent smart technologies include portable bioprinters, electro sprayers, in situ 3D printing, and in situ hydrogels. In addition, several cellular therapies such as treatment of stromal vascular fraction, micro RNA (miRNA), immunomodulation, and small interfering RNA (siRNA) charged skin therapies are also effective wound healing techniques (Chouhan et al., 2019). These kinds of novel research will contribute more specificity, patient compliance, better preventive measures in critical wound infections like burns and cost effectiveness in wound care management.

Conflicts of interest

All authors declare no conflicts of interest.

References

Abbaszadeh, A., Tehmasebi-Foolad, A., Rajabzadeh, A., Beigi-Brojeni, N., Zarei, L., 2019. Effects of chitosan/nano selenium biofilm on infected wound healing in rats; an experimental study. Bull. Emerg. Trauma 7 (3), 284–291.

Ahmed, A., Niazi, M.B.K., Jahan, Z., Ahmad, T., Hussain, A., Pervaiz, E., Janjua, H.A., Hussain, Z., 2020. In-vitro and in-vivo study of superabsorbent PVA/starch/g-C3N4/Ag@TiO_2 NPs hydrogel membranes for wound dressing. Eur. Polym. J. 130, 1–14.

Arantes, V.T., Faraco, A.A., Ferreira, F.B., Oliveira, C.A., Martins-Santos, E., Cassini-Vieira, P., Barcelos, L.S., Ferreira, L.A., Goulart, G.A., 2020. Retinoic acid-loaded solid lipid nanoparticles surrounded by chitosan film support diabetic wound healing in in vivo study. Colloids Surf. B: Biointerfaces 188, 1–9.

Arshad, R., Sohail, M.F., Sarwar, H.S., Saeed, H., Ali, I., Akhtar, S., Hussain, S.Z., Afzal, I., Jahan, S., Shahnaz, G., 2019. ZnO-NPs embedded biodegradable thiolated bandage for post-operative surgical site infection; in vitro and in vivo evaluation. PLoS One 14 (6), 1–18.

Bakhsheshi-Rad, H.R., Ismail, A.F., Aziz, M., Akbari, M., Hadisi, Z., Daroonparvar, M., Chen, X.B., 2019. Antibacterial activity and in vivo wound healing evaluation of polycaprolactone-gelatin methacryloyl-cephalexin electrospun nanofibrous. ACS Mater. Lett. 256, 1–4.

Bakhsheshi-Rad, H.R., Hadisi, Z., Ismail, A.F., Aziz, M., Akbari, M., Berto, F., Chen, X.B., 2020. In vitro and in vivo evaluation of chitosan-alginate/gentamicin wound dressing nanofibrous with high antibacterial performance. Polym. Test. 82, 1–28.

Barna, M., Kucera, A., Hladícova, M., Kucera, M., 2007. Der wundheilende Effekt einer Symphytum-Herba-Extrakt-Creme (Symphytum× uplandicum Nyman); Ergebnisse einer randomisierten, kontrollierten Doppelblindstudie. Wien. Med. Wochenschr. 157 (21 – 22), 569–574.

Buss, N., Ryan, P., Baughman, T., Roy, D., Patterson, C., Gordon, C., Dixit, R., 2018. Nonclinical safety and pharmacokinetics of Miglyol 812; a medium chain triglyceride in exenatide once weekly suspension. J. Appl. Toxicol. 38 (10), 1293–1301.

Canpolat, I., Alper, B., 2017. Wound healing and current treatment techniques. J. Agric. Vet. Sci. 1 (3), 180–184.

Carlson, G.A., Dragoo, J.L., Samimi, B., Bruckner, D.A., Bernard, G.W., Hedrick, M., Benhaim, P., 2004. Bacteriostatic properties of biomatrices against common orthopaedic pathogens. Biochem. Biophys. Res. Commun. 321 (2), 472–478.

Chen, J., Cheng, D., Li, J., Wang, Y., Guo, J.X., Chen, Z.P., Cai, B.C., Yang, T., 2013. Influence of lipid composition on the phase transition temperature of liposomes composed of both DPPC and HSPC. Drug Dev. Ind. Pharm. 39 (2), 197–204.

Chen, W.Y., Chang, H.Y., Lu, J.K., Huang, Y.C., Harroun, S.G., Tseng, Y.T., Li, Y.J., Huang, C.C., Chang, H.T., 2015. Self-assembly of antimicrobial peptides on gold nanodots; against multidrug-resistant bacteria and wound-healing application. Adv. Funct. Mater. 25 (46), 7189–7199.

Chen, K., Wang, F., Liu, S., Wu, X., Xu, L., Zhang, D., 2020. In situ reduction of silver nanoparticles by sodium alginate to obtain silver-loaded composite wound dressing with enhanced mechanical and antimicrobial property. Int. J. Biol. Macromol. 148, 501–509.

Chereddy, K.K., Her, C.H., Comune, M., Moia, C., Lopes, A., Porporato, P.E., Vanacker, J., Lam, M.C., Steinstraesser, L., Sonveaux, P., Zhu, H., 2014. PLGA nanoparticles loaded with host defense peptide LL37 promote wound healing. J. Control. Release 194, 138–147.

Chiellini, E., Corti, A., D'Antone, S., Solaro, R., 2003. Biodegradation of poly (vinyl alcohol) based materials. Prog. Polym. Sci. 28 (6), 963–1014.

Cho, K.Y., Chung, T.W., Kim, B.C., Kim, M.K., Lee, J.H., Wee, W.R., Cho, C.S., 2003. Release of ciprofloxacin from poloxamer-graft-hyaluronic acid hydrogels in vitro. Int. J. Pharm. 260 (1), 83–91.

Chouhan, D., Dey, N., Bhardwaj, N., Mandal, B.B., 2019. Emerging and innovative approaches for wound healing and skin regeneration; current status and advances. Biomaterials 216, 119–267.

Comune, M., Rai, A., Chereddy, K.K., Pinto, S., Aday, S., Ferreira, A.F., Zonari, A., Blersch, J., Cunha, R., Rodrigues, R., Lerma, J., 2017. Antimicrobial peptide-gold nanoscale therapeutic formulation with high skin regenerative potential. J. Control. Release 262, 58–71.

Croisier, F., Jérôme, C., 2013. Chitosan-based biomaterials for tissue engineering. Eur. Polym. J. 49 (4), 780–792.

Değim, Z., Çelebi, N., Alemdaroğlu, C., Deveci, M., Öztürk, S., Özoğul, C., 2011. Evaluation of chitosan gel containing liposome-loaded epidermal growth factor on burn wound healing. Int. Wound J. 8 (4), 343–354.

Demidova-Rice, T.N., Hamblin, M.R., Herman, I.M., 2012. Acute and impaired wound healing: pathophysiology and current methods for drug delivery, part 1; normal and chronic wounds: biology, causes, and approaches to care. Adv. Skin Wound Care 25 (7), 304–314.

Devlin, J.J., Kircher, S., Kozen, B.G., Littlejohn, L.F., Johnson, A.S., 2011. Comparison of ChitoFlex®, CELOX™, and QuikClot® in control of hemorrhage. J. Emerg. Med. 41 (3), 237–245.

Drumright, R.E., Gruber, P.R., Henton, D.E., 2000. Polylactic acid technology. Adv. Mater. 12 (23), 1841–1846.

Dudhani, A.R., Kosaraju, S.L., 2010. Bioadhesive chitosan nanoparticles; preparation and characterization. Carbohydr. Polym. 81 (2), 243–251.

Eglin, D., Mortisen, D., Alini, M., 2009. Degradation of synthetic polymeric scaffolds for bone and cartilage tissue repairs. Soft Matter 5 (5), 938–947.

Ehlers, E.M., Behrens, P., Wünsch, L., Kühnel, W., Russlies, M., 2001. Effects of hyaluronic acid on the morphology and proliferation of human chondrocytes in primary cell culture. Ann. Anat. 183 (1), 13–17.

Enoch, S., Price, P., 2004. Cellular, molecular and biochemical differences in the pathophysiology of healing between acute wounds, chronic wounds and wounds in the aged. World Wide Wounds 13, 1–17.

Fang, Y., Zhu, X., Wang, N., Zhang, X., Yang, D., Nie, J., Ma, G., 2019. Biodegradable core-shell electrospun nanofibers based on PLA and γ-PGA for wound healing. Eur. Polym. J. 116, 30–37.

Ferreira, H., Matamá, T., Silva, R., Silva, C., Gomes, A.C., Cavaco-Paulo, A., 2013. Functionalization of gauzes with liposomes entrapping an anti-inflammatory drug; a strategy to improve wound healing. React. Funct. Polym. 73, 1328–1334.

Fischer, M., Gebhard, F., Hammer, T., Zurek, C., Meurer, G., Marquardt, C., Hoefer, D., 2017. Microbial alginate dressings show improved binding capacity for pathophysiological factors in chronic wounds compared to commercial alginate dressings of marine origin. J. Biomater. Appl. 31 (9), 1267–1276.

Galliard, H. von T., 1987. 151 Seiten, zahlr. Abb. und Tab. John Wiley & Sons, Chichester u. a. 1987. Food / Nahrung 32 (8), 782. https://doi.org/10.1002/food.19880320816.

Garcia-Orue, I., Gainza, G., Garcia-Garcia, P., Gutierrez, F.B., Aguirre, J.J., Hernandez, R.M., Delgado, A., Igartua, M., 2019. Composite nanofibrous membranes of PLGA/Aloe vera containing lipid nanoparticles for wound dressing applications. Int. J. Pharm. 556, 320–329.

George, M., Abraham, T.E., 2006. Polyionic hydrocolloids for the intestinal delivery of protein drugs; alginate and chitosan—a review. J. Control. Release 114 (1), 1–14.

Ghodrati, M., Farahpour, M.R., Hamishehkar, H., 2019. Encapsulation of peppermint essential oil in nanostructured lipid carriers; in-vitro antibacterial activity and accelerative effect on infected wound healing. Colloids. Surf. A Physicochem. Eng. Asp. 564, 161–169.

Ghosh, K., Clark, R.A.F., 2007. Wound repair. In: Principles of Tissue Engineering. Elsevier, pp. 1149–1166, https://doi.org/10.1016/B978-012370615-7/50080-9.

Gunatillake, P.A., Adhikari, R., 2003. Biodegradable synthetic polymers for tissue engineering. Eur. Cell. Mater. 5 (1), 1–16.

Hajji, S., Khedir, S.B., Hamza-Mnif, I., Hamdi, M., Jedidi, I., Kallel, R., Boufi, S., Nasri, M., 2019. Biomedical potential of chitosan-silver nanoparticles with special reference to antioxidant, antibacterial, hemolytic and in vivo cutaneous wound healing effects. Biochim. Biophys. Acta Gen. Subj. 1863 (1), 241–254.

Halbleib, M., Skurk, T., de Luca, C., von Heimburg, D., Hauner, H., 2003. Tissue engineering of white adipose tissue using hyaluronic acid-based scaffolds. I; in vitro differentiation of human adipocyte precursor cells on scaffolds. Biomaterials 24 (18), 3125–3132.

Hamdan, S., Pastar, I., Drakulich, S., Dikici, E., Tomic-Canic, M., Deo, S., Daunert, S., 2017. Nanotechnology-driven therapeutic interventions in wound healing; potential uses and applications. ACS Cent. Sci. 3 (3), 163–175.

Hivechi, A., Bahrami, S.H., Siegel, R.A., Milan, P.B., Amoupour, M., 2020. In vitro and in vivo studies of biaxially electrospun poly (caprolactone)/gelatin nanofibers, reinforced with cellulose nanocrystals, for wound healing applications. Cellulose 1–18.

Homaeigohar, S., Boccaccini, A.R., 2020. Antibacterial biohybrid nanofibers for wound dressings. Acta Biomater. 107, 25–49.

Horakova, J., Mikes, P., Saman, A., Svarcova, T., Jencova, V., Suchy, T., Heczkova, B., Jakubkova, S., Jirousova, J., Prochazkova, R., 2018. Comprehensive assessment of electrospun scaffolds hemocompatibility. Mater. Sci. Eng. C 82, 330–335.

Hu, L., Sun, Y., Wu, Y., 2013. Advances in chitosan-based drug delivery vehicles. Nanoscale 5 (8), 3103–3111.

Jeschke, M.G., van Baar, M.E., Choudhry, M.A., Chung, K.K., Gibran, N.S., Logsetty, S., 2020. Burn injury. Nat. Rev. Dis. Primers 6 (1), 1–25.

Kaushik, M., Niranjan, R., Thangam, R., Madhan, B., Pandiyarasan, V., Ramachandran, C., Oh, D.H., Venkatasubbu, G.D., 2019. Investigations on the antimicrobial activity and wound healing potential of ZnO nanoparticles. Appl. Surf. Sci. 479, 1169–1177.

Khezri, K., Farahpour, M.R., Rad, S.M., 2020. Efficacy of *Mentha pulegium* essential oil encapsulated into nanostructured lipid carriers as an in vitro antibacterial and infected wound healing agent. Colloids Surf. A Physicochem. Eng. Asp. 589, 124414.

Kim, I.Y., Seo, S.J., Moon, H.S., Yoo, M.K., Park, I.Y., Kim, B.C., Cho, C.S., 2008. Chitosan and its derivatives for tissue engineering applications. Biotechnol. Adv. 26 (1), 1–21.

Kim, H.S., Sun, X., Lee, J.H., Kim, H.W., Fu, X., Leong, K.W., 2019. Advanced drug delivery systems and artificial skin grafts for skin wound healing. Adv. Drug Deliv. Rev. 146, 209–239.

Krausz, A.E., Adler, B.L., Cabral, V., Navati, M., Doerner, J., Charafeddine, R.A., Chandra, D., Liang, H., Gunther, L., Clendaniel, A., Harper, S., 2015. Curcumin-encapsulated nanoparticles as innovative antimicrobial and wound healing agent. Nanomedicine 11 (1), 195–206.

Kundu, B., Rajkhowa, R., Kundu, S.C., Wang, X., 2013. Silk fibroin biomaterials for tissue regenerations. Adv. Drug Deliv. Rev. 65 (4), 457–470.

Lee, J.E., Park, J.C., Kim, J.G., Suh, H., 2001. Preparation of collagen modified hyaluronan microparticles as antibiotics carrier. Yonsei Med. J. 42 (3), 291–298.

Lee, Y.S., Kang, S.U., Lee, M.H., Kim, H.J., Han, C.H., Won, H.R., Park, Y.U., Kim, C.H., 2019. GnRH impairs diabetic wound healing through enhanced NETosis. Cell. Mol. Immunol. 17 (8), 856–864.

Li, X., Chen, S., Zhang, B., Li, M., Diao, K., Zhang, Z., Li, J., Xu, Y., Wang, X., Chen, H., 2012. In situ injectable nano-composite hydrogel composed of curcumin, N, O-carboxymethyl chitosan and oxidized alginate for wound healing application. Int. J. Pharm. 437 (1–2), 110–119.

Liu, Y., Shu, X.Z., Prestwich, G.D., 2005. Biocompatibility and stability of disulfide-crosslinked hyaluronan films. Biomaterials 26 (23), 4737–4746.

Losi, P., Briganti, E., Magera, A., Spiller, D., Ristori, C., Battolla, B., Balderi, M., Kull, S., Balbarini, A., Di Stefano, R., Soldani, G., 2010. Tissue response to poly (ether) urethane-polydimethylsiloxane-fibrin composite scaffolds for controlled delivery of pro-angiogenic growth factors. Biomaterials 31 (20), 5336–5344.

Mahmoud, A.A., Salama, A.H., 2016. Norfloxacin-loaded collagen/chitosan scaffolds for skin reconstruction; preparation, evaluation and in-vivo wound healing assessment. Eur. J. Pharm. Sci. 83, 155–165.

Mahmoud, N.N., Hikmat, S., Ghith, D.A., Hajeer, M., Hamadneh, L., Qattan, D., Khalil, E.A., 2019. Gold nanoparticles loaded into polymeric hydrogel for wound healing in rats; effect of nanoparticles shape and surface modification. Int. J. Pharm. 565, 174–186.

Majeed, Z., Ramli, N.K., Binti Mansor, N., Man, Z., 2014. Lignin loading effect on biodegradability and nitrogen release properties of urea modified tapioca starch in wet soil. Key Eng. Mater. 594-595, 798–802.

Masood, N., Ahmed, R., Tariq, M., Ahmed, Z., Masoud, M.S., Ali, I., Asghar, R., Andleeb, A., Hasan, A., 2019. Silver nanoparticle impregnated chitosan-PEG hydrogel enhances wound healing in diabetes induced rabbits. Int. J. Pharm. 559, 23–36.

Milella, E., Brescia, E., Massaro, C., Ramires, P.A., Miglietta, M.R., Fiori, V., Aversa, P., 2002. Physico-chemical properties and degradability of non-woven hyaluronan benzylic esters as tissue engineering scaffolds. Biomaterials 23 (4), 1053–1063.

Mitragotri, S., Burke, P.A., Langer, R., 2014. Overcoming the challenges in administering biopharmaceuticals: formulation and delivery strategies. Nat. Rev. Drug Discov. 13, 655–672.

Movahedi, M., Asefnejad, A., Rafienia, M., Khorasani, M.T., 2020. Potential of novel electrospun core-shell structured polyurethane/starch (hyaluronic acid) nanofibers for skin tissue engineering; in vitro and in vivo evaluation. Int. J. Biol. Macromol. 146, 627–637.

Mulinti, P., Brooks, J., Lervick, B., Pullan, J., Brooks, A., 2018. Strategies to improve the hemocompatibility of biodegradable biomaterials. In: Hemocompatibility of Biomaterials for Clinical Applications. Woodhead Publishing, pp. 53–278.

Naeem, M., Tetlow, I.J., Emes, M.J., 1997. Starch synthesis in amyloplasts purified from developing potato tubers. Plant J. 11 (5), 1095–1103.

Naseri, N., Valizadeh, H., Zakeri-Milani, P., 2015. Solid lipid nanoparticles and nanostructured lipid carriers; structure, preparation and application. Adv. Pharm. Bull. 5 (3), 305–313.

Natarajan, J., Sanapalli, B.K.R., Bano, M., Singh, S.K., Gulati, M., Karri, V.V.S.R., 2019. Nanostructured lipid carriers of pioglitazone loaded collagen/chitosan composite scaffold for diabetic wound healing. Adv. Wound Care 8 (10), 499–513.

Nguyen, T.D., Nguyen, T.T., Ly, K.L., Tran, A.H., Nguyen, T.T.N., Vo, M.T., Ho, H.M., Dang, N.T.N., Vo, V.T., Nguyen, D.H., Nguyen, T.T.H., 2019. In vivo study of the antibacterial chitosan/polyvinyl alcohol loaded with silver nanoparticle hydrogel for wound healing applications. Int. J. Polym. Sci. 1-10.

Padalhin, A.R., Thuy Ba Linh, N., Ki Min, Y., Lee, B.T., 2014. Evaluation of the cytocompatibility hemocompatibility in vivo bone tissue regenerating capability of different PCL blends. J. Biomater. Sci. Polym. Ed. 25 (5), 487–503.

Park, S.H., Park, S.R., Chung, S.I., Pai, K.S., Min, B.H., 2005. Tissue-engineered cartilage using fibrin/hyaluronan composite gel and it's in vivo implantation. Artif. Organs 29 (10), 838–845.

Poonguzhali, R., Basha, S.K., Kumari, V.S., 2018. Fabrication of asymmetric nanostarch reinforced chitosan/PVP membrane and its evaluation as an antibacterial patch for in vivo wound healing application. Int. J. Biol. Macromol. 114, 204–213.

Pozza, M., Millner, R.W., 2011. Celox (chitosan) for haemostasis in massive traumatic bleeding; experience in Afghanistan. Eur. J. Emerg. Med. 18 (1), 31–33.

Reis, R.L., Cunha, A.M., 2001. Starch and starch-based thermoplastics. In: Jurgen, K.H., Buschow, R., Cahn, W., Flemings, M.C., Ilschner, B., Kramer, E.J., Mahajan, S. (Eds.), Encyclopedia of Materials Science and Technology (11 Volumes). Volume on Biological and Biomimetic Materials, vol. 11. Pergamon-Elsevier Science, Amsterdam, pp. 8810–8816.

Rodriguez, M.J., Brown, J., Giordano, J., Lin, S.J., Omenetto, F.G., Kaplan, D.L., 2017. Silk based bioinks for soft tissue reconstruction using 3-dimensional (3D) printing with in vitro and in vivo assessments. Biomaterials 117, 105–115.

Saghazadeh, S., Rinoldi, C., Schot, M., Kashaf, S.S., Sharifi, F., Jalilian, E., Nuutila, K., Giatsidis, G., Mostafalu, P., Derakhshandeh, H., Yue, K., 2018. Drug delivery systems and materials for wound healing applications. Adv. Drug Deliv. Rev. 127, 138–166.

Samavedi, S., Poindexter, L.K., Van Dyke, M., Goldstein, A.S., 2014. Synthetic biomaterials for regenerative medicine applications. In: Regenerative Medicine Applications in Organ Transplantation. Elsevier, pp. 81–99.
Sandhiya, S., Dkhar, S.A., Surendiran, A., 2009. Emerging trends of nanomedicine–an overview. Fundam. Clin. Pharmacol. 23 (3), 263–269.
Sarhan, W.A., Azzazy, H.M., El-Sherbiny, I.M., 2016. Honey/chitosan nanofiber wound dressing enriched with *Allium sativum* and *Cleome droserifolia*; enhanced antimicrobial and wound healing activity. ACS Appl. Mater. Interfaces 8 (10), 6379–6390.
Sarker, B., Singh, R., Silva, R., Roether, J.A., Kaschta, J., Detsch, R., Schubert, D.W., Cicha, I., Boccaccini, A.R., 2014. Evaluation of fibroblasts adhesion and proliferation on alginate-gelatin crosslinked hydrogel. PLoS One 9 (9), 107952.
Semenova, M.V., Osadchenko, S.V., Mezhuev, Y.O., Shtil'man, M.I., Semenova, I.N., 2016. Synthesis of hemocompatible materials based on branched polyvinyl alcohol. Russ. J. Appl. Chem. 89 (8), 1286–1291.
Shao, J., Wang, B., Li, J., Jansen, J.A., Walboomers, X.F., Yang, F., 2019. Antibacterial effect and wound healing ability of silver nanoparticles incorporation into chitosan-based nanofibrous membranes. Mater. Sci. Eng. C 98, 1053–1063.
Shefa, A.A., Amirian, J., Kang, H.J., Bae, S.H., Jung, H.I., Choi, H.J., Lee, S.Y., Lee, B.T., 2017. In vitro and in vivo evaluation of effectiveness of a novel TEMPO-oxidized cellulose nanofiber-silk fibroin scaffold in wound healing. Carbohydr. Polym. 177, 284–296.
Shende, P., Gupta, H., 2020. Formulation and comparative characterization of nanoparticles of curcumin using natural, synthetic and semi-synthetic polymers for wound healing. Life Sci. 253, 117588.
Shou, Y., Zhang, J., Yan, S., Xia, P., Xu, P., Li, G., Zhang, K., Yin, J., 2020. Thermoresponsive chitosan/DOPA-based hydrogel as an injectable therapy approach for tissue-adhesion and hemostasis. ACS Biomater. Sci. Eng. 6 (6), 3619–3629.
Shu, X.Z., Liu, Y., Palumbo, F., Prestwich, G.D., 2003. Disulfide-crosslinked hyaluronan-gelatin hydrogel films: a covalent mimic of the extracellular matrix for in vitro cell growth. Biomaterials 24 (21), 3825–3834.
Shu, X.Z., Liu, Y., Palumbo, F.S., Luo, Y., Prestwich, G.D., 2004. In situ crosslinkable hyaluronan hydrogels for tissue engineering. Biomaterials 25 (7–8), 1339–1348.
Solchaga, L.A., Temenoff, J.S., Gao, J., Mikos, A.G., Caplan, A.I., Goldberg, V.M., 2005. Repair of osteochondral defects with hyaluronan-and polyester-based scaffolds. Osteoarthr. Cartil. 13 (4), 297–309.
Sonker, A.K., Teotia, A.K., Kumar, A., Nagarale, R.K., Verma, V., 2017. Development of polyvinyl alcohol based high strength biocompatible composite films. Macromol. Chem. Phys. 218 (15), 1700130.
Tan, H., Chu, C.R., Payne, K.A., Marra, K.G., 2009. Injectable in situ forming biodegradable chitosan–hyaluronic acid-based hydrogels for cartilage tissue engineering. Biomaterials 30 (13), 2499–2506.
Thapa, R.K., Kiick, K.L., Sullivan, M.O., 2020. Encapsulation of collagen mimetic peptide-tethered vancomycin liposomes in collagen-based scaffolds for infection control in wounds. Acta Biomater. 103, 115–128.
Tian, J., Wong, K.K., Ho, C.M., Lok, C.N., Yu, W.Y., Che, C.M., Chiu, J.F., Tam, P.K., 2007. Topical delivery of silver nanoparticles promotes wound healing. ChemMedChem 2 (1), 129–136.
VandeVord, P.J., Matthew, H.W., DeSilva, S.P., Mayton, L., Wu, B., Wooley, P.H., 2002. Evaluation of the biocompatibility of a chitosan scaffold in mice. J. Biomed. Mater. Res. 59 (3), 585–590.
Wang, W., Lu, K.J., Yu, C.H., Huang, Q.L., Du, Y.Z., 2019. Nano-drug delivery systems in wound treatment and skin regeneration. J. Nanobiotechnol. 17 (1), 1–15.

Wang, C.H., Hsieh, D.J., Periasamy, S., Chuang, C.T., Tseng, F.W., Kuo, J.C., Tarng, Y.W., 2020. Regenerative porcine dermal collagen matrix developed by supercritical carbon dioxide extraction technology; role in accelerated wound healing. Materialia 9, 100576.
Wentao, W., Tao, Z., Bulei, S., Tongchang, Z., Qicheng, Z., Fan, W., Ninglin, Z., Jian, S., Ming, Z., Yi, S., 2019. Functionalization of polyvinyl alcohol composite film wrapped in am-ZnO@ CuO@ Au nanoparticles for antibacterial application and wound healing. Appl. Mater. Today 17, 36–44.
Whang, H.S., Kirsch, W., Zhu, Y.H., Yang, C.Z., Hudson, S.M., 2005. Hemostatic agents derived from chitin and chitosan. Polym. Rev. (Phila Pa) 45 (4), 309–323.
WHO, 2020a. Burns. WHO. https://www.who.int/news-room/fact-sheets/detail/burns. (Viewed 29 August 2020).
WHO, 2020b. Wound Management. WHO. https://www.who.int/hac/techguidance/tools/guidelines_prevention_and_management_wound_infection.pdf?ua=1#:~:text=to%20water%20quality),1.,away%20damaged%20and%20dead%20tissue. (Viewed 29 August 2020).
Xia, J., Zhang, H., Yu, F., Pei, Y., Luo, X., 2020. Super clear, porous cellulose membranes with chitosan-coated nanofibers for visualized cutaneous wound healing dressing. ACS Appl. Mater. Interfaces 12 (21), 24370–24379.
Zeplin, P.H., Maksimovikj, N.C., Jordan, M.C., Nickel, J., Lang, G., Leimer, A.H., Römer, L., Scheibel, T., 2014. Spider silk coatings as a bioshield to reduce periprosthetic fibrous capsule formation. Adv. Funct. Mater. 24 (18), 2658–2666.
Zepon, K.M., Marques, M.S., Hansen, A.W., Pucci, C.D.A.F., Morisso, F.D.P., Ziulkoski, A.L., do Nascimento, J.H.O., Magnago, R.F., Kanis, L.A., 2020. Polymer-based wafers containing in situ synthesized gold nanoparticles as a potential wound-dressing material. Mater. Sci. Eng. C 109, 110630.
Zhang, Y., Zhang, M., 2001. Microstructural and mechanical characterization of chitosan scaffolds reinforced by calcium phosphates. J. Non-Cryst. Solids 282 (2–3), 159–164.
Zulkifli, F.H., Hussain, F.S.J., Zeyohannes, S.S., Rasad, M.S.B.A., Yusuff, M.M., 2017. A facile synthesis method of hydroxyethyl cellulose-silver nanoparticle scaffolds for skin tissue engineering applications. Mater. Sci. Eng. C 79, 151–160.

CHAPTER 6

Nanobiomaterials for regenerative medicine

Anjali Pandya, Prashant Upadhaya, Shruti Lohakare, Tishya Srivastava, Susmit Mhatre, Sreeranjini Pulakkat, and Vandana B. Patravale
Department of Pharmaceutical Sciences and Technology, Institute of Chemical Technology, Mumbai, Maharashtra, India

6.1 Introduction

With the recent advancements in the biotechnological arena, a multidisciplinary science namely tissue engineering and regenerative medicine (RM) has emerged with enormous potential and has been gaining interest in the medical fraternity. RM is a transformational link between tissue engineering and its clinical applications encompassing innumerable approaches which include the use of biomaterials and de novo produced cells or both to replace the damaged tissues both anatomically and functionally, thereby causing tissue healing and organ restoration (Bajaj et al., 2014). Today, RM is looked on as a potential field to reconcile or replace tissues/organs damaged owing to age, medical condition, trauma, congenital imperfections, etc. It is evident from the current data of preclinical and clinical studies that RM can be a promising alternative for the treatment of chronic and acute medical conditions (Bailey et al., 2014; Jaklenec et al., 2012). Further, RM can also be looked on as a strategy to repair damaged organs owing to cardiovascular diseases, certain types of cancer, topical wounds, trauma wounds, etc. as the success rate in the currently used transplant therapy is minimal mainly because of immunity complications and unavailability of donors (Mendelson and Frenette, 2014; Vacanti et al., 2014). With such promising potentials, the market of RM is continuously growing, and a number of FDA-approved products have made their place in the global market (Table 6.1).

With the progressive and enormous growth in the sector of nanotechnology, a lot of expectations have emerged from the fields of biology and medicine to solve the mysteries concerning the human biological systems

Nanotechnology in Medicine and Biology
https://doi.org/10.1016/B978-0-12-819469-0.00007-1

Table 6.1 Representative list of FDA-approved products in regenerative medicine.

Brand name	Source	Application	Approval date	References
Allocord	Allogeneic	Treatment of unrelated donor hematopoietic cell transplantation	May 2013	(Research, C. for B.E, 2019a)
Carticel	Autologous	Treatment of cartilage defects from acute or repetitive trauma	August 1997	(Mao and Mooney, 2015)
Celution	Autologous	Transfer of autologous adipose stem cells	September 2006	(Mao and Mooney, 2015)
Clevecord	Allogeneic	Treatment of unrelated donor hematopoietic cell transplantation	September 2016	(Research, C. for B.E, 2019b)
HPC, Cord Blood	Allogenic	Treatment of unrelated donor hematopoietic cell transplantation	January 2019	(Research, C. for B.E, 2019c)
Dermagraft	Allogenic	Treatment of diabetic foot ulcer	September 2001	(Mao and Mooney, 2015)
Ducord	Allogeneic	Treatment of unrelated donor hematopoietic cell transplantation	October 2012	(Research, C. for B.E, 2019d)
GEM 125	Allogenic	Treatment of periodontal defects	August 2015	(Mao and Mooney, 2015)
GINTUIT	Allogenic	Treatment of topical mucogingival conditions, leg, and diabetic foot ulcers	March 2012	(Research, C. for B.E, 2019e)

Hemacord	Allogeneic	Treatment of unrelated donor hematopoietic cell transplantation	November 2011	(Research, C. for B.E, 2019f)
Laviv	Autologous	Improves nasolabial fold appearance	June 2011	(Research, C. for B.E, 2019g)
Imlygic	Oncolytic	Local treatment of nodal lesions in melanoma patients	October 2015	(Research, C. for B.E, 2019h)
Infuse	Allogenic	Treatment of tibia fracture and non-union, and lower spine fusion	September 2002	(Mao and Mooney, 2015)
Kymriah (Tisagenlecleucel)	Autologous T-cells	Treatment of acute lymphoblastic leukemia (ALL)	August 2017	(Research, C. for B.E, 2019i)
MACI	Autologous	Treatment of cartilage defects	December 2013	(Research, C. for B.E, 2019j)
Provenge	Autologous	Treatment of prostate cancer	April 2010	(Research, C. for B.E, 2019k)
Regranex	Allogenic	Treatment of lower extremity diabetic ulcers	December 1997	(Mao and Mooney, 2015)
Yescrata (Axicabtageneciloleucel)	Autologous T-cells	Treatment of diffuse large B-cell lymphoma	October 2017	(Research, C. for B.E, 2020)

which are known to function at the nanoscale level. Hence, various approaches at the nanoscale have been used in biomedical applications and are continuously drawing attention. The use of nanobiomaterials in the area of tissue engineering and RM is one such approach that is currently being explored. Given that the sizes of these functional biomaterials lie in the nanorange, they interact efficiently with the biological system and thereby present an excellent outcome in the arena of RM. These nanobiomaterials, apart from being nontoxic, are expected to be physically stable and have the potential to interact with proteins and cells without altering their biological activities (Solanki et al., 2008). The nanomaterials used in RM are generally fabricated by a bottom-up or top-down approach. The bottom-up technique is strongly used for the synthesis of novel materials behaving contrarily in their nanoscale version than bulk materials. These include inorganic and polymeric nanoparticles, quantum dots, dendrimers, nanotubes, self-assembled materials, layer-by-layer structures, etc. The top-down approach includes the amendment at the nanoscale of polymeric and other materials which further generates nanoengineered systems such as nanopatterns with structures influencing cell behavior and ensuing tissue development (Verma et al., 2011). The major use of the aforementioned nanobiomaterials in the field of RM as of now extends to the use of scaffolds for cell growth, delivery devices for drugs, genes and growth factors, cellular tracking, isolation and modification, biosensors, bone void fillers, wound healing, etc. However, the future looks bright and may witness tissue and organ printing, organ regeneration, tissue restoration, etc., with the aid of nanobiomaterials.

Just like nanomaterials, stems cells also play an important part in the field of RM. Stem cells are characterized by their ability to self-reintroduce and propagate along multiple lineage alleyways. These intrinsic properties of stem cells make them a striking candidate for applications in the RM field (Brunt et al., 2012). Human stem cells can broadly be classified into different categories with respect to their origin and differentiating capabilities. The basic types include embryonic stem cells, induced pluripotent stem cells, hematopoietic stem cells, mesenchymal stem cells (MSCs), endothelial progenitor cells, and organ-specific precursors such as cardiac stem cells, neural stem cells, etc. Ideally, the stem cells for an RM purpose are expected to meet certain criteria such as availability in abundance, extraction with a minimal invasive procedure, reproducibility, safe and effective transplantation in allogenic and autologous hosts, the feasibility of manufacturing according to the GMP guidelines, etc. As discussed earlier, an interest in modern techniques in biology has recently increased since isolating living and healthy cells from the body, expanding them, and combining with a biocompatible material to re-transplant in the body has become feasible. Tissue engineering thus demands a prerequisite of the abundance of tissue-specific cells without the morbidity of the donor site. As a result, much attention is currently being given to multipotential progenitor cells, for example, periosteal, embryonic, and MSCs (Brunt et al., 2012; Kolios and Moodley, 2013; Ringe et al., 2002).

6.2 Properties of nanobiomaterials

The properties of nanobiomaterials are significantly different than the parent biomaterials, mainly because of their characteristic nanosize and higher surface area-to-volume ratio (Adaya et al., 2016). Although it is difficult to define a perfect nanobiomaterial, there are some ideal properties that these materials should possess for being better candidates in the context of tissue regeneration. Physical properties play a major role in governing the role and function of nanomaterials (Yang et al., 2019). The size and shape are important parameters that are to be considered in the physical properties. The surface properties of nanomaterials also have to be considered since several cellular functions are directly corelated to the surface morphology (Mitragotri and Lahann, 2009).

6.2.1 Size

The size of nanobioparticles determines their ability to bypass physiological barriers in the body (Schreiber and Witte, 2017). In neural tissue regeneration, these carriers should pass the blood-brain barrier effectively and a particle size less than 100 nm, usually between 15 and 50 nm for metal nanoparticles, like gold nanoparticles (AuNPs), are suggested for this purpose (Gao and Jiang, 2006; Sonavane et al., 2008). A particle size of around 50 nm is targeted for polymeric nanomaterials functioning as immunomodulators. The size range for magnetic nanoparticles varies from 15 nm to as high as 1500 nm, depending on the type of material and the application intended (Markides et al., 2012). For the efficient uptake of nanobioparticles, the recommended particle size is between 5 and 50 nm, since those below 5 nm fail to provide enough area for sufficient binding to the membrane receptors followed by cellular uptake whereas those above 50 nm can bind to the membrane receptors but at a cost of inhibition of the further binding of nanoparticles (Albanese et al., 2012).

6.2.2 Shape

Nanomaterials can be found in a variety of shapes ranging from 0-dimensional nanostructures like metal ions, metal complexes like sulfides and oxides quantum dots and nanocomposites, to three-dimensional (3D) materials like scaffolds, hydrogels, electrospun nanofibers, and microneedle patches. In the context of the regeneration of tissues, usually nanobiomaterials with higher dimensions are preferred (Liu et al., 2019). An ideal nanobiomaterial must possess the ability to encapsulate stem cells (Koutsopoulos, 2012). Shape has a direct impact on the mechanical and biological properties of nanobiomaterials. For example, filomicelles having two dimensions at the nanolevel have a considerably better half-life of circulation than micrometer-sized counterparts (Sahoo et al., 2013). The shape of nanobiomaterials is usually engineered to mimic the shape of the extracellular matrix (ECM) based on the application for improved regeneration and compatibility (Meyer and Green, 2016).

6.2.3 Surface morphology

The surface properties of a biomaterial dictate cell orientation, cell differentiation, and cell adhesion (Engel et al., 2008). The biomaterial needs to have properties that are compatible with the site of application (Koutsopoulos, 2012). Stiff materials with a porous nature need to be used for applications in bone regeneration (Ruhé et al., 2005). For neural regeneration, a soft biomaterial should be used whereas for applications in the spinal cord, the biomaterial should be compatible with white and gray matter (Friedman et al., 2002). The growth of dorsal root ganglion neurons can be enhanced if the surface of the biomaterial has grooves and ridges (Wieringa et al., 2012). Similarly, for skin regeneration, materials with elastic properties should be used (Sieminski et al., 2007).

6.2.4 Chemical properties

The surface area-to-volume ratio is significantly higher for nanoparticles and hence their surface properties are crucial in determining other chemical properties like solubility and catalytic activity and biological properties like adhesion, cell growth, and cell differentiation (Boles et al., 2016; Han et al., 2015). The surface charge needs to be considered in the fabrication of scaffolds using nanobiomaterials. Usually, positively charged materials are subjected to cellular uptake efficiently due to desired electrostatic interactions with negatively charged cellular membranes (Albanese et al., 2012). For this reason, surfaces of nanobiomaterials can be modified to enhance cell adhesion, biocompatibility, and interactions with cells (Jiao and Cui, 2007).

This can be done by physical approaches like adsorption, the Langmuir-Blodgett method, and chemical approaches like pulsed laser deposition, plasma treatment, covalent immobilization, and acid etching (Rana et al., 2016). Nanobiomaterials which are formed by a bottom-up approach, such as self-assembly, demonstrate the formation of ionic and hydrogen bonds as well as other noncovalent interactions (Zhang, 2003). Such materials can form a matrix forming a scaffold for applications in the regeneration of tissue (Zhang et al., 1993). One such application of self-assembling molecules is peptide nanofibers used in myocardial infarction which capture paracrine molecules (Webber et al., 2010). These scaffolds represent the structure of the ECM with high water content and small internal pores, enabling gradual diffusion of growth factors (Zhang, 2003).

6.2.5 Biological properties

The most important property for biomaterial use in RM is biocompatibility. Materials derived from natural sources like collagen, fibrin, alginate laminin, and chitosan are made of nanofibers with less compatibility issues. However, synthetic materials should display nontoxicity and solubility to be biocompatible. Based on the application of the nanobiomaterials, the pathways by which these materials can interact with the immune system should be considered (Adaya et al., 2016).

6.2.6 Electromagnetic properties

Electromagnetic properties are significant for biomaterials including metals like gold, iron, nickel, and carbon-based materials like graphene, carbon nanotubes, etc. Superparamagnetic iron oxide nanoparticles show a peculiar application in tissue regeneration via stem cell tracking and cell surface receptor actuation owing to their ability to not agglomerate due to a lack of mutual attraction (Markides et al., 2012). Another advantage of using biomaterials with magnetic properties is their ability to attach to the cell membrane and activate ion channels in the magnetic field, thereby controlling the cellular processes (Dobson, 2008). In cardiac tissue regeneration, biomaterials with electrical conductivity are critical since they modulate the activity of the stem cells affecting the electrochemical signaling pathway (Severs et al., 2008). Similarly in neural applications, materials like graphene and carbon nanotubes show electrical conductivity that promote interneural signal transmission (Engel et al., 2008). Graphene-like nanomaterials have been shown to promote neural outgrowth and branching by forming conductive scaffolds (John et al., 2015).

6.3 Scaffolds

The field of RM relies extensively on the use of porous scaffolds (generally 3D) to simulate an environment conducive for the regeneration of tissues and organs in vitro or in vivo. The scaffolds serve as templates onto which tissue formation is conducted by seeding cells along with all the necessary growth factors or with the help of bioreactors for providing biophysical stimuli or via mechanical or chemical induction of cell growth and support (O'Brien, 2011). In addition, they enable enhanced oxygen transport to seeded cells and can also facilitate the delivery of relevant therapeutic agents to aid in the tissue formation and/or regeneration of compromised tissue functions. In in vitro procedures, cells are cultured in the scaffolds, allowed to grow to the desired stage, and then implanted into the injured site. On the other hand, the in vivo procedure involves direct implantation of the scaffolds at the site of injury, thereby enabling the regeneration of tissues or organs by utilizing nutrition from the host environment. Cell-laden scaffolds are most widely used and typically involve 3D porous structures as well as hydrogel-based scaffolds which allow for the growth of cells and mimic the natural ECM of the tissues or organs. The design of these 3D structures has to be such that they effectively fulfill the purpose of ECM development in vitro, after which they degrade in a predetermined manner via resorption or metabolism, once implanted. The criticality of this process makes it imperative to deeply study and understand the nanobiomaterials used for the construction of these 3D porous scaffolds. Close regulation of the scaffold properties like porosity, pore size, pore interconnectivity, tensile strength, surface area, and degradation profile, governs the functionality of the scaffolds. A good porosity ensures appropriate cell infiltration and favorable conditions for ECM growth. Interconnectivity within the porous structure aids in cell growth, proliferation, and migration of the cells to enable ECM growth further leading to better vascularization (Pina et al., 2019). Microporosity helps in attaining cell adhesion and growth and to further maintain the scaffold tissue interaction.

6.3.1 Nanobiomaterials for scaffolds in RM

Scaffolds for use in RM are expected to be biomimetic to the native ECM of the host with respect to both their mechanical properties and the chemical composition. A wide range of biomaterials comprised of natural and synthetic polymers, inorganic biomaterials, and hybrids of these have been in use for tissue engineering and RM applications. Natural and synthetic polymers include proteins, polysaccharides, lactic, and glycolic acid derivatives, etc.; they are preferred for their biosimilarity and low immunogenicity. Also, polymers like poly-lactic acid (PLA), poly-lactic-*co*-glycolic acid (PLGA), poly-ε-caprolactone (PCL), and collagen, have been already approved by the FDA, making them feasible alternatives. Inorganic biomaterials include ceramics like alumina, calcium phosphate cements, zirconia, silicates, calcium carbonates, glass-ceramics, and many more which are generally used for orthopedic applications owing to their bioresorbable nature (Pina et al., 2019). Metals are another category of inorganic biomaterials wherein stainless steel, cobalt, and titanium alloys are the ideal candidates for scaffold production. Composite or hybrid scaffolds utilize a combination of polymers (natural or synthetic), ceramics, and metals. These composite scaffolds have an upper edge over conventional biomaterials in terms of their superior abilities to exhibit biocompatibility and suitable biodegradation along with mechanical strength. Their versatility makes them applicable for the fabrication of scaffolds for both hard and soft tissue regeneration (Dolcimascolo et al., 2019).

6.3.2 Factors for consideration while designing scaffolds

6.3.2.1 Biocompatibility

As discussed earlier, biocompatibility is the first and very basic criterion that is to be considered while designing scaffolds for RM applications that aim at utilizing tissue engineering to re-establish normal tissue or organ function. Biocompatibility is important for functions like cell adhesion, restoration of normal cellular functions, cell proliferation, cell migration from the scaffold to the host environment, and establishment of a new tissue matrix (O'Brien, 2011). Apart from serving these functions, biocompatibility plays an important role to avoid the occurrence of any untoward immune response post scaffold implantation. Any incident of immunogenicity would trigger implant rejection or incomplete tissue healing.

6.3.2.2 Bioactivity

Bioactivity is the measure of how well the scaffolds can adapt to the host environment and enable the healing process. The ability of the biomaterial to induce cell adhesion, proliferation, and their ultimate migration defines the bioactivity of the scaffold as a whole. Biocompatibility is a vital factor for the scaffold to be bioactive because the more the simulation of the host environment by the scaffold, the higher the cellular recognition which would evoke optimal tissue growth (Dolcimascolo et al., 2019). Enhancement of bioactivity can therefore be achieved when the biomaterials are designed in a way so that they generate a better simulated biomimetic microenvironment at the site of scaffold implantation. Materials like collagen, fibronectin, and laminin have been observed to serve as an important addition to the biomaterial composition due to their ability to favorably modulate the tissue microenvironment.

6.3.2.3 Biodegradability

Biodegradability is a property which allows the scaffolds to serve as a one-time implant without the need for its removal from the host. Since scaffolds are implanted with an aim to restore the body's ability to regenerate the lost or injured tissues, it is important that they maintain a temporary profile inside the body. Once the implanted cells gain the power to produce their own ECM, biodegradation of scaffolds must commence. During the dissociation of the scaffold biomaterial, it is important that the by-products produced during this process are non-toxic and are easily eliminated without host tissue interference. Along with this, the degradation kinetics of the biomaterial plays a vital role in the process of biodegradation. The rate of in vivo biodegradation needs to be considered while designing the scaffolds for a desired application and the time for which it is to be retained. Biodegradation will therefore define functions of both bioactivity and biocompatibility.

6.3.2.4 Mechanical properties

Mechanical strength is a significant parameter while designing and selecting biomaterials for the fabrication of scaffolds for RM applications. Adequacy of the mechanical strength of the scaffold is important due to the need for high accuracy and specificity of RM. The implant needs to stay intact in the host bioenvironment throughout the remodeling process of the cells to form tissues. The strength of the scaffold would be defined by its ability to hold together without deforming upon implantation in vivo, be it because of the process of cellular growth or the implantation procedure itself. The scaffolds must therefore be fabricated in accordance with the exact site of implantation, to make them practically viable and rugged. It has been observed that cells respond to the stiffness of scaffolds in the form of ion channel activation or unfolding of cellular proteins, further impacting the cell proliferation and differentiation processes (Dolcimascolo et al., 2019). This becomes vital while designing scaffolds for the regeneration of bones and cartilage since these tissues demand superior mechanical strength to get re-established in their natural milieu. Another factor here is the difference in the rate of healing of different individuals depending on the severity of wounds, age, underlying physiological conditions, etc. For a scaffold to exhibit its function in full capacity, it must be able to allow complete vascularization of the tissue while also providing mechanical support. Citing the importance of mechanical properties, the focus has further shifted on the scaffold architecture, design, and execution.

The porous nature of scaffolds is an essential property which provides an ideal environment for the growth, proliferation, and infiltration of the seeded cells on implantation. Regulation of factors like scaffold stiffness and permeability, optimal architecture with distinct topology and desired mechanobiological properties can be obtained. The subcellular structures of the tissues control the intercellular interactions whereas the supracellular scale structures build the functional tissue units (Chen et al., 2010). To maintain these properties, the 3D modalities of scaffolds must be optimized, majorly the micro-architecture including porosity, pore size, pore network, and tortuosity (Hutmacher, 2001).

6.3.3 Fabrication of scaffolds

The various techniques for fabricating 3D scaffolds can be broadly divided into conventional or rapid prototyping methods. Conventional techniques involve the fabrication of porous polymer structures for supporting cell growth; however, it is difficult to tune the microscale and macroscale features using these methods. Rapid prototyping techniques provide potential opportunities for independent control of macroscale and microscale features characteristic of the ECM and multicellular structures, development of 3D vascular beds and possibly, the development of customized scaffolds and their large-scale production.

6.3.3.1 Conventional techniques for the fabrication of scaffolds

Scaffold fabrication using solvent casting and particulate leaching involves dissolving a polymer in a solvent combined with uniformly distributed salt particles followed by solvent evaporation that leaves a matrix containing salt particles. On submerging this matrix in water, the salt leaches away to form a highly porous structure. This method provides control over the scaffold shape and pore size but is limited in terms of connectivity of the void space. It has been employed with several modifications to make porous nanocomposite scaffolds using synthetic and biopolymers for applications in mostly bone and cartilage tissue engineering (Liao et al., 2002;

Prasad et al., 2017; Thanh et al., 2016). Another method of fabrication is freeze-drying or lyophilization, which involves cooling of a polymer solution under the freezing point and subsequent sublimation of the solvent resulting in a solid scaffold with numerous interconnected pores. The fabricated scaffolds need to be washed repeatedly and dried to remove the solvent and minimize cell death. This technique is widely adopted for scaffold fabrication for use in tissue engineering, cell or drug delivery, and membranes (Aranaz et al., 2014; Autissier et al., 2010; Dragusin et al., 2012; Guex et al., 2017; Lu et al., 2013).

Another major fabrication method for nanofibrous scaffolds is electrospinning, in which a polymer solution, when charged under high voltage, causes droplets on a spinneret to erupt and stretch. This results in a liquid jet being continuously extended and whipped owing to electrostatic repulsion before getting deposited on the grounded collector to form a nonwoven fibrous membrane that can mimic the ECM. Electrospinning has been employed for the preparation of nanofibers of several synthetic polymers, biopolymers and their blends, and even nanoparticle/drug-loaded composite fibers for applications in wound healing and regeneration of dermal, neural, orthopedic tissues, etc. (Balusamy et al., 2019; Braghirolli et al., 2014; Mortimer, 2018). Thermal-induced phase separation involves forced phase separation of a homogeneous polymer solution into a polymer-rich and a polymer-less phase by a change in temperature. A well-interconnected porous scaffold structure can be achieved after the solvent is removed by freeze-drying. This method is mostly employed for the construction of the thermoplastic crystalline polymer scaffolds like that of PLA, polyurethane (PU), PCL, etc. (Jing et al., 2014; Ruggiero et al., 2015; Salerno and Domingo, 2015). Another technique used is gas foaming that uses relatively inert gas foaming agents like carbon dioxide and nitrogen to pressurize biodegradable polymers with water or fluoroform until they are saturated or full of gas bubbles. This technique usually produces sponge-like structures with up to 85% porosity (Harris et al., 1998). The advantages and disadvantages of conventional scaffold fabrication techniques are listed in Table 6.2.

Rapid prototyping technologies or solid free-form fabrication are a set of manufacturing processes that can generate scaffolds with precise spatial control using computer-aided design (CAD) models. These techniques enable the production of customized and patient-specific scaffolds suitable for the tissues and organs in question. Common rapid prototyping techniques include 3D printing, fused deposition modeling, laser bioprinting, stereolithography, etc.

Table 6.2 Advantages and disadvantages of conventional scaffold fabrication techniques.

Fabrication technique	Advantages	Disadvantages
Solvent casting and particle leaching	Suitable for thin membranes of 3D specimens High porosity (50%–90%) Lost cost technique	Time consuming since thin membranes only are used Widespread use of very toxic solvents
Freeze-drying	Capability of avoiding high temperatures The pore size is manageable by changing the freezing method	High energy and time consumption Use of cytotoxic solvents Generation of small irregular sized pores
Gas foaming	High porosity up to 85%	Possibility of obtaining products with closed pore structures or a solid polymeric skin
Electrospinning	Efficient, simple procedure and inexpensive setup Ability to control many factors, such as the fiber diameter, orientation, and composition Possibility of the fabrication of polymer blends and composite nanofibers	Use of organic solvents Limited control of porosity
Thermal-induced phase separation	Low temperature enables integration of bioactive molecules Very high porosity (~98%) and a higher surface-to-volume ratio	Can be used only for thermoplastic polymers

Adapted from Eltom, A., Zhong, G., Muhammad, A., 2019. Scaffold techniques and designs in tissue engineering functions and purposes: a review. Adv. Mater. Sci. Eng. 2019, 3429527. https://doi.org/10.1155/2019/3429527, an open access article under CC BY-NC-ND 4.0).

6.3.3.2 3D printing

Nanostructured biomaterials (including nanocrystals, nanofibers, nanocomposites, etc.) have been explored for their applications in RM due to their favorable physicochemical properties (Thomas et al., 2006). 3D printing technology has been on a rise for its applications in the tissue engineering arena because of its cutting edge design and allied specificity. The emphasis on personalized therapy is the driving force behind the extensive research in the field of cell biology to understand the interface between cells and implanted biomaterials. Nanobiomaterials have emerged as a boon in this regard because they enable achievement of a greater level of control over cellular arrangements in a predefined manner along with a better material geometry. 3D printing offers an effective way of fabricating a suitable nanobiomaterial-based scaffold according to the desired application. 3D printing has been accepted as a versatile technology by the manufacturing industry because it enables rapid prototyping of the precisely formulated computer-aided design (O'Brien et al., 2015). 2D cellular arrays were developed from adhesion protein based cellular templates by Robert Klebe in 1988, giving rise to a bioprinting approach called "cytoscribing." Cytoscribing involves the use of either a computer-based inkjet printer or a graphics plotter for the deposition of adhesion proteins and monoclonal antibodies on the substratum for the formation of 2D tissue constructs (Klebe, 1988). This process underwent multiple modifications and in 2003, Wilson and Boland were the first to report modification of a conventional inkjet printer to a bioprinter hardware which could dispense protein or cell solutions instead of ink for the manufacturing of proteins and cell arrays (Wilson and Boland, 2003). The emergence of bioprinters and 3D bioprinting has proved to be a boon to medical science because of the escalating incidents of organ shortage and organ donors, globally, which demands the use of allografts. RM addresses this issue by fulfilling the unmet need for artificial tissues and organs; a field which has now culminated into regenerative engineering. Regenerative engineering is the convergence of materials science, stem cell science, physics, developmental biology, and clinical translation for enabling the fabrication of tissues and organs of complex nature. Matai et al. described 3D bioprinting as a promising biofabrication technique which is extremely precise with biologics like living cells and components of the ECM and can lead to the formation of pre-defined 3D hierarchies for developing desired tissues or organs (Matai et al., 2020). The schematic diagram depicting the processes involved in bioprinting is given in Fig. 6.1.

Bioprinters have emerged as the next big thing in the field of biotechnology after the first patent for the bioprinting technique was granted to Thomas Boland and co-workers at Clemson University, in the year 2003, entitled "Ink-jet printing of viable cells" (patent US7051654B2). This was followed by a series of minor modifications and a major breakthrough came in the year 2009 with the introduction of the first commercial bioprinter called NovoGen MMX Bioprinter by the company Oranovo and

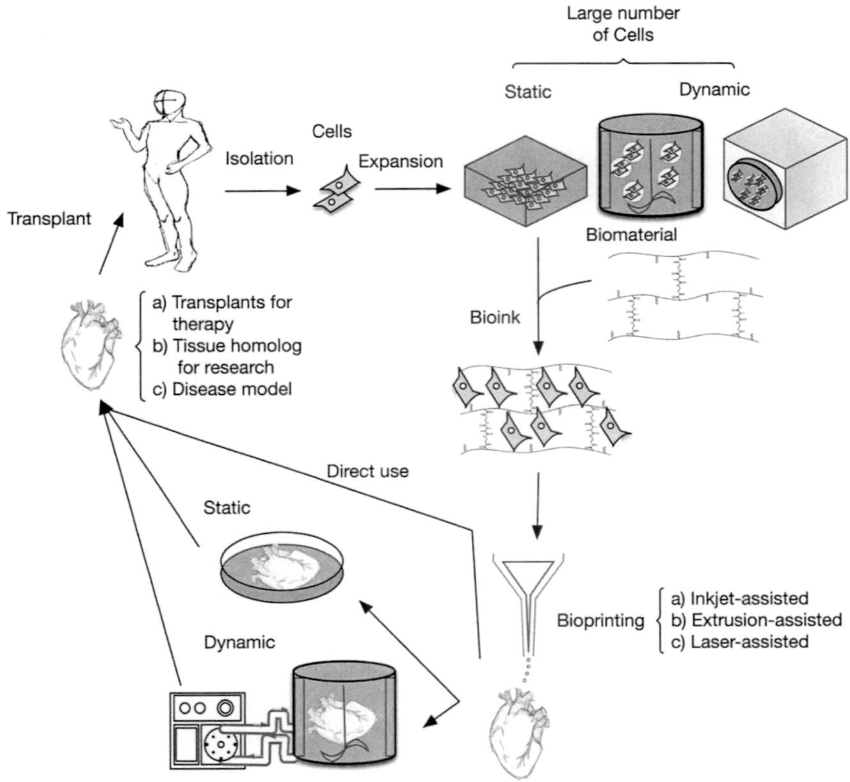

Fig. 6.1 Schematic representation of the bioprinting process. *(Reproduced with permission from Angelopoulos, I., Allenby, M.C., Lim, M., Zamorano, M., 2020. Engineering inkjet bioprinting processes toward translational therapies. Biotechnol. Bioeng. https://doi.org/10.1002/bit.27176.)*

Invetech (https://www.invetechgroup.com/case-studies/organovo-novogen-mmx-bioprinter/). This led to numerous research outcomes in the form of printed skin constructs, ear-shaped constructs and Organovo produced world's first commercial liver tissue model (Jose et al., 2016). Overall, printing techniques based on inkjet printers, extrusion, laser-assisted bioprinting, and stereolithography have been reported along with continuous modifications made in each of these methods (Correia Carreira et al., 2019).

- Inkjet printing

Inkjet printing is a bioprinting technique which is capable of fabricating 3D structures with a drop-by-drop approach. It is a non-contact reprographic method where digital data is fed in the form of an image or character which is then reproduced onto the substrate of choice using ink drops (Boland et al., 2006). The drop-by-drop methodology is further characterized into thermal, piezoelectric, and electromagnetic printing on the basis of the force applied to generate the compression on the printing nozzle (Angelopoulos et al., 2020; Kačarević et al., 2018). Inkjet bioprinting is a high-speed (upto 1–10,000 droplets/*sec*) and economic process which can achieve a resolution of around 50–75 μm in width and is capable of producing approximately 10^6 cells/mL of cell densities with a viability of more than 85% (Angelopoulos et al., 2020).

- Extrusion printing or fused deposition modeling

Extrusion based bioprinting is a pressure-based technology where the bioink is extruded from a nozzle via pneumatic or mechanical forces and deposited on the pre-determined 3D design (Kačarević et al., 2018; Xia et al., 2018). This type of printing process produces filaments instead of the droplets that are seen in an inkjet type of a printer. This demands for biomaterials to possess a high elastic modulus and adequate loss modulus so as to facilitate an efficient extrusion from the nozzle (Xia et al., 2018). The process is also referred to as melt extrusion or fused deposition modeling wherein the material exits the extruder in a molten state and immediately hardens on contacting the substrate due to its thermoplastic nature (Melchels et al., 2012). It is thereby important to closely monitor the solidification point of the biomaterial to assure its optimum layering on the substrate. The technique can be utilized when a high viscosity cell suspension has to be bioprinted. Despite these features, the technology has some disadvantages including a limited resolution (feature size greater than 100 μm), this limits precise patterning of the cells. Also, the peculiar requirement for a thermoplastic bioink which can follow gelation and solidification cycle limits the applications of this process (Ozbolat and Hospodiuk, 2016). The high viscosity of the cell suspension makes it difficult for extrusion process to optimize the number of living cells being extruded during the process (Chang et al., 2008).

- Stereolithography (SLA)

SLA is a process of bioprinting where an ultraviolet laser is used to photopolymerize the polymer surface. The procedure involves multiple layering via selective photoinitiated cure reaction of the polymer to develop 3D objects (Melchels et al., 2012). SLA-based 3D bioprinting has emerged as a promising strategy for the fabrication of complex tissues and organs. With the advent of novel cytocompatible photoinitiators which can operate over a wide range of UV and visible light spectrums, explorations of SLA have been carried out for bone and neural tissue engineering along with the development of controlled microenvironments for studying cell behavior (Kumar and Kim, 2020). First of its kind cell-attachable and visible light crosslinkable gelatinmethacrylolyl (GelMA) bioinks using Eosin Y as the photoinitiator were developed recently for SLA based bioprinting (Wang et al., 2018a). GelMA and methacrylated hyaluronic acid was explored with SLA to create artificial cartilage in vitro with varying cell differentiation patterns and ECM organization (Lam et al., 2019). The researchers further suggest multimaterial blended bioinks-based bioprinting as an ideal alternative to fabricating complex tissues like cartilage and also in repairing patient specific cartilage defects by adjusting dimensions of the hydrogel being printed (Lam et al., 2019). Overall, SLA has been regarded as a versatile and flexible bioprinting approach which is constantly evolving to cater to a plethora of possibilities in the field of RM.

- Laser-Assisted Bioprinting (LAB)

The process of high resolution patterning of metals using the fabrication of computer chips has been the starting point for the introduction of LAB as a method for bioprinting of 3D structures for tissue engineering applications. LAB involves utilization of laser pulses through a ribbon of bioink supported by a gold or titanium layer for energy transfer (Bishop et al., 2017). The cells along with the bioink are suspended on the ribbon when the laser pulse leads to their vaporization creating a high pressure bubble which propels the droplets toward the substrate placed below the ribbon. A continuous cycle of this process is required to form the desired 3D structures. A superior level of precision and resolution, automation, better reproducibility, and high throughput are some of the major advantages of LAB making it an industrially feasible bioprinting alternative (Devillard et al., 2014). This technique of bioprinting enables bioprinting of micropatterned peptides, DNA, cell arrays, in situ bioprinting of mesenchymal stromal cells, bone regeneration, etc. (Bishop et al., 2017; Guillotin et al., 2010; Hakobyan et al., 2020; Keriquel et al., 2017). This method of 3D bioprinting is continuously undergoing newer explorations and is set to open new avenues in the years to come. Fig. 6.2 depicts a schematic representation of the commonly used 3D bioprinting methods.

In the following sections, a glimpse into some of the applications of nanobiomaterials in RM like cardiovascular, orthopedic, dental, neural, and skin regenerative applications is presented.

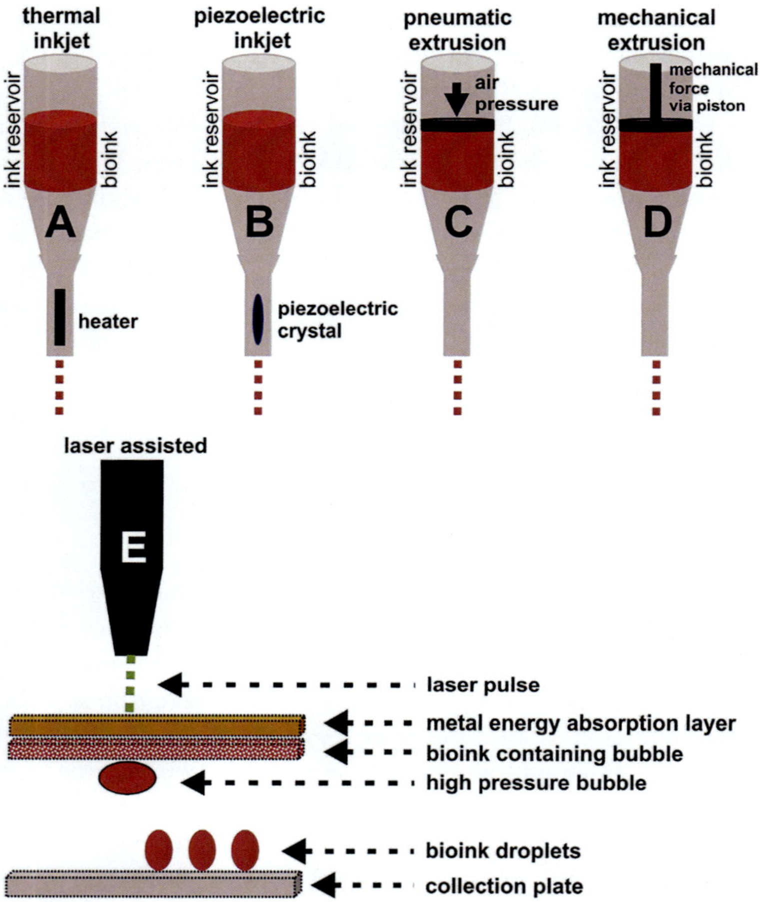

Fig. 6.2 Schematic representation of the most commonly used 3D bioprinting methods. *(Reproduced from Bishop, E.S., Mostafa, S., Pakvasa, M., Luu, H.H., Lee, M.J., Wolf, J.M., Ameer, G.A., He, T.C., Reid, R.R., 2017. 3-D bioprinting technologies in tissue engineering and regenerative medicine: current and future trends. Genes Dis. https://doi.org/10.1016/j.gendis.2017.10.002, an open access article under CC BY-NC-ND 4.0.)*

6.4 Applications of nanobiomaterials in regenerative medicine

6.4.1 Cardiac regeneration

Cardiovascular diseases remain one of the leading cause of deaths from the last few decades accounting for more than 30% of all deaths worldwide as per the WHO (World Health Organization, 2020). Poor availability of donors as well as a criticality in operative procedures are two important reasons for deaths caused by cardiovascular failures. Newer technology approaches to resolve the earlier-mentioned issues involves tissue regeneration aspects.

The success of cardiac tissue regenerative therapy is largely depended on the use of materials which possess similar properties to that of ECM with reference to mechanical, topological as well as electrical aspects (Ciofani et al., 2011). Common cardiac regenerative therapy can be classified into two parts: (1) conductive patches (3D printed, nanomolded mainly using a polypyrrole base) and (2) nonconductive patches [structured scaffolds, injectable hydrogels, etc. (Stout et al., 2011)].

The use of electrically conductive nanomaterials like carbon nanotubes, graphene oxide nanomaterials, silicon (Si) nanowires, and magnetic nanomaterials, like iron oxide nanoparticles in 3D scaffolds, have also increased in the field of cardiac tissue regeneration. For instance, Martinelli et al. studied the influence of carbon nanotubes on cardiomyocytes and cardiac fibroblasts. Cardiomyocytes showed enhanced proliferation and electrophysiological properties when grown in carbon nanotube coated substrates as compared with controls (gelatin coated). The carbon nanotubes also resulted in the upregulation of normal cardiac-specific genes and the suppression of genes related to pathological hypertrophy. However, similar observations were not seen for cardiac fibroblasts (Martinelli et al., 2012, 2013). Another study demonstrated that the incorporation of carbon nanotubes in gelatin methacrylate hydrogels aided in the elongation of cardiomyocytes and homogenous formation of cell-to-cell junctions, in addition to the enhanced spontaneous beating of matured cardiomyocytes (Shin et al., 2013b). Similarly, graphene oxide nanoflakes were found to adsorb ECM proteins, induce proangiogenic growth factors, and improve the viability and retention of transplanted MSCs in an in vitro infarcted myocardium and an in vivo myocardial ischemia reperfusion model (Park et al., 2015a, 2015b). Reduced graphene oxide added into gelatin methacrylate hydrogels has also been shown to enhance cell attachment and spreading of fibroblast cells (Shin et al., 2013a). Si nanowires also provide electrically conducting microenvironments that enhance the maturation and electrophysiological response of human induced pluripotent stem cell-derived cardiomyocytes (Richards et al., 2016). In another study, iron oxide nanoparticle incorporated liposomes were added into rat cardiomyocytes grown on a cell-repellant substrate. These cardiac cells formed a sheet-like structure in the presence of an external magnetic field while spherical cell structures were formed in the absence of magnetic field. These scaffold-free cardiac cell sheets could be then used for cardiac tissue regeneration studies (Shimizu et al., 2007).

In Table 6.3, we have summarized some of the recent advances in cardiovascular regenerative therapy with respect to the use of polymeric materials, their fabrication and their properties.

Table 6.3 Representative examples of polymeric and decullarized biomaterials used in cardiac regenerative therapy.

Biomaterial	Fabrication methods	Properties	References
Polycaprolactone (PCL)	Electrospinning technology to obtain nanofiber scaffolds, and myocardial patches, laser sintering scaffolds, trilayer nanofibrous patches	Biocompatibility, high structural integrity, improved cellular adhesion in combination with other, impart hydrophobicity to patch improving its durability	(Mousa et al., 2020; Silvestri et al., 2014; Tillman et al., 2009; Yeong et al., 2010)
Poly-L-lactic acid (PLLA)	Electro spun fiber-based scaffolds, nanofibrous scaffolds, cardiac patches, heart valve leaflet construct	Biocompatibility, biodegradation, cellular adhesion, biomimicking ECM	(Breuer et al., 1996; Liu et al., 2017; Santoro et al., 2016; Zong et al., 2005)
Poly-(lactic-*co*-glycolic) acid (PLGA)	Nanofiber composite micro capsulated injectable scaffolds, electro spun nanofibers	Electroconductivity, cytocompatibility, good rheological properties, FDA approved	(Kang et al., 2009; Miller et al., 2004; Stout et al., 2011; Zamani et al., 2015)
Polyethylene glycol-based polymers (PEG)	Nano molded scaffolds, 3D-encapsulated hydrogels, myocardial patches, nanopillar array hydrogels	Biocompatibility, improved cell adhesion, biodegradability, high elastomeric properties	(Grover et al., 2014; Kang et al., 2009; Kim et al., 2006; Silvestri et al., 2014)
Decellularized myocardial scaffolds	Platform technology in the form of scaffolds, 3D printed complex tissue constructs, cardiac cell patches, injectable hydrogels	Higher tissue regeneration, stronger cellular adhesion, mimicking biorelevant microenvironment, improved vascularization and differentiating ability of cells	(Godier-furemont Amandine et al., 2011; Jang et al., 2017; Nguyen et al., 2015)

There are other technologies, such as injectable biomaterials and bulking biomaterials, which also help in bringing the regeneration of delicate tissue within the myocardium. Although this technology uses more conventional approaches, that is, hydrogel-based compositions, it gives prominent results and also can be combined with various inorganic nanoparticles and/or with protein moieties further facilitating regeneration procedures. Such materials comprise of alginates, chitosan, collagen, fibrin, methacrylate, hyaluronic acid, polyethylene glycol, etc. (Lewis and et al., 2016). The use of nano-enabled strategies for cardiac regeneration is still premature and several concerns exist in terms of cytotoxicity and the long-term fate of nanomaterials, especially carbon-based nanomaterials which need to be studied in detail.

6.4.2 Orthopedic applications

Biomaterials show high potential in mimicking/replicating the constitute organs in orthopedic applications. Nanomaterials not only serve as the structural backbone as in the case of nanostructured scaffolds but also facilitate cell growth, differentiation as well as migration. In orthopedic applications, biomaterials are in demand to treat irreversible damage caused to the natural structure of bones. Biomaterials used in orthopedics can be roughly categorized under metallic and nonmetallic origin. Nanomaterials are preferred over other conventional materials due to their high strength and compatibility and tunable surface morphology (Rezwan et al., 2006). Metallic biomaterials as implants show certain limitations such as corrosion on prolonged use, reaction toward hydrogen, requirement of removal surgeries. Due to these, polymer and composite-based biomaterials are dominating the field of research (Kumar et al., 2020). Some of the natural proteins that have been extensively evaluated for bone tissue engineering include collagen, gelatin, silk fibroin, and fibrin, which have been fabricated as 3D scaffolds in the form of films, sponges, or nanofibers (Ansari, 2019; Sayin et al., 2014). Natural polymers explored for bone regeneration also include polysaccharides like hyaluronic acid (Zhai et al., 2020; Zhu et al., 2017), chitosan (Levengood and Zhang, 2014; Saravanan et al., 2016), alginate (Kaczmarek-Pawelska and Pereira, 2020; Sun and Tan, 2013), cellulose, (Hickey and Pelling, 2019), etc. However, the mechanical strength, toughness, and load bearing capability of these natural materials are limited and hence, several composite or bioceramic materials have been envisioned and tested as scaffolds for orthopedic applications. A host of synthetic bioceramic materials which can be broadly classified into bioinert (alumina), bioresorbable (α-tricalcium phosphate, calcium oxide, calcium carbonate), and bioactive (bioactive glasses, hydroxyapatite) categories have been studied alone or mostly in combination with natural materials for bone regeneration. Some of the synthetic polymers widely studied for bone regeneration owing to their controllable biodegradability and feasibility of surface functionalization include PLGA, poly(glycolic acid) (PGA), PLA, PCL, polyethylene glycol (PEG), polyvinyl alcohol (PVA), PU, etc. (Donnaloja et al., 2020; Qu et al., 2019). Nanoparticles have also been employed to enhance physiochemical, mechanical, and biological properties of scaffolds so as to improve osteocompatibility and osseointegration of implants or to deliver drugs, biomolecules, or growth factors (Eivazzadeh-Keihan et al., 2020; Walmsley et al., 2015).

The following Table 6.4 gives representative examples of applications of nano-biomaterials for orthopedic applications.

For enhancing the properties of scaffolds, such as elasticity, tensile strength, durability, etc., various additives and combinations are used in the fabrication (Liao et al., 2005). Nowadays, nano-coatings over conventional implants to improve its properties are taken into consideration. Various anti-microbial coatings, for example, Ag nanoparticles, chitosan microspheres, PEG and Si-based coatings to improve adhesion properties, PLGA-based nanocoatings for obtaining a desired sustain release profile, have been developed and studied in detail (Kumar et al., 2020). In the case of cartilage tissue recovery, an agarose polymer is commonly used due to its cell adhesion abilities and higher hydrophilicity aiding in cell growth, differentiation, and migration (Eftekhari et al., 2020).

6.4.3 Dental applications

Dental tissues are highly prone to damage due to bacterial infections and/or trauma due to accidents. Owing to the limited ability of pulp tissue for self-healing, dental fillings with the help of biomaterials will accelerate the process of regeneration and provide structural advances (Kishen, 2015). While considering dental applications, periodontal tissue engineering is also important as inflammation in gums and gingiva and degradation in cementum lead to the failing of teeth. Designing tissue regenerative scaffolds for this application is a little tricky as it needs materials favorable in generating hard as well as soft muscle tissue. It mainly involves guided tissue regeneration (Jang et al., 2017). Due to complex and smaller areas of application, injectable scaffolds, and in situ hydrogels are favored instead of predesigned scaffolds. Tricalcium phosphate or nanohydroxyapatite nanostructures have been often added in the form of filling powders or within hydrogels to

Table 6.4 Representative examples of nanobiomaterials used in orthopedic applications.

Biomaterial	Fabrication	Properties	References
Hydroxyapatite (HA) (Most commonly used as a raw material for the preparation of artificial bone)	Injectable hydrogels, foam scaffolds, nano-coatings thin films, nanoparticular formulations	Biocompatibility, mimics composition of bone, acts as a slow release matrix when combined with growth regulatory moieties (proteins, hormones, enzymes), antimicrobial properties	(Arcos and Vallet-Regí, 2020; Thomson et al., 1998; Thorwarth et al., 2005)
Collagen (Commonly used as it mimics the matrix structure in bone)	Electrospun nanofiber composite, hydrogel for injections, aerogels	Biocompatibility, mimics the microenvironment of chondral cells, i.e., ECM, osteogenesis, elastomeric properties, anisotropic growth of cells, collagen-based scaffold in combination with hyaluronic acids are most commonly used for cartilage recoveries	(Eftekhari et al., 2020; Kim et al., 2006; Shih et al., 2006; Van Duong et al., 2018)
Carbon nanotubes (Carbon nanotubes are proven to promote osteoblast formation and hence, commonly used in osteogenic scaffolds)	Multiwalled carbon nanotubes-based 3D scaffolds, single-walled carbon nanotubes, nanofibers-based nanocomposites	Biocompatibility, improved tensile strength, no hindrance to normal cell regeneration, improved durability, flexibility, osteoblast formation	(Aoki et al., 2020; Gutiérrez-Hernández et al., 2017; Shimizu et al., 2012)
Chitosan	Nanocomposite films, hydrogels, scaffolds, nanofibers, nanoparticulate coatings	Biocompatibility, antimicrobial action, mimics ECM, durability, cartilage recovery, regeneration of hyaline-like tissue, mucoadhesion	(De Witte et al., 2020; Eftekhari et al., 2020; Jahed et al., 2020; Khan et al., 2020)
Poly-L-lactic acid (PLLA)	Laser fritter scaffolds, nanofiber membranes	Improved tensile strength, durability, improved cell viabilities when used in combination, biocompatibility	(Santos et al., 2017; Cijun et al., 2020)
Fibrin	Nanofibrous, microporous scaffolds, hydrogel	Stimulation of spontaneous repair, proinflammatory, structure mimics the ECM	(Osathanon et al., 2008; Sanchez-Casanova et al., 2020)

promote remineralization, protein absorption, and cellular responses (Al-Sanabani et al., 2013; Chen et al., 2005; Zhang et al., 2010). Stem cells incorporated into nanofibrous composite scaffolds prepared by the electrospinning of PLLA, PCL, gelatin, etc., and hydroxyapatite have been also studied for dental regeneration (Deng et al., 2007; Xu et al., 2007; Yang et al., 2010).

The following Table 6.5 compiles the most commonly used biomaterials for treating dental deformities.

Fibrin-based hydrogels are another commonly used material in the case of dental tissue regeneration (Ahmed et al., 2008; Haugen et al., 2020). Many inorganic materials such as zeolite, Si, titanium oxide as well as silver also play crucial roles in treating defects in dental as well as periodontal tissues (Kishen, 2015; Mohandesnezhad et al., 2020).

6.4.4 Neural tissue engineering

The nervous system in the human body consists of two important elements; the central nervous system (CNS) is made up of the brain, spinal cord, and nerves, while the peripheral nervous system (PNS) consists of sensory neurons, ganglia (clusters of neurons) and nerves that connect to one another and to the CNS. Self-regeneration and healing of the system of nerves start after the injury caused due to trauma, disorder, or any other diseases. The different players in the self-regeneration process are listed in Fig. 6.3.

Although the auto-repair mode of the PNS system works immediately, it is not in the capacity to combat the Wallerian degeneration when coupled with fibrosis of the endoneurium. The CNS unfortunately does not undergo the self-reconstruction process as it is devoid of Schwann cells.

The introduction of biomaterial-based strategies is therefore very important as they help in the reduction of the risks associated with the traditional methods such as autografting, which requires two surgeries and allografting that may lead to loss of functionality permanently. RM strategies involving the use of biomaterials provide a therapeutic advantage by itself or act as a delivery vehicle for growth factors and ECM proteins at the target site. They facilitate tissue regeneration at the spot. For PNS regeneration, the bioengineered nerve implants should simulate longitudinally orientated conduits that can not only provide support and guide the growth of neurons but also maintain their biological and functional viability. Self-assembled peptide nanofiber scaffolds incorporated with neural stem cells and Schwann cells have been extensively studied for nerve tissue regeneration (Pugliese and Gelain, 2017). In a pioneering study by Ellis-Behnke et al.,

Table 6.5 Representative examples of biomaterials used for treating dental deformities.

Biomaterial	Fabrication	Properties	References
Hydroxyapatite (It is one of the components of enamel present in dental tissue, commonly used in dental fixtures)	Scaffolds, coatings, dental cements	Biocompatibility, structural similarity to dental tissue, bioactive, conductivity	(Hosseinzade et al., 2016; Reshma and Khan, 2020; Yang et al., 2010)
Chitosan	Nanofibers, nano-scaffolds, hydrogels, films	Biocompatible, antimicrobial action, potent osteogenic response when combined with other biomaterials, osteoconduct properties, biodegradation, mucoadhesion	(Haugen et al., 2020; In et al., 2009; Khoroushi et al., 2018)
Bioactive glass	Scaffolds, bio-cements, nanofibrous composites, membranes	Biocompatibility, high cellular binding ability, good conductive properties, stimulates induction of ossification, remineralization of dentin	(Bae et al., 2012; Erol-Taygun et al., 2013; Khoroushi et al., 2018; Mota et al., 2012)

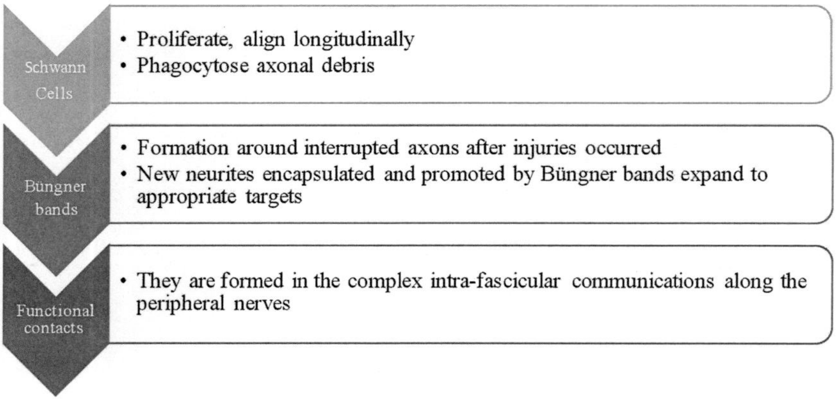

Fig. 6.3 Self-repair of the PNS (Ribeiro-Resende et al., 2009).

it was demonstrated that RADA16-I, a representative self-assembled peptide nanofiber scaffold, aided in axonal growth through the treated lesions and resulted in partial restoration of the optic tract and functional vision in brachium transected Syrian hamsters (Ellis-Behnke et al., 2006). Another study reported the use of the RADA16-I self-assembled peptide nanofiber scaffold to regenerate the injury gap inflicted in the sensory-motor cortex (Guo et al., 2009). The same group also reported the use of a self-assembled peptide nanofiber scaffold for the delivery of a cell-permeable RhoA inhibitor, CT04, that can improve the regeneration of an injured spinal cord with significant axonal regeneration and motor functionality (Zhang et al., 2012). Another major technique employed for fabricating nanofibrous scaffolds for nerve regeneration is electrospinning. Nerve conduits made of natural and synthetic elctrospinnable polymers like chitosan, collagen, PLLA, PCL, blends of PLGA/PCL, and poly(propylene glycol) have been investigated for PNS regeneration (Amini et al., 2020; Carvalho et al., 2019; Wang et al., 2008; Zhu et al., 2011).

Table 6.6 consolidates some of the major recent advancements in the use of polymers in the field of neural tissue re-engineering.

There are a lot of new strategies that are being adopted for regeneration in neural tissue engineering. Along with the traditional scaffolds which we saw in Table 6.6, hydrogels are being widely accepted now-a-days due to the flexibility provided by them in the shape which is beneficial in an irregularly shaped cavity. Another prominent technology which has been noticed is the *co*-plantation and seeding of vital stem cells and growth factors into the polymer scaffold to promote regeneration at the target site

Table 6.6 Representative list of biomaterials used for neural tissue engineering.

Biomaterials	Additive	Method	References
Polycaprolactone (PCL)	Chitosan	Nanofibers: Electrospinning	
	Poly(2-hydroxyethyl methacrylate) (pHEMA)	Hydrogels: Fiber templating	(Flynn et al., 2003)
	Gelatin	Electrospun Nanofibers Scaffolds	(KarbalaeiMahdi et al., 2017; Vatankhah et al., 2014)
	Hyaluronic acid	Nanofibers: Electrospinning	(Entekhabi et al., 2016)
	Collagen	Fibers: Electrospinning	(Ebrahimi-Barough et al., 2017)
	Lignin	Nanofibers: solvent free ring-opening polymerization	(Wang et al., 2018b)
Poly-L-lactic acid (PLLA)	–	Aligned PLLA nano/micro fibrous scaffolds	(Yang et al., 2005)
	Gelatin	Co-electro spun fibers	(Binan et al., 2014)
	Lysine-doped polypyrrole/regenerated spider silk protein/PLLA/nerve growth factor (L-PRPN)	Scaffold: co-axial electro spraying and electrospinning	(Zhang et al., 2015)
	4-methoxyphenyl	Biocompatible porous scaffold by electrospinning	(Vicentini et al., 2015)
	–	Single-walled carbon-nanotube (SWCNT): electrospinning	(Kabiri et al., 2015)
	Collagen matrix with Schwann Cells	Conduits: Injected the matrix and seeded with Schwann cells	(Evans et al., 2002)
	Poly 3,4-ethylenedioxythiophene (PEDOT) + hyaluronic acid	Conductive composite films	(Wang et al., 2017)

Continued

Table 6.6 Representative list of biomaterials used for neural tissue engineering—cont'd

Biomaterials	Additive	Method	References
Poly-(lactic-*co*-glycolic) acid (PLGA)	Hydrophobin II (HFBI)	Film: microcontact printing (μCP)	(Li et al., 2009)
	Co-transplantation of neural stem cells and Schwann cells	Seeded scaffolds	(Xia et al., 2013)
	Poly-D-lysine with laminin, fibronectin or collagen	Films with coated materials for surface modification	(Han et al., 2005)
	Hyaluronic acid (HA)	HA hydrogel/PLGA microsphere systems	(Wang et al., 2011)
	Bone marrow MSCs with chitosan	Neural scaffold with autologous MSCs	(Ding et al., 2010)
	Polypyrrole (PPy)	Mesh: Electrospinning	(Lee et al., 2009)

(Xia et al., 2013). In a specific case study to consider the most appropriate polymer for nerve regeneration, biocompatibility tests were performed and found PLGA as the most appropriate polymer for the task (Bhang et al., 2007). Another advancement observed in the field is plasma treatment of the polymers to increase their surface characteristics; the hydrophilicity increased greatly after an O_2 plasma treatment of PLLA. There was better cell attachment with the B65 nervous cells due to the combination of surface chemistry and wettability due to the plasma treatment (Khorasani et al., 2008). In another experiment, PLGA surface was modified with TiO_2 using magnetron sputtering to improve the PLGA surface/cell interaction (Ryu et al., 2005). Although huge strides have been undertaken in the field of nerve regeneration, functional integration of host-implant and complete restoration of neurological function still need to be addressed.

6.4.5 Skin regeneration

Skin, the largest organ in our body performs vital functions like offering a barrier against external injuries and regulating temperature. Although skin wounds heal naturally, therapies that would enhance wound healing might be required in cases where healing is impaired, for example, in diabetic patients with deficient vascular supply or burn patients (Boyce and Lalley, 2018). Tissue-engineered skin scaffolds can be classified as epidermal, dermal, and dermoepidermal and the ECM structure can be mimicked to an extent by using 3D scaffolds incorporated with drugs, growth factors, and skin cells. In addition to biomaterial selection, other factors which potentially influence the skin regeneration process like the damaged skin's condition, immunological status, and age also play a key role in designing tissue-engineered skin scaffolds. Natural, synthetic, and composite biomaterials have been used for the preparation of skin scaffolds so far. Natural polymers like chitosan, collagen, alginate, silk fibroin, and gelatin have been extensively used for skin regeneration as they promote wound healing and have the potential to mimic ECM properties. However, they do possess some disadvantages in terms of possible immunological and inflammatory reactions. Synthetic polymers, on the other hand, are cost-effective, easy to modify and sterilize, and pose minimal immunogenicity risks. However, only a few of them like PLA, PGA, and PLGA are FDA approved for use in biomedical applications (Mohamed and Xing, 2012).

None of the traditional skin grafts were developed to regenerate wound injuries, including xenografts, allografts, and autografts, nor have successfully satisfied the requirements of fully functional skin. It could be due to the insufficient healthy donor skin, immune reactions after allografting, scarring, or any other specific adverse effects associated with surgery (Dai et al., 2020; Kallis et al., 2018). The research to develop an ideal skin substitute that supports optimal wound healing is ongoing and nanotechnology has played a key role in that race for the most suited biocompatible scaffolds for skin regeneration. The most commonly employed techniques for controlling the surface topography of a scaffold for skin regeneration at the nanometer level include self-assembly, phase separation, electrospinning, and 3D printing. Further, the compositions and mechanical properties of these scaffolds can be tuned by blending natural and synthetic biomaterials and can be incorporated with drugs, growth factors, antibacterial molecules, or proteins also. The common types of scaffolds utilized in skin regeneration are given in Table 6.7.

Porous scaffolds in the form of sponges or foam can be fabricated from both natural and synthetic biodegradable materials by using porogens, prototyping, 3D printing, etc. (Chan and Leong, 2008). Most of the porous scaffolds in skin tissue engineering have a collagen base with keratinocytes or fibroblasts seeded into the scaffold. For instance, Orcel (Ortec International, New York, NY, USA) is an FDA approved, bilayered tissue engineered skin construct with a porous type I bovine collagen sponge as its base and a nonporous collagen-gel. The keratinocytes are added to the non-porous gel while the fibroblasts are seeded into the porous collagen sponge (Shevchenko et al., 2010; Still et al., 2003). Another example is that of a dermal substitute, Terudermis which consists of a bovine collagen sponge bound to a silicone layer and is used for the treatment of deep burns and trauma-induced deformities (Choi et al., 1999). Pelnac (Gunze Ltd., Kyoto, Japan) is a porous sponge scaffold made of porcine collagen (Suzuki et al., 2000). In addition, several preclinical studies involving the development of sponge scaffolds using natural and synthetic biomaterials like chitosan, gelatin, PVA, keratin, silk fibroin have been reported for applications in skin regeneration (Chen et al., 2006; Jinno et al., 2016; Mahnama et al., 2017; Rnjak-Kovacina et al., 2015; Yeo et al., 2000).

Fibrous scaffolds are also a type of porous scaffold, except that they are composed of nanofibers. For tissue regeneration, nanofiber scaffolds with highly interconnected porosity are inevitable and have been found beneficial for cell seeding and supply of nutrients and growth factors to regulate cell behavior. Electrospinning is the most widely employed technique for fabricating fibrous scaffolds of various materials (Dias et al., 2016; Mulholland, 2020). There have been several studies to develop dermal and epidermal substitutes that mimic

Table 6.7 Advantages and disadvantages of different scaffolds used in skin regeneration.

Scaffold type	Advantages	Disadvantages	Future prospects
Porous scaffolds	High porosity favoring ECM secretion and nutrient supply to the cells Pore sizes specific to cell types prevent clustering of the cells and avoids the formation of a necrotic center	Porosity limits the homogenous distribution of the cells Varying requirements of pore sizes for different cell types make scaffold design challenging and time consuming	Improvement in the interconnectivity of pores in the scaffold structure
Fibrous scaffolds	Highly microporous structure most suited for cell adhesion, proliferation, and differentiation Low inflammatory response upon implantation	Surface functionalization/additional design modifications to create nanofeatures in these scaffolds	Incorporation and sustained release of drugs and biomolecules like proteins, genes, growth factors, etc.
Hydrogel scaffolds	Highly biocompatible with a controlled biodegradation rate	Limited mechanical strength due to soft structures	Lacks well-defined degradation behavior and tenability Sustained release of growth factors to facilitate cell differentiation
Microsphere scaffolds	Ease of fabrication with a controlled release property Enhanced cell attachment and migration	Microsphere sintering methods not compatible to the cells may reduce cell viability	Target specific delivery of drugs including antibiotics and anticancer drugs
Composite scaffolds	High biodegradability, absorbability, and better mechanical strength	Tedious fabrication methods Generation of acidic degradation byproducts Poor cell affinity	Development of nano-bioceramic and polymer composites with faster degradation
Acellular scaffolds	The native ECM is retained resulting in normal anatomical features Less inflammatory and immune response with higher mechanical strength	Incomplete decellularization is required to avoid immune responses	Promising candidates for developing artificial organs

Adapted from Chaudhari, A.A., Vig, K., Baganizi, D.R., Sahu, R., Dixit, S., Dennis, V., Singh, S.R., Pillai, S.R., 2016. Future prospects for scaffolding methods and biomaterials in skin tissue engineering: a review. Int. J. Mol. Sci. 17. https://doi.org/10.3390/ijms17121974, an open access article under CC BY-NC-ND 4.0.

them in terms of matrix composition, mechanical properties, and functionalities. Acellular scaffolds like Biobrane and Integra and cellular scaffolds like Apligraf and Transcyte, are examples of commercial fibrous scaffolds (Falanga et al., 2014; Garfein, 2009). Development of nanofiber scaffolds seeded with stem cells that play an important role in all stages of wound healing is another promising approach for skin tissue regeneration. A host of research in the field of biodegradable hydrogels comprising synthetic polymers and natural macromolecules have demonstrated their utility in controlled delivery and RM applications. Typically, hydrogel encapsulating cells, drugs or biomolecules for RM applications are prepared by ionic or covalent crosslinking of biomaterials capable of self-assembling into a solid polymeric network on the influence of stimuli like pH and temperature. In the case of RM applications, balancing the degradation rate and cell adhesion and growth in the scaffold is vital (Budama-Kilinc, 2018). Preclinical studies of hydrogels made of natural polymers like hyaluronic acid (da Silva et al., 2019; Hong et al., 2018; Khunmanee et al., 2017), chitosan (Jiao et al., 2019; Liu et al., 2018), gelatin (Zhao et al., 2016), fibronectin (Trujillo et al., 2020), collagen (Bacakova et al., 2019; Helary et al., 2012), alginate (Kaczmarek-Pawelska and Pereira, 2020), dextran (Catoira et al., 2019; Sun et al., 2011) and their blends with synthetic polymers like PEG, PVA, PLGA (Bahadoran et al., 2020; Chen et al., 2018; Lee et al., 2007; Wall et al., 2018) have been extensively reported for wound healing skin regeneration. Bilayered scaffolds, hydrogels in combination with a fibrous or porous scaffold, have also been reported (Jaiswal et al., 2013), for instance, a bilayered scaffold having a PEG-chitosan hydrogel seeded with fibroblasts and a porous chitosan-alginate scaffold seeded with keratinocytes have been developed (Tsao et al., 2014). Self-assembling peptide-based hydrogels have also been recently proposed for dermal tissue regeneration (Bradshaw et al., 2014; Kim et al., 2017). Further, the use of microsphere scaffolds, specifically with the nanoparticle-based microspheres has facilitated the controlled release of actives that would augment skin regeneration like growth factors, anti-bacterial agents, and even stem cells (Gupta et al., 2017; Huang et al., 2012). Bioceramics, specifically bioactive glasses, have also garnered interest recently owing to their angiogenic and antibacterial potential. Nanosized 45S5 Bioglass incorporated scaffolds have been found to induce in vitro and in vivo neovascularization, accelerate blood clot time and, thus, improve wound healing. The most widely studied category of bioactives glasses, mesoporous bioactive glasses, and their biocomposites have emerged as suitable candidates for the controlled delivery of bioactives for the regeneration of wound injuries (Jia et al., 2011; Kargozar et al., 2019; Li et al., 2019).

6.5 Conclusions and future perspectives

Advancements in the biomedical field of tissue engineering and RM has led to the advent of newer technologies for attaining superior outcomes with respect to tissue regeneration and allied healing. The past decade has witnessed a multitude of growth in the research of nanobiomaterial fabrication and design for applications in RM. With an ever-increasing demand for tissues and organs for multiple modalities, it is imperative to use advanced technology-based approaches to cater to these critical healthcare needs. Currently applied technologies engineer tissues with a low speed of vascularization post-implantation, thereby limiting their applications to structurally simple tissues like skin, cartilage, and the bladder. Another fact remains that the tissues formed by the present techniques do not completely simulate the native tissues or organs being replaced, necessitating a dire need for advanced technological platforms with higher specificity and accuracy. This dawns the need for nanoscale and microscale biomaterials for effectively utilizing upcoming fabrication technologies. Engineering 3D tissues has not seen that much success yet clinically because of the intricacies involved in accomplishing the process. The introduction of new nanobiomaterials has enabled researchers to bridge this gap between virtual theories and reality by exploring the potential of these materials for RM development.

References

Adaya, D.S., Aguirre-Cruz, L., Guevara, J., Ortiz-Islas, E., 2016. Nanobiomaterials applications in neurodegenerative diseases. J. Biomater. Appl. https://doi.org/10.1177/0885328216659032.

Ahmed, T.A.E., Dare, E.V., Hincke, M., 2008. Fibrin: a versatile scaffold for tissue engineering applications. Tissue Eng. Part B Rev. 14, 199–215. https://doi.org/10.1089/ten.teb.2007.0435.

Albanese, A., Tang, P.S., Chan, W.C.W., 2012. The effect of nanoparticle size, shape, and surface chemistry on biological systems. Annu. Rev. Biomed. Eng. 14, 1–16. https://doi.org/10.1146/annurev-bioeng-071811-150124.

Al-Sanabani, J.S., Madfa, A.A., Al-Sanabani, F.A., 2013. Application of calcium phosphate materials in dentistry. Int. J. Biomater. 2013, 876132. https://doi.org/10.1155/2013/876132.

Amini, S., Saudi, A., Amirpour, N., Jahromi, M., Najafabadi, S.S., Kazemi, M., Rafienia, M., Salehi, H., 2020. Application of electrospun polycaprolactone fibers embedding lignin nanoparticle for peripheral nerve regeneration: In vitro and in vivo study. Int. J. Biol. Macromol. 159, 154–173. https://doi.org/10.1016/j.ijbiomac.2020.05.073.

Angelopoulos, I., Allenby, M.C., Lim, M., Zamorano, M., 2020. Engineering inkjet bioprinting processes toward translational therapies. Biotechnol. Bioeng. https://doi.org/10.1002/bit.27176.

Ansari, M., 2019. Bone tissue regeneration: biology, strategies and interface studies. Prog. Biomater. 8, 223–237. https://doi.org/10.1007/s40204-019-00125-z.

Aoki, K., Haniu, H., Kim, Y.A., Saito, N., 2020. The use of electrospun organic and carbon nanofibers in bone regeneration. Nanomaterials 10. https://doi.org/10.3390/nano10030562.

Aranaz, I., Gutiérrez, M.C., Ferrer, M.L., del Monte, F., 2014. Preparation of chitosan nanocomposites with a macroporous structure by unidirectional freezing and subsequent freeze-drying. Mar. Drugs 12, 5619–5642. https://doi.org/10.3390/md12115619.

Arcos, D., Vallet-Regí, M., 2020. Substituted hydroxyapatite coatings of bone implants. J. Mater. Chem. B 8, 1781–1800. https://doi.org/10.1039/c9tb02710f.

Autissier, A., Visage, C.L., Pouzet, C., Chaubet, F., Letourneur, D., 2010. Fabrication of porous polysaccharide-based scaffolds using a combined freeze-drying/cross-linking process. Acta Biomater. 6, 3640–3648. https://doi.org/10.1016/j.actbio.2010.03.004.

Bacakova, M., Pajorova, J., Broz, A., Hadraba, D., Lopot, F., Zavadakova, A., Vistejnova, L., Beno, M., Kostic, I., Jencova, V., Bacakova, L., 2019. A two-layer skin construct consisting of a collagen hydrogel reinforced by a fibrin-coated polylactide nanofibrous membrane. Int. J. Nanomedicine 14, 5033–5050. https://doi.org/10.2147/IJN.S200782.

Bae, W.J., Min, K.S., Kim, J.J., Kim, J.J., Kim, H.W., Kim, E.C., 2012. Odontogenic responses of human dental pulp cells to collagen/nanobioactive glass nanocomposites. Dent. Mater. 28, 1271–1279. https://doi.org/10.1016/j.dental.2012.09.011.

Bahadoran, M., Shamloo, A., Nokoorani, Y.D., 2020. Development of a polyvinyl alcohol/sodium alginate hydrogel-based scaffold incorporating bFGF-encapsulated microspheres for accelerated wound healing. Sci. Rep. 10, 7342. https://doi.org/10.1038/s41598-020-64480-9.

Bailey, A.M., Mendicino, M., Au, P., 2014. An FDA perspective on preclinical development of cell-based regenerative medicine products. Nat. Biotechnol. 32, 721–723.

Bajaj, P., Schweller, R.M., Khademhosseini, A., West, J.L., Bashir, R., 2014. 3D biofabrication strategies for tissue engineering and regenerative medicine. Annu. Rev. Biomed. Eng. 16, 247–276.

Balusamy, B., Senthamizhan, A., Uyar, T., 2019. Design and development of electrospun nanofibers in regenerative medicine. In: Tekinay, A.B. (Ed.), Nanomaterials for Regenerative Medicine. Springer International Publishing, Cham, pp. 47–79, https://doi.org/10.1007/978-3-030-31202-2_2.

Bhang, S.H., Lim, J.S., Choi, C.Y., Kwon, Y.K., Kim, B.-S., 2007. The behavior of neural stem cells on biodegradable synthetic polymers. J. Biomater. Sci. Polym. Ed. 18, 223–239. https://doi.org/10.1163/156856207779116711.

Binan, L., Tendey, C., De Crescenzo, G., El Ayoubi, R., Ajji, A., Jolicoeur, M., 2014. Differentiation of neuronal stem cells into motor neurons using electrospun poly-l-lactic acid/gelatin scaffold. Biomaterials 35, 664–674. https://doi.org/10.1016/j.biomaterials.2013.09.097.

Bishop, E.S., Mostafa, S., Pakvasa, M., Luu, H.H., Lee, M.J., Wolf, J.M., Ameer, G.A., He, T.C., Reid, R.R., 2017. 3-D bioprinting technologies in tissue engineering and regenerative medicine: current and future trends. Genes Dis. https://doi.org/10.1016/j.gendis.2017.10.002.

Boland, T., Xu, T., Damon, B., Cui, X., 2006. Application of inkjet printing to tissue engineering. Biotechnol. J. https://doi.org/10.1002/biot.200600081.

Boles, M.A., Ling, D., Hyeon, T., Talapin, D.V., 2016. The surface science of nanocrystals. Nat. Mater. 15, 141–153. https://doi.org/10.1038/nmat4526.

Boyce, S.T., Lalley, A.L., 2018. Tissue engineering of skin and regenerative medicine for wound care. Burns & Trauma 6, 4. https://doi.org/10.1186/s41038-017-0103-y.

Bradshaw, M., Ho, D., Fear, M.W., Gelain, F., Wood, F.M., Iyer, K.S., 2014. Designer self-assembling hydrogel scaffolds can impact skin cell proliferation and migration. Sci. Rep. 4, 6903. https://doi.org/10.1038/srep06903.

Braghirolli, D.I., Steffens, D., Pranke, P., 2014. Electrospinning for regenerative medicine: a review of the main topics. Drug Discov. Today 19, 743–753. https://doi.org/10.1016/j.drudis.2014.03.024.

Breuer, C.K., Shin'oka, T., Tanel, R.E., Zund, G., Mooney, D.J., Ma, P.X., Miura, T., Colan, S., Langer, R., Mayer, J.E., Vacanti, J.P., 1996. Tissue engineering lamb heart valve leaflets. Biotechnol. Bioeng. 50, 562–567. https://doi.org/10.1002/(SICI)1097-0290(19960605)50:5<562::AID-BIT11>3.0.CO;2-L.

Brunt, K.R., Weisel, R.D., Li, R.-K., 2012. Stem cells and regenerative medicine—future perspectives. Can. J. Physiol. Pharmacol. 90, 327–335.

Budama-Kilinc, Y., 2018. Hydrogels in regenerative medicine. Burcu Özkan (Tran.), In: Cakir-Koc, R. (Ed.), Biomaterials in Regenerative Medicine. IntechOpen, Rijeka, https://doi.org/10.5772/intechopen.70409. Ch. 12.

Carvalho, C.R., Oliveira, J.M., Reis, R.L., 2019. Modern trends for peripheral nerve repair and regeneration: beyond the hollow nerve guidance conduit. Front. Bioeng. Biotechnol. 7, 337. https://doi.org/10.3389/fbioe.2019.00337.

Catoira, M.C., Fusaro, L., Di Francesco, D., Ramella, M., Boccafoschi, F., 2019. Overview of natural hydrogels for regenerative medicine applications. J. Mater. Sci. Mater. Med. 30, 115. https://doi.org/10.1007/s10856-019-6318-7.

Chan, B.P., Leong, K.W., 2008. Scaffolding in tissue engineering: general approaches and tissue-specific considerations. Eur. Spine J. 17 (Suppl 4), 467–479. https://doi.org/10.1007/s00586-008-0745-3.

Chang, R., Nam, J., Sun, W., 2008. Effects of dispensing pressure and nozzle diameter on cell survival from solid freeform fabrication-based direct cell writing. Tissue Eng. Part A 14, 41–48. https://doi.org/10.1089/ten.a.2007.0004.

Chen, Y.H., Cadman, J., Li, Q., 2010. Effect of scaffold architecture on tissue regeneration. In: IFMBE Proceedings. Springer, Berlin, Heidelberg, pp. 815–818, https://doi.org/10.1007/978-3-642-14515-5_207.

Chen, H., Clarkson, B.H., Sun, K., Mansfield, J.F., 2005. Self-assembly of synthetic hydroxyapatite nanorods into an enamel prism-like structure. J. Colloid Interface Sci. 288, 97–103. https://doi.org/10.1016/j.jcis.2005.02.064.

Chen, Y., Dong, W., Xiao, Y., Zhao, B., Hu, G., An, L., 2006. Preparation and bioactivity of human hair keratin-collagen sponge, a new type of dermal analogue. Nan Fang Yi Ke Da Xue Xue Bao 26, 131–138.

Chen, S.-L., Fu, R.-H., Liao, S.-F., Liu, S.-P., Lin, S.-Z., Wang, Y.-C., 2018. A PEG-based hydrogel for effective wound care management. Cell Transplant. 27, 275–284. https://doi.org/10.1177/0963689717749032.

Choi, M.H., Yi, S.B., Hwang, J.W., Yang, W.S., Lee, K.K., 1999. Treatment of bone and tendon-exposed wounds using-Terudermis. J. Korean Soc. Plast. Reconstr. Surg. 26, 491–497.

Cijun, S., Li, Y., Yang, W., Peng, S., 2020. Phosphonic acid coupling agent modification of HAP nanoparticles: interfacial effects in PLLA/HAP bone scaffold. Polymers 12.

Ciofani, G., Ricotti, L., Menciassi, A., Mattoli, V., 2011. Preparation, characterization and in vitro testing of poly (lactic-co-glycolic) acid/barium titanate nanoparticle composites for enhanced cellular proliferation. Biomed. Microdevices. https://doi.org/10.1007/s10544-010-9490-6.

Correia Carreira, S., Begum, R., Perriman, A.W., 2019. 3D bioprinting: the emergence of programmable biodesign. Adv. Healthc. Mater. https://doi.org/10.1002/adhm.201900554, 1900554.

Dai, C., Shih, S., Khachemoune, A., 2020. Skin substitutes for acute and chronic wound healing: an updated review. J. Dermatolog. Treat. 31, 639–648. https://doi.org/10.1080/09546634.2018.1530443.

De Witte, T.M., Wagner, A.M., Fratila-Apachitei, L.E., Zadpoor, A.A., Peppas, N.A., 2020. Immobilization of nanocarriers within a porous chitosan scaffold for the sustained delivery of growth factors in bone tissue engineering applications. J. Biomed. Mater. Res. A 108, 1122–1135. https://doi.org/10.1002/jbm.a.36887.

Deng, X.L., Xu, M.M., Li, D., Sui, G., Hu, X.Y., Yang, X.P., 2007. Electrospun PLLA/MWNTs/HA hybrid nanofiber scaffolds and their potential in dental tissue engineering. Key Eng. Mater. 330–332, 393–396. https://doi.org/10.4028/www.scientific.net/KEM.330-332.393.

Devillard, R., Pagès, E., Correa, M.M., Kériquel, V., Rémy, M., Kalisky, J.Ô., Ali, M., Guillotin, B., Guillemot, F., 2014. Cell patterning by laser-assisted bioprinting. In: Methods in Cell Biology. Academic Press Inc, pp. 159–174, https://doi.org/10.1016/B978-0-12-416742-1.00009-3.

Dias, J.R., Granja, P.L., Bártolo, P.J., 2016. Advances in electrospun skin substitutes. Prog. Mater. Sci. 84, 314–334. https://doi.org/10.1016/j.pmatsci.2016.09.006.

Ding, F., Wu, J., Yang, Y., Hu, W., Zhu, Q., Tang, X., Liu, J., Gu, X., 2010. Use of tissue-engineered nerve grafts consisting of a chitosan/poly (lactic-co-glycolic acid)-based scaffold included with bone marrow mesenchymal cells for bridging 50-mm dog sciatic nerve gaps. Tissue Eng. A 16, 3779–3790. https://doi.org/10.1089/ten.tea.2010.0299.

Dobson, J., 2008. Remote control of cellular behaviour with magnetic nanoparticles. Nat. Nanotechnol. 3, 139–143. https://doi.org/10.1038/nnano.2008.39.

Dolcimascolo, A., Calabrese, G., Conoci, S., Parenti, R., 2019. Innovative biomaterials for tissue engineering, in: biomaterial-supported tissue reconstruction or regeneration. IntechOpen. https://doi.org/10.5772/intechopen.83839.

Donnaloja, F., Jacchetti, E., Soncini, M., Raimondi, M.T., 2020. Natural and synthetic polymers for bone scaffolds optimization. Polymers 12. https://doi.org/10.3390/polym12040905.

Dragusin, D.-M., Van Vlierberghe, S., Dubruel, P., Dierick, M., Van Hoorebeke, L., Declercq, H.A., Cornelissen, M.M., Stancu, I.-C., 2012. Novel gelatin–PHEMA porous scaffolds for tissue engineering applications. Soft Matter 8, 9589–9602. https://doi.org/10.1039/C2SM25536G.

Ebrahimi-Barough, S., Hoveizi, E., Yazdankhah, M., Ai, J., Khakbiz, M., Faghihi, F., Tajerian, R., Bayat, N., 2017. Inhibitor of PI3K/Akt signaling pathway small molecule promotes motor neuron differentiation of human endometrial stem cells cultured on electrospun biocomposite polycaprolactone/collagen scaffolds. Mol. Neurobiol. 54, 2547–2554. https://doi.org/10.1007/s12035-016-9828-z.

Eftekhari, A., Dizaj, S.M., Sharifi, S., Salatin, S., Saadat, Y.R., Vahed, S.Z., Samiei, M., Ardalan, M., Rameshrad, M., Ahmadian, E., Cucchiarini, M., 2020. The use of nanomaterials in tissue engineering for cartilage regeneration; current approaches and future perspectives. Int. J. Mol. Sci. https://doi.org/10.3390/ijms21020536.

Eivazzadeh-Keihan, R., Bahojb Noruzi, E., Khanmohammadi Chenab, K., Jafari, A., Radinekiyan, F., Hashemi, S.M., Ahmadpour, F., Behboudi, A., Mosafer, J., Mokhtarzadeh, A., Maleki, A., Hamblin, M.R., 2020. Metal-based nanoparticles for bone tissue engineering. J. Tissue Eng. Regen. Med. https://doi.org/10.1002/term.3131.

Ellis-Behnke, R.G., Liang, Y.-X., You, S.-W., Tay, D.K.C., Zhang, S., So, K.-F., Schneider, G.E., 2006. Nano neuro knitting: peptide nanofiber scaffold for brain repair and axon regeneration with functional return of vision. Proc. Natl. Acad. Sci. U. S. A. 103, 5054. https://doi.org/10.1073/pnas.0600559103.

Engel, E., Michiardi, A., Navarro, M., Lacroix, D., Planell, J.A., 2008. Nanotechnology in regenerative medicine: the materials side. Trends Biotechnol. 26, 39–47. https://doi.org/10.1016/j.tibtech.2007.10.005.

Entekhabi, E., Haghbin Nazarpak, M., Moztarzadeh, F., Sadeghi, A., 2016. Design and manufacture of neural tissue engineering scaffolds using hyaluronic acid and polycaprolactone nanofibers with controlled porosity. Mater. Sci. Eng. C 69, 380–387. https://doi.org/10.1016/j.msec.2016.06.078.

Erol-Taygun, M., Zheng, K., Boccaccini, A.R., 2013. Nanoscale bioactive glasses in medical applications. Int. J. Appl. Glas. Sci. 4, 136–148. https://doi.org/10.1111/ijag.12029.
Evans, G.R.D., Brandt, K., Katz, S., Chauvin, P., Otto, L., Bogle, M., Wang, B., Meszlenyi, R.K., Lu, L., Mikos, A.G., Patrick, C.W., 2002. Bioactive poly(l-lactic acid) conduits seeded with Schwann cells for peripheral nerve regeneration. Biomaterials 23, 841–848. https://doi.org/10.1016/S0142-9612(01)00190-9.
Falanga, V., Faria, K., Bollenbach, T., 2014. Chapter 77—bioengineered skin constructs. In: Lanza, R., Langer, R., Vacanti, J. (Eds.), Principles of Tissue Engineering, Fourth ed. Academic Press, Boston, pp. 1619–1643, https://doi.org/10.1016/B978-0-12-398358-9.00077-X.
Flynn, L., Dalton, P.D., Shoichet, M.S., 2003. Fiber templating of poly(2-hydroxyethyl methacrylate) for neural tissue engineering. Biomaterials 24, 4265–4272. https://doi.org/10.1016/S0142-9612(03)00334-X.
Friedman, J.A., Windebank, A.J., Moore, M.J., Spinner, R.J., Currier, B.L., Yaszemski, M.J., 2002. Biodegradable polymer grafts for surgical repair of the injured spinal cord. Neurosurgery 51, 742–752. https://doi.org/10.1227/00006123-200209000-00024.
Gao, K., Jiang, X., 2006. Influence of particle size on transport of methotrexate across blood brain barrier by polysorbate 80-coated polybutylcyanoacrylate nanoparticles. Int. J. Pharm. 310, 213–219. https://doi.org/10.1016/j.ijpharm.2005.11.040.
Garfein, E., 2009. 2—skin replacement products and markets. In: Orgill, D., Blanco, C. (Eds.), Biomaterials for Treating Skin Loss. Woodhead Publishing, pp. 9–17, https://doi.org/10.1533/9781845695545.1.9.
Godier-furemont Amandine, F.G., et al., 2011. Composite scaffold provides a cell delivery platform for cadiovascular repair. PNAS 108, 7974–7979.
Grover, G.N., Rao, N., Christman, K.L., 2014. Myocardial matrix-polyethylene glycol hybrid hydrogels for tissue engineering. Nanotechnology 25. https://doi.org/10.1088/0957-4484/25/1/014011.
Guex, A.G., Puetzer, J.L., Armgarth, A., Littmann, E., Stavrinidou, E., Giannelis, E.P., Malliaras, G.G., Stevens, M.M., 2017. Highly porous scaffolds of PEDOT:PSS for bone tissue engineering. Acta Biomater. 62, 91–101. https://doi.org/10.1016/j.actbio.2017.08.045.
Guillotin, B., Souquet, A., Catros, S., Duocastella, M., Pippenger, B., Bellance, S., Bareille, R., Rémy, M., Bordenave, L., Amédée, J., Guillemot, F., 2010. Laser assisted bioprinting of engineered tissue with high cell density and microscale organization. Biomaterials 31, 7250–7256. https://doi.org/10.1016/j.biomaterials.2010.05.055.
Guo, J., Leung, K.K.G., Su, H., Yuan, Q., Wang, L., Chu, T.-H., Zhang, W., Pu, J.K.S., Ng, G.K.P., Wong, W.M., Dai, X., Wu, W., 2009. Self-assembling peptide nanofiber scaffold promotes the reconstruction of acutely injured brain. Nanomedicine 5, 345–351. https://doi.org/10.1016/j.nano.2008.12.001.
Gupta, V., Khan, Y., Berkland, C.J., Laurencin, C.T., Detamore, M.S., 2017. Microsphere-based scaffolds in regenerative engineering. Annu. Rev. Biomed. Eng. 19, 135–161. https://doi.org/10.1146/annurev-bioeng-071516-044712.
Gutiérrez-Hernández, J.M., Escobar-García, D.M., Escalante, A., Flores, H., González, F.J., Gatenholm, P., Toriz, G., 2017. In vitro evaluation of osteoblastic cells on bacterial cellulose modified with multi-walled carbon nanotubes as scaffold for bone regeneration. Mater. Sci. Eng. C 75, 445–453. https://doi.org/10.1016/j.msec.2017.02.074.
Hakobyan, D., Kerouredan, O., Remy, M., Dusserre, N., Medina, C., Devillard, R., Fricain, J.C., Oliveira, H., 2020. Laser-assisted bioprinting for bone repair. In: Methods in Molecular Biology. Humana Press Inc, pp. 135–144, https://doi.org/10.1007/978-1-0716-0520-2_8.
Han, J., Park, J., Kim, B.-S., 2015. Integration of mesenchymal stem cells with nanobiomaterials for the repair of myocardial infarction. Adv. Drug Deliv. Rev. 95, 15–28. https://doi.org/10.1016/j.addr.2015.09.002.

Han, D.-W., Sub Lee, M., Park, B.J., Kim, J.K., Park, J.-C., 2005. Enhanced neurite outgrowth of rat neural cortical cells on surface-modified films of poly(lactic-co-glycolic acid). Biotechnol. Lett. 27, 53–58. https://doi.org/10.1007/s10529-004-6585-2.

Harris, L.D., Kim, B.-S., Mooney, D.J., 1998. Open pore biodegradable matrices formed with gas foaming. J. Biomed. Mater. Res. 42, 396–402. https://doi.org/10.1002/(SICI)1097-4636(19981205)42:3<396::AID-JBM7>3.0.CO;2-E.

Haugen, H.J., Basu, P., Sukul, M., Mano, F., 2020. Injectable biomaterials for dental tissue regeneration. Int. J. Mol. Sci. 21.

Helary, C., Zarka, M., Giraud-Guille, M.M., 2012. Fibroblasts within concentrated collagen hydrogels favour chronic skin wound healing. J. Tissue Eng. Regen. Med. 6, 225–237. https://doi.org/10.1002/term.420.

Hickey, R.J., Pelling, A.E., 2019. Cellulose biomaterials for tissue engineering. Front. Bioeng. Biotechnol. 7, 45. https://doi.org/10.3389/fbioe.2019.00045.

Hong, L., Shen, M., Fang, J., Wang, Y., Bao, Z., Bu, S., Zhu, Y., 2018. Hyaluronic acid (HA)-based hydrogels for full-thickness wound repairing and skin regeneration. J. Mater. Sci. Mater. Med. 29, 150. https://doi.org/10.1007/s10856-018-6158-x.

Hosseinzade, M., Soflou, R.K., Valian, A., Nojehdehian, H., 2016. Physicochemical properties of MTA, CEM, hydroxyapatite and nano hydroxyapatite-chitosan dental cements. Biomed. Res. 27.

Huang, S., Lu, G., Wu, Y., Jirigala, E., Xu, Y., Ma, K., Fu, X., 2012. Mesenchymal stem cells delivered in a microsphere-based engineered skin contribute to cutaneous wound healing and sweat gland repair. J. Dermatol. Sci. 66, 29–36. https://doi.org/10.1016/j.jdermsci.2012.02.002.

Hutmacher, D.W., 2001. Scaffold design and fabrication technologies for engineering tissues—state of the art and future perspectives. J. Biomater. Sci. Polym. Ed. 12, 107–124. https://doi.org/10.1163/156856201744489.

In, K.S., Won, H.S., Sang, Y.L., Sang, H.L., Seong, J.H., Myung, C.L., Lee, S.J., 2009. Chitosan nano−/microfibrous double-layered membrane with rolled-up three-dimensional structures for chondrocyte cultivation. J. Biomed. Mater. Res. A 90, 595–602. https://doi.org/10.1002/jbm.a.32109.

Jahed, V., Vasheghani-Farahani, E., Bagheri, F., Zarrabi, A., Jensen, H.H., Larsen, K.L., 2020. Quantum dots-βcyclodextrin-histidine labeled human adipose stem cells-laden chitosan hydrogel for bone tissue engineering. Nanomedicine 27, 102217. https://doi.org/10.1016/j.nano.2020.102217.

Jaiswal, M., Gupta, A., Agrawal, A.K., Jassal, M., Dinda, A.K., Koul, V., 2013. Bi-layer composite dressing of gelatin nanofibrous mat and poly vinyl alcohol hydrogel for drug delivery and wound healing application: in-vitro and in-vivo studies. J. Biomed. Nanotechnol. 9, 1495–1508. https://doi.org/10.1166/jbn.2013.1643.

Jaklenec, A., Stamp, A., Deweerd, E., Sherwin, A., Langer, R., 2012. Progress in the tissue engineering and stem cell industry "are we there yet?". Tissue Eng. Part B Rev. 18, 155–166.

Jang, J., Park, H.J., Kim, S.W., Kim, H., Park, J.Y., Na, S.J., Kim, H.J., Park, M.N., Choi, S.H., Park, S.H., Kim, S.W., Kwon, S.M., Kim, P.J., Cho, D.W., 2017. 3D printed complex tissue construct using stem cell-laden decellularized extracellular matrix bioinks for cardiac repair. Biomaterials 112, 264–274. https://doi.org/10.1016/j.biomaterials.2016.10.026.

Jia, T., Chen, J., Feng, X., Chang, J., 2011. Symbolfabrication and characterization of chitosan/mesoporous bioactive glasses porous films. J. Clin. Rehab. Tissue Eng. Res. 15, 7877–7880.

Jiao, Y.-P., Cui, F.-Z., 2007. Surface modification of polyester biomaterials for tissue engineering. Biomed. Mater. 2, R24–R37. https://doi.org/10.1088/1748-6041/2/4/R02.

Jiao, J., Huang, J., Zhang, Z., 2019. Hydrogels based on chitosan in tissue regeneration: how do they work? A mini review. J. Appl. Polym. Sci. 136, 47235. https://doi.org/10.1002/app.47235.

Jing, X., Mi, H.-Y., Salick, M.R., Cordie, T., Crone, W.C., Peng, X.-F., Turng, L.-S., 2014. Morphology, mechanical properties, and shape memory effects of poly(lactic acid)/thermoplastic polyurethane blend scaffolds prepared by thermally induced phase separation. J. Cell. Plast. 50, 361–379. https://doi.org/10.1177/0021955X14525959.

Jinno, C., Morimoto, N., Ito, R., Sakamoto, M., Ogino, S., Taira, T., Suzuki, S., 2016. A comparison of conventional collagen sponge and collagen-gelatin sponge in wound healing. Biomed. Res. Int. 2016, 4567146. https://doi.org/10.1155/2016/4567146.

John, A.A., Subramanian, A.P., Vellayappan, M.V., Balaji, A., Mohandas, H., Jaganathan, S.K., 2015. Carbon nanotubes and graphene as emerging candidates in neuroregeneration and neurodrug delivery. Int. J. Nanomedicine 10, 4267–4277. https://doi.org/10.2147/IJN.S83777.

Jose, R.R., Rodriguez, M.J., Dixon, T.A., Omenetto, F., Kaplan, D.L., 2016. Evolution of bioinks and additive manufacturing technologies for 3D bioprinting. ACS Biomater Sci. Eng. https://doi.org/10.1021/acsbiomaterials.6b00088.

Kabiri, M., Oraee-Yazdani, S., Dodel, M., Hanaee-Ahvaz, H., Soudi, S., Seyedjafari, E., Salehi, M., Soleimani, M., 2015. Cytocompatibility of a conductive nanofibrous carbon nanotube/poly (L-lactic acid) composite scaffold intended for nerve tissue engineering. EXCLI J. 14, 851–860. https://doi.org/10.17179/excli2015-282.

Kačarević, Ž.P., Rider, P.M., Alkildani, S., Retnasingh, S., Smeets, R., Jung, O., Ivanišević, Z., Barbeck, M., 2018. An introduction to 3D bioprinting: possibilities, challenges and future aspects. Materials. https://doi.org/10.3390/ma11112199.

Kaczmarek-Pawelska, A., Pereira, L., 2020. Alginate-based hydrogels in regenerative medicine. In: Alginates. IntechOpen, Rijeka, https://doi.org/10.5772/intechopen.88258. Ch. 5.

Kallis, P.J., Friedman, A.J., Lev-Tov, H., 2018. A guide to tissue-engineered skin substitutes. J. Drugs Dermatol. 17, 57–64.

Kang, S.W., La, W.G., Kim, B.S., 2009. Open macroporous poly(lactic-co-glycolic acid) microspheres as an injectable scaffold for cartilage tissue engineering. J. Biomater. Sci. Polym. Ed. 20, 399–409. https://doi.org/10.1163/156856209X412236.

KarbalaeiMahdi, A., Shahrousvand, M., Javadi, H.R., Ghollasi, M., Norouz, F., Kamali, M., Salimi, A., 2017. Neural differentiation of human induced pluripotent stem cells on polycaprolactone/gelatin bi-electrospun nanofibers. Mater. Sci. Eng. C 78, 1195–1202. https://doi.org/10.1016/j.msec.2017.04.083.

Kargozar, S., Mozafari, M., Hamzehlou, S., Baino, F., 2019. Using bioactive glasses in the management of burns. Front. Bioeng. Biotechnol. 7, 62. https://doi.org/10.3389/fbioe.2019.00062.

Keriquel, V., Oliveira, H., Rémy, M., Ziane, S., Delmond, S., Rousseau, B., Rey, S., Catros, S., Amédée, J., Guillemot, F., Fricain, J.C., 2017. In situ printing of mesenchymal stromal cells, by laser-assisted bioprinting, for in vivo bone regeneration applications. Sci. Rep. 7, 1–10. https://doi.org/10.1038/s41598-017-01914-x.

Khan, S., Garg, M., Chockalingam, S., Gopinath, P., Kundu, P.P., 2020. TiO2 doped chitosan/poly (vinyl alcohol) nanocomposite film with enhanced mechanical properties for application in bone tissue regeneration. Int. J. Biol. Macromol. https://doi.org/10.1016/j.ijbiomac.2019.11.246. Elsevier B.V.

Khorasani, M.T., Mirzadeh, H., Irani, S., 2008. Plasma surface modification of poly (l-lactic acid) and poly (lactic-co-glycolic acid) films for improvement of nerve cells adhesion. Radiat. Phys. Chem. 77, 280–287. https://doi.org/10.1016/j.radphyschem.2007.05.013.

Khoroushi, M., Foroughi, M.R., Karbasi, S., Hashemibeni, B., Khademi, A.A., 2018. Effect of Polyhydroxybutyrate/chitosan/bioglass nanofiber scaffold on proliferation and differentiation of stem cells from human exfoliated deciduous teeth into odontoblast-like cells. Mater. Sci. Eng. C 89, 128–139. https://doi.org/10.1016/j.msec.2018.03.028.

Khunmanee, S., Jeong, Y., Park, H., 2017. Crosslinking method of hyaluronic-based hydrogel for biomedical applications. J. Tissue Eng. 8. https://doi.org/10.1177/2041731417726464, 2041731417726464.

Kim, D.H., Kim, P., Song, I., Cha, J.M., Lee, S.H., Kim, B., Suh, K.Y., 2006. Guided three-dimensional growth of functional cardiomyocytes on polyethylene glycol nanostructures. Langmuir 22, 5419–5426. https://doi.org/10.1021/la060283u.

Kim, J.E., Lee, J.H., Kim, S.H., Jung, Y., 2017. Skin regeneration with self-assembled peptide hydrogels conjugated with substance P in a diabetic rat model. Tissue Eng. A 24, 21–33. https://doi.org/10.1089/ten.tea.2016.0517.

Kishen, A., 2015. Nanotechnology in Endodontics: Current and Potential Clinical Applications. Nanotechnology in Endodontics: Current and Potential Clinical Applications, pp. 1–199, https://doi.org/10.1007/978-3-319-13575-5.

Klebe, R.J., 1988. Cytoscribing: a method for micropositioning cells and the construction of two- and three-dimensional synthetic tissues. Exp. Cell Res. 179, 362–373. https://doi.org/10.1016/0014-4827(88)90275-3.

Kolios, G., Moodley, Y., 2013. Introduction to stem cells and regenerative medicine. Respiration 85, 3–10.

Koutsopoulos, S., 2012. Molecular fabrications of smart nanobiomaterials and applications in personalized medicine. Adv. Drug Deliv. Rev. 64, 1459–1476. https://doi.org/10.1016/j.addr.2012.08.002.

Kumar, H., Kim, K., 2020. Stereolithography 3D bioprinting. In: Methods in Molecular Biology. Humana press Inc, pp. 93–108, https://doi.org/10.1007/978-1-0716-0520-2_6.

Kumar, S., Nehra, M., Kedia, D., Dilbaghi, N., Tankeshwar, K., Kim, K.H., 2020. Nanotechnology-based biomaterials for orthopaedic applications: recent advances and future prospects. Mater. Sci. Eng. C. https://doi.org/10.1016/j.msec.2019.110154. Elsevier.

Lam, T., Dehne, T., Krüger, J.P., Hondke, S., Endres, M., Thomas, A., Lauster, R., Sittinger, M., Kloke, L., 2019. Photopolymerizable gelatin and hyaluronic acid for stereolithographic 3D bioprinting of tissue-engineered cartilage. J. Biomed. Mater. Res. B Appl. Biomater. 107, 2649–2657. https://doi.org/10.1002/jbm.b.34354.

Lee, J.Y., Bashur, C.A., Goldstein, A.S., Schmidt, C.E., 2009. Polypyrrole-coated electrospun PLGA nanofibers for neural tissue applications. Biomaterials 30, 4325–4335. https://doi.org/10.1016/j.biomaterials.2009.04.042.

Lee, P.Y., Cobain, E., Huard, J., Huang, L., 2007. Thermosensitive hydrogel PEG–PLGA–PEG enhances engraftment of muscle-derived stem cells and promotes healing in diabetic wound. Mol. Ther. 15, 1189–1194. https://doi.org/10.1038/sj.mt.6300156.

Levengood, S.K.L., Zhang, M., 2014. Chitosan-based scaffolds for bone tissue engineering. J. Mater. Chem. B 2, 3161–3184. https://doi.org/10.1039/C4TB00027G.

Lewis, R.A., et al., 2016. Biomaterials in myocardial tissue engineering. J. Tissue Eng. Regen. Med. 10, 11–28.

Li, X., Hou, S., Feng, X., Yu, Y., Ma, J., Li, L., 2009. Patterning of neural stem cells on poly(-lactic-co-glycolic acid) film modified by hydrophobin. Colloids Surf. B Biointerfaces 74, 370–374. https://doi.org/10.1016/j.colsurfb.2009.07.039.

Li, H., Wu, Z., Zhou, Y., Chang, J., 2019. 8—bioglass for skin regeneration. In: García-Gareta, E. (Ed.), Biomaterials for Skin Repair and Regeneration. Woodhead Publishing, pp. 225–250, https://doi.org/10.1016/B978-0-08-102546-8.00008-X.

Liao, C.-J., Chen, C.-F., Chen, J.-H., Chiang, S.-F., Lin, Y.-J., Chang, K.-Y., 2002. Fabrication of porous biodegradable polymer scaffolds using a solvent merging/particulate leaching method. J. Biomed. Mater. Res. 59, 676–681. https://doi.org/10.1002/jbm.10030.

Liao, S., Wang, W., Uo, M., Ohkawa, S., Akasaka, T., Tamura, K., Cui, F., Watari, F., 2005. A three-layered nano-carbonated hydroxyapatite/collagen/PLGA composite membrane for guided tissue regeneration. Biomaterials 26, 7564–7571. https://doi.org/10.1016/j.biomaterials.2005.05.050.

Liu, H., Wang, C., Li, C., Qin, Y., Wang, Z., Yang, F., Li, Z., Wang, J., 2018. A functional chitosan-based hydrogel as a wound dressing and drug delivery system in the treatment of wound healing. RSC Adv. 8, 7533–7549. https://doi.org/10.1039/C7RA13510F.

Liu, Y., Wang, S., Zhang, R., 2017. Composite poly(lactic acid)/chitosan nanofibrous scaffolds for cardiac tissue engineering. Int. J. Biol. Macromol. 103, 1130–1137. https://doi.org/10.1016/j.ijbiomac.2017.05.101.

Liu, Y., Yu, Q., Chang, J., Wu, C., 2019. Nanobiomaterials: from 0D to 3D for tumor therapy and tissue regeneration. Nanoscale 11, 13678–13708. https://doi.org/10.1039/c9nr02955a.

Lu, T., Li, Y., Chen, T., 2013. Techniques for fabrication and construction of three-dimensional scaffolds for tissue engineering. Int. J. Nanomedicine 8, 337–350. https://doi.org/10.2147/IJN.S38635.

Mahnama, H., Dadbin, S., Frounchi, M., Rajabi, S., 2017. Preparation of biodegradable gelatin/PVA porous scaffolds for skin regeneration. Artif. Cells Nanomed. Biotechnol. 45, 928–935. https://doi.org/10.1080/21691401.2016.1193025.

Mao, A.S., Mooney, D.J., 2015. Regenerative medicine: current therapies and future directions. PNAS 112, 14452–14459. https://doi.org/10.1073/pnas.1508520112.

Markides, H., Rotherham, M., El Haj, A.J., 2012. Biocompatibility and toxicity of magnetic nanoparticles in regenerative medicine (WWW document). J. Nanomater. https://doi.org/10.1155/2012/614094.

Martinelli, V., Cellot, G., Toma, F.M., Long, C.S., Caldwell, J.H., Zentilin, L., Giacca, M., Turco, A., Prato, M., Ballerini, L., Mestroni, L., 2012. Carbon nanotubes promote growth and spontaneous electrical activity in cultured cardiac myocytes. Nano Lett. 12, 1831–1838. https://doi.org/10.1021/nl204064s.

Martinelli, V., Cellot, G., Toma, F.M., Long, C.S., Caldwell, J.H., Zentilin, L., Giacca, M., Turco, A., Prato, M., Ballerini, L., Mestroni, L., 2013. Carbon nanotubes instruct physiological growth and functionally mature syncytia: nongenetic engineering of cardiac myocytes. ACS Nano 7, 5746–5756. https://doi.org/10.1021/nn4002193.

Matai, I., Kaur, G., Seyedsalehi, A., McClinton, A., Laurencin, C.T., 2020. Progress in 3D bioprinting technology for tissue/organ regenerative engineering. Biomaterials. https://doi.org/10.1016/j.biomaterials.2019.119536.

Melchels, F.P.W., Domingos, M.A.N., Klein, T.J., Malda, J., Bartolo, P.J., Hutmacher, D.W., 2012. Additive manufacturing of tissues and organs. Prog. Polym. Sci. https://doi.org/10.1016/j.progpolymsci.2011.11.007.

Mendelson, A., Frenette, P.S., 2014. Hematopoietic stem cell niche maintenance during homeostasis and regeneration. Nat. Med. 20, 833.

Meyer, R.A., Green, J.J., 2016. Shaping the future of nanomedicine: anisotropy in polymeric nanoparticle design. Wiley Interdiscip. Rev. Nanomed. Nanobiotechnol. 8, 191–207. https://doi.org/10.1002/wnan.1348.

Miller, D.C., Thapa, A., Haberstroh, K.M., Webster, T.J., 2004. Endothelial and vascular smooth muscle cell function on poly(lactic-co-glycolic acid) with nano-structured surface features. Biomaterials 25, 53–61. https://doi.org/10.1016/S0142-9612(03)00471-X.

Mitragotri, S., Lahann, J., 2009. Physical approaches to biomaterial design. Nat. Mater. 8, 15–23. https://doi.org/10.1038/nmat2344.

Mohamed, A., Xing, M.M., 2012. Nanomaterials and nanotechnology for skin tissue engineering. Int. J. Burns Trauma 2, 29–41.

Mohandesnezhad, S., Alizadeh, E., Pilehvar-Soltanahmadi, Y., 2020. In Vitro Evaluation of Novel Zeolite-Hydroxyapatite Blended Scaffold for Dental Tissue Engineering.

Mortimer, C.J., 2018. Electrospinning of functional nanofibers for regenerative medicine: from bench to commercial scale. In: Widdowson, J.P. (Ed.), Novel Aspects of Nanofibers. IntechOpen, Rijeka, https://doi.org/10.5772/intechopen.73677. Ch. 6.

Mota, J., Yu, N., Caridade, S.G., Luz, G.M., Gomes, M.E., Reis, R.L., Jansen, J.A., Frank Walboomers, X., Mano, J.F., 2012. Chitosan/bioactive glass nanoparticle composite membranes for periodontal regeneration. Acta Biomater. 8, 4173–4180. https://doi.org/10.1016/j.actbio.2012.06.040.

Mousa, H.M., Hussein, K.H., Sayed, M.M., El-Aassar, M.R., Mohamed, I.M.A., Kwak, H.H., Woo, H.M., Abdal-hay, A., 2020. Development of biocompatible tri-layered nanofibers patches with endothelial cells for cardiac tissue engineering. Eur. Polym. J. 129, 109630. https://doi.org/10.1016/j.eurpolymj.2020.109630.

Mulholland, E.J., 2020. Electrospun biomaterials in the treatment and prevention of scars in skin wound healing. Front. Bioeng. Biotechnol. 8, 481. https://doi.org/10.3389/fbioe.2020.00481.

Nguyen, M.M., Gianneschi, N.C., Christman, K.L., 2015. Developing injectable nanomaterials to repair the heart current opinion in biotechnology, (34) nanobiotechnology 2015. Curr. Opin. Biotechnol. 34, 225–231. https://doi.org/10.1586/14737175.2015.1028369.Focused.

O'Brien, F.J., 2011. Biomaterials & scaffolds for tissue engineering. Mater. Today 14, 88–95. https://doi.org/10.1016/S1369-7021(11)70058-X.

O'Brien, C.M., Holmes, B., Faucett, S., Zhang, L.G., 2015. Three-dimensional printing of nanomaterial scaffolds for complex tissue regeneration. Tissue Eng. Part B Rev. 21, 103–114. https://doi.org/10.1089/ten.teb.2014.0168.

Osathanon, T., Linnes, M.L., Rajachar, R.M., Ratner, B.D., Somerman, M.J., Giachelli, C.M., 2008. Microporous nanofibrous fibrin-based scaffolds for bone tissue engineering. Biomaterials 29, 4091–4099. https://doi.org/10.1016/j.biomaterials.2008.06.030.

Ozbolat, I.T., Hospodiuk, M., 2016. Current advances and future perspectives in extrusion-based bioprinting. Biomaterials. https://doi.org/10.1016/j.biomaterials.2015.10.076.

Park, J., Kim, B., Han, J., Oh, J., Park, S., Ryu, S., Jung, S., Shin, J.-Y., Lee, B.S., Hong, B.H., Choi, D., Kim, B.-S., 2015a. Graphene oxide flakes as a cellular adhesive: prevention of reactive oxygen species mediated death of implanted cells for cardiac repair. ACS Nano 9, 4987–4999. https://doi.org/10.1021/nn507149w.

Park, J., Kim, Y.S., Ryu, S., Kang, W.S., Park, S., Han, J., Jeong, H.C., Hong, B.H., Ahn, Y., Kim, B.-S., 2015b. Graphene potentiates the myocardial repair efficacy of mesenchymal stem cells by stimulating the expression of Angiogenic growth factors and gap junction protein. Adv. Funct. Mater. 25, 2590–2600. https://doi.org/10.1002/adfm.201500365.

Pina, S., Ribeiro, V.P., Marques, C.F., Maia, F.R., Silva, T.H., Reis, R.L., Oliveira, J.M., 2019. Regenerative medicine applications. Materials 12.

Prasad, A., Sankar, M.R., Katiyar, V., 2017. State of art on solvent casting particulate leaching method for orthopedic scaffolds fabrication. Mater. Today Proc. 4, 898–907. https://doi.org/10.1016/j.matpr.2017.01.101.

Pugliese, R., Gelain, F., 2017. Peptidic biomaterials: from self-assembling to regenerative medicine. Trends Biotechnol. 35, 145–158. https://doi.org/10.1016/j.tibtech.2016.09.004.

Qu, H., Fu, H., Han, Z., Sun, Y., 2019. Biomaterials for bone tissue engineering scaffolds: a review. RSC Adv. 9, 26252–26262. https://doi.org/10.1039/C9RA05214C.

Rana, D., Ramasamy, K., Leena, M., Jiménez, C., Campos, J., Ibarra, P., Haidar, Z.S., Ramalingam, M., 2016. Surface functionalization of nanobiomaterials for application in stem cell culture, tissue engineering, and regenerative medicine. Biotechnol. Prog. 32, 554–567. https://doi.org/10.1002/btpr.2262.

Research, C. for B.E, 2019a. ALLOCORD (HPC Cord Blood). FDA.

Research, C. for B.E, 2019b. CLEVECORD (HPC Cord Blood). FDA.

Research, C. for B.E, 2019c. HPC, Cord Blood. FDA.

Research, C. for B.E, 2019d. DUCORD (HPC Cord Blood). FDA.

Research, C. for B.E, 2019e. GINTUIT (Allogeneic Cultured Keratinocytes and Fibroblasts in Bovine Collagen). FDA.

Research, C. for B.E, 2019f. HEMACORD (HPC, Cord Blood). FDA.

Research, C. for B.E, 2019g. LAVIV (Azficel-T). FDA.

Research, C. for B.E, 2019h. IMLYGIC (talimogene laherparepvec). FDA.

Research, C. for B.E, 2019i. KYMRIAH (tisagenlecleucel). FDA.

Research, C. for B.E, 2019j. MACI (Autologous Cultured Chondrocytes on a Porcine Collagen Membrane). FDA.

Research, C. for B.E, 2019k. PROVENGE (sipuleucel-T). FDA.

Research, C. for B.E, 2020.YESCARTA (axicabtagene ciloleucel). FDA.

Reshma, J., Khan, A., 2020. Bioactive *Phoenix dactylifera* seeds incorporated chitosan/hydroxyapatite nanoconjugate for prospective bone tissue engineering applications: a bio-synergistic approach. Mater. Sci. Eng. C 109.

Rezwan, K., Chen, Q.Z., Blaker, J.J., Boccaccini, A.R., 2006. Biodegradable and bioactive porous polymer/inorganic composite scaffolds for bone tissue engineering. Biomaterials 27, 3413–3431. https://doi.org/10.1016/j.biomaterials.2006.01.039.

Ribeiro-Resende, V.T., Koenig, B., Nichterwitz, S., Oberhoffner, S., Schlosshauer, B., 2009. Strategies for inducing the formation of bands of Büngner in peripheral nerve regeneration. Biomaterials 30, 5251–5259. https://doi.org/10.1016/j.biomaterials.2009.07.007.

Richards, D.J., Tan, Y., Coyle, R., Li, Y., Xu, R., Yeung, N., Parker, A., Menick, D.R., Tian, B., Mei, Y., 2016. Nanowires and electrical stimulation synergistically improve functions of hiPSC cardiac spheroids. Nano Lett. 16, 4670–4678. https://doi.org/10.1021/acs.nanolett.6b02093.

Ringe, J., Kaps, C., Burmester, G.-R., Sittinger, M., 2002. Stem cells for regenerative medicine: advances in the engineering of tissues and organs. Naturwissenschaften 89, 338–351.

Rnjak-Kovacina, J., Wray, L.S., Burke, K.A., Torregrosa, T., Golinski, J.M., Huang, W., Kaplan, D.L., 2015. Lyophilized silk sponges: a versatile biomaterial platform for soft tissue engineering. ACS Biomater Sci. Eng. 1, 260–270. https://doi.org/10.1021/ab500149p.

Ruggiero, F., Netti, P.A., Torino, E., 2015. Experimental investigation and thermodynamic assessment of phase equilibria in the PLLA/Dioxane/water ternary system for applications in the biomedical field. Langmuir 31, 13003–13010. https://doi.org/10.1021/acs.langmuir.5b02460.

Ruhé, P.Q., Hedberg, E.L., Padron, N.T., Spauwen, P.H.M., Jansen, J.A., Mikos, A.G., 2005. Biocompatibility and degradation of poly(DL-lactic-co-glycolic acid)/calcium phosphate cement composites. J. Biomed. Mater. Res. A 74, 533–544. https://doi.org/10.1002/jbm.a.30341.

Ryu, G.H., Yang, W.-S., Roh, H.-W., Lee, I.-S., Kim, J.K., Lee, G.H., Lee, D.H., Park, B.J., Lee, M.S., Park, J.-C., 2005. Plasma surface modification of poly (d,l-lactic-co-glycolic acid) (65/35) film for tissue engineering. In: Surface and Coatings Technology, Asian-European International Conference on Plasma Surface Engineering 2003 193, pp. 60–64, https://doi.org/10.1016/j.surfcoat.2004.07.062.

Sahoo, N.G., Pan, Y.Z., Li, L., He, C.B., 2013. Nanocomposites for bone tissue regeneration. Nanomedicine (Lond.) 8, 639–653. https://doi.org/10.2217/nnm.13.44.

Salerno, A., Domingo, C., 2015. Pore structure properties of scaffolds constituted by aggregated microparticles of PCL and PCL-HA processed by phase separation. J. Porous. Mater. 22, 425–435. https://doi.org/10.1007/s10934-015-9911-2.

Sanchez-Casanova, S., Martin-Saavedra, F.M., Escudero-Duch, C., Falguera Uceda, M.I., Prieto, M., Arruebo, M., Acebo, P., Fabiilli, M.L., Franceschi, R.T., Vilaboa, N., 2020. Local delivery of bone morphogenetic protein-2 from near infrared-responsive hydrogels for bone tissue regeneration. Biomaterials 241, 119909. https://doi.org/10.1016/j.biomaterials.2020.119909.

Santoro, M., Shah, S.R., Walker, J.L., Mikos, A.G., 2016. Poly(lactic acid) nanofibrous scaffolds for tissue engineering. Adv. Drug Deliv. Rev. 107, 206–212. https://doi.org/10.1016/j.addr.2016.04.019.

Santos, D., Silva, D.M., Gomes, P.S., Fernandes, M.H., Santos, J.D., Sencadas, V., 2017. Multifunctional PLLA-ceramic fiber membranes for bone regeneration applications. J. Colloid Interface Sci. 504, 101–110. https://doi.org/10.1016/j.jcis.2017.05.032.

Saravanan, S., Leena, R.S., Selvamurugan, N., 2016. Chitosan based biocomposite scaffolds for bone tissue engineering. Int. J. Biol. Macromol. 93, 1354–1365. https://doi.org/10.1016/j.ijbiomac.2016.01.112.

Sayin, E., Baran, E.T., Hasirci, V., 2014. Protein-based materials in load-bearing tissue-engineering applications. Regen. Med. 9, 687–701. https://doi.org/10.2217/rme.14.52.

Schreiber, A., Witte, F., 2017. 13—immune response to nanobiomaterials. In: Razavi, M., Thakor, A. (Eds.), Nanobiomaterials Science, Development and Evaluation. Woodhead Publishing, pp. 249–260, https://doi.org/10.1016/B978-0-08-100963-5.00013-6.

Severs, N.J., Bruce, A.F., Dupont, E., Rothery, S., 2008. Remodelling of gap junctions and connexin expression in diseased myocardium. Cardiovasc. Res. 80, 9–19. https://doi.org/10.1093/cvr/cvn133.

Shevchenko, R.V., James, S.L., James, S.E., 2010. A review of tissue-engineered skin bioconstructs available for skin reconstruction. J. R. Soc. Interface 7, 229–258. https://doi.org/10.1098/rsif.2009.0403.

Shih, Y.-R.V., Chen, C.-N., Tsai, S.-W., Wang, Y.J., Lee, O.K., 2006. Growth of mesenchymal stem cells on electrospun type I collagen nanofibers. Stem Cells 24, 2391–2397. https://doi.org/10.1634/stemcells.2006-0253.

Shimizu, K., Ito, A., Lee, J.-K., Yoshida, T., Miwa, K., Ishiguro, H., Numaguchi, Y., Murohara, T., Kodama, I., Honda, H., 2007. Construction of multi-layered cardiomyocyte sheets using magnetite nanoparticles and magnetic force. Biotechnol. Bioeng. 96, 803–809. https://doi.org/10.1002/bit.21094.

Shimizu, M., Kobayashi, Y., Mizoguchi, T., Nakamura, H., Kawahara, I., Narita, N., Usui, Y., Aoki, K., Hara, K., Haniu, H., Ogihara, N., Ishigaki, N., Nakamura, K., Kato, H., Kawakubo, M., Dohi, Y., Taruta, S., Kim, Y.A., Endo, M., Ozawa, H., Udagawa, N., Takahashi, N., Saito, N., 2012. Carbon nanotubes induce bone calcification by bidirectional interaction with osteoblasts. Adv. Mater. 24, 2176–2185. https://doi.org/10.1002/adma.201103832.

Shin, S.R., Aghaei-Ghareh-Bolagh, B., Dang, T.T., Topkaya, S.N., Gao, X., Yang, S.Y., Jung, S.M., Oh, J.H., Dokmeci, M.R., Tang, X.S., Khademhosseini, A., 2013a. Cell-laden microengineered and mechanically tunable hybrid hydrogels of gelatin and graphene oxide. Adv. Mater. 25, 6385–6391. https://doi.org/10.1002/adma.201301082.

Shin, S.R., Jung, S.M., Zalabany, M., Kim, K., Zorlutuna, P., Kim, S.B., Nikkhah, M., Khabiry, M., Azize, M., Kong, J., Wan, K.-T., Palacios, T., Dokmeci, M.R., Bae, H., Tang, X.S., Khademhosseini, A., 2013b. Carbon-nanotube-embedded hydrogel sheets for engineering cardiac constructs and bioactuators. ACS Nano 7, 2369–2380. https://doi.org/10.1021/nn305559j.

Sieminski, A.L., Was, A.S., Kim, G., Gong, H., Kamm, R.D., 2007. The stiffness of three-dimensional ionic self-assembling peptide gels affects the extent of capillary-like network formation. Cell Biochem. Biophys. 49, 73–83. https://doi.org/10.1007/s12013-007-0046-1.

da Silva, L.P., Reis, R.L., Correlo, V.M., Marques, A.P., 2019. Hydrogel-based strategies to advance therapies for chronic skin wounds. Annu. Rev. Biomed. Eng. 21, 145–169. https://doi.org/10.1146/annurev-bioeng-060418-052422.

Silvestri, A., Sartori, S., Boffito, M., Mattu, C., Di Rienzo, A.M., Boccafoschi, F., Ciardelli, G., 2014. Biomimetic myocardial patches fabricated with poly(ε-caprolactone) and polyethylene glycol-based polyurethanes. J. Biomed. Mater. Res. B Appl. Biomater. 102, 1002–1013. https://doi.org/10.1002/jbm.b.33081.

Solanki, A., Kim, J.D., Lee, K.-B., 2008. Nanotechnology for regenerative medicine: nanomaterials for stem cell imaging. Nanomedicine (Lond) 3, 567–578.

Sonavane, G., Tomoda, K., Makino, K., 2008. Biodistribution of colloidal gold nanoparticles after intravenous administration: effect of particle size. Colloids Surf. B Biointerfaces 66, 274–280. https://doi.org/10.1016/j.colsurfb.2008.07.004.

Still, J., Glat, P., Silverstein, P., Griswold, J., Mozingo, D., 2003. The use of a collagen sponge/living cell composite material to treat donor sites in burn patients. Burns 29, 837–841. https://doi.org/10.1016/S0305-4179(03)00164-5.

Stone II, R., Wall, J.T., Natesan, S., Christy, R.J., 2018. PEG-plasma hydrogels increase epithelialization using a human ex vivo skin model. Int. J. Mol. Sci. 19, 3156. https://doi.org/10.3390/ijms19103156.

Stout, D.A., Basu, B., Webster, T.J., 2011. Poly(lactic-co-glycolic acid): carbon nanofiber composites for myocardial tissue engineering applications. Acta Biomater. 7, 3101–3112. https://doi.org/10.1016/j.actbio.2011.04.028.

Sun, J., Tan, H., 2013. Alginate-based biomaterials for regenerative medicine applications. Materials (Basel) 6, 1285–1309. https://doi.org/10.3390/ma6041285.

Sun, G., Zhang, X., Shen, Y.-I., Sebastian, R., Dickinson, L.E., Fox-Talbot, K., Reinblatt, M., Steenbergen, C., Harmon, J.W., Gerecht, S., 2011. Dextran hydrogel scaffolds enhance angiogenic responses and promote complete skin regeneration during burn wound healing. Proc. Natl. Acad. Sci. U. S. A. 108, 20976–20981. https://doi.org/10.1073/pnas.1115973108.

Suzuki, S., Kawai, K., Ashoori, F., Morimoto, N., Nishimura, Y., Ikada, Y., 2000. Long-term follow-up study of artificial dermis composed of outer silicone layer and inner collagen sponge. Br. J. Plast. Surg. 53, 659–666. https://doi.org/10.1054/bjps.2000.3426.

Thanh, D.T.M., Trang, P.T.T., Thom, N.T., Phuong, N.T., Nam, P.T., Trang, N.T.T., Seo-Park, J., Hoang, T., 2016. Effects of porogen on structure and properties of poly lactic acid/hydroxyapatite nanocomposites (PLA/HAp). J. Nanosci. Nanotechnol. 16, 9450–9459. https://doi.org/10.1166/jnn.2016.12032.

Thomas, V., Dean, D.R., Vohra, Y.K., 2006. Nanostructured biomaterials for regenerative medicine. Curr. Nanosci. 2.

Thomson, R.C., Yaszemski, M.J., Powers, J.M., Mikos, A.G., 1998. Hydroxyapatite fiber reinforced poly(α-hydroxy ester) foams for bone regeneration. Biomaterials 19, 1935–1943. https://doi.org/10.1016/S0142-9612(98)00097-0.

Thorwarth, M., Schultze-Mosgau, S., Kessler, P., Wiltfang, J., Schlegel, K.A., 2005. Bone regeneration in osseous defects using a resorbable nanoparticular hydroxyapatite. J. Oral Maxillofac. Surg. 63, 1626–1633. https://doi.org/10.1016/j.joms.2005.06.010.

Tillman, B.W., Yazdani, S.K., Lee, S.J., Geary, R.L., Atala, A., Yoo, J.J., 2009. The in vivo stability of electrospun polycaprolactone-collagen scaffolds in vascular reconstruction. Biomaterials 30, 583–588. https://doi.org/10.1016/j.biomaterials.2008.10.006.

Trujillo, S., Gonzalez-Garcia, C., Rico, P., Reid, A., Windmill, J., Dalby, M.J., Salmeron-Sanchez, M., 2020. Engineered 3D hydrogels with full-length fibronectin that sequester and present growth factors. Biomaterials 252, 120104. https://doi.org/10.1016/j.biomaterials.2020.120104.

Tsao, C.-T., Leung, M., Chang, J.Y.-F., Zhang, M., 2014. A simple material model to generate epidermal and dermal layers in vitro for skin regeneration. J. Mater. Chem. B 2, 5256–5264. https://doi.org/10.1039/C4TB00614C.

Vacanti, J.P., Otte, J.-B., Wertheim, J.A., 2014. Introduction: regenerative medicine and solid organ transplantation from a historical perspective. In: Regenerative Medicine Applications in Organ Transplantation. Elsevier, pp. 1–15.

Van Duong, H., Chau, T.T.L., Dang, N.T.T., Van Nguyen, D., Le, S.L., Ho, T.S., Vu, T.P., Van Tran, T.T., Nguyen, T.D., 2018. Self-aggregation of water-dispersible nanocollagen helices. Biomater. Sci. 6, 651–660. https://doi.org/10.1039/c7bm01141e.

Vatankhah, E., Semnani, D., Prabhakaran, M.P., Tadayon, M., Razavi, S., Ramakrishna, S., 2014. Artificial neural network for modeling the elastic modulus of electrospun polycaprolactone/gelatin scaffolds. Acta Biomater. 10, 709–721. https://doi.org/10.1016/j.actbio.2013.09.015.

Verma, S., Domb, A.J., Kumar, N., 2011. Nanomaterials for regenerative medicine. Nanomedicine 6, 157–181.

Vicentini, N., Gatti, T., Salice, P., Scapin, G., Marega, C., Filippini, F., Menna, E., 2015. Covalent functionalization enables good dispersion and anisotropic orientation of multi-walled carbon nanotubes in a poly(l-lactic acid) electrospun nanofibrous matrix boosting neuronal differentiation. Carbon 95, 725–730. https://doi.org/10.1016/j.carbon.2015.08.094.

Walmsley, G.G., McArdle, A., Tevlin, R., Momeni, A., Atashroo, D., Hu, M.S., Feroze, A.H., Wong, V.W., Lorenz, P.H., Longaker, M.T., Wan, D.C., 2015. Nanotechnology in bone tissue engineering. Nanomedicine 11, 1253–1263. https://doi.org/10.1016/j.nano.2015.02.013.

Wang, S., Guan, S., Wang, J., Liu, H., Liu, T., Ma, X., Cui, Z., 2017. Fabrication and characterization of conductive poly (3,4-ethylenedioxythiophene) doped with hyaluronic acid/poly (l-lactic acid) composite film for biomedical application. J. Biosci. Bioeng. 123, 116–125. https://doi.org/10.1016/j.jbiosc.2016.07.010.

Wang, W., Itoh, S., Matsuda, A., Aizawa, T., Demura, M., Ichinose, S., Shinomiya, K., Tanaka, J., 2008. Enhanced nerve regeneration through a bilayered chitosan tube: the effect of introduction of glycine spacer into the CYIGSR sequence. J. Biomed. Mater. Res. A 85, 919–928. https://doi.org/10.1002/jbm.a.31522.

Wang, Z., Kumar, H., Tian, Z., Jin, X., Holzman, J.F., Menard, F., Kim, K., 2018a. Visible light photoinitiation of cell-adhesive gelatin methacryloyl hydrogels for stereolithography 3D bioprinting. ACS Appl. Mater. Interfaces 10, 26859–26869. https://doi.org/10.1021/acsami.8b06607.

Wang, J., Tian, L., Luo, B., Ramakrishna, S., Kai, D., Loh, X.J., Yang, I.H., Deen, G.R., Mo, X., 2018b. Engineering PCL/lignin nanofibers as an antioxidant scaffold for the growth of neuron and Schwann cell. Colloids Surf. B Biointerfaces 169, 356–365. https://doi.org/10.1016/j.colsurfb.2018.05.021.

Wang, Y., Wei, Y.T., Zu, Z.H., Ju, R.K., Guo, M.Y., Wang, X.M., Xu, Q.Y., Cui, F.Z., 2011. Combination of hyaluronic acid hydrogel scaffold and PLGA microspheres for supporting survival of neural stem cells. Pharm. Res. 28, 1406. https://doi.org/10.1007/s11095-011-0452-3.

Webber, M.J., Han, X., Murthy, S.N.P., Rajangam, K., Stupp, S.I., Lomasney, J.W., 2010. Capturing the stem cell paracrine effect using heparin-presenting nanofibres to treat cardiovascular diseases. J. Tissue Eng. Regen. Med. 4, 600–610. https://doi.org/10.1002/term.273.

Wieringa, P., Tonazzini, I., Micera, S., Cecchini, M., 2012. Nanotopography induced contact guidance of the F11 cell line during neuronal differentiation: a neuronal model cell line for tissue scaffold development. Nanotechnology 23, 275102. https://doi.org/10.1088/0957-4484/23/27/275102.

Wilson, W.C., Boland, T., 2003. Cell and organ printing 1: protein and cell printers. Anat. Rec. A: Discov. Mol. Cell. Evol. Biol. 272, 491–496. https://doi.org/10.1002/ar.a.10057.

World Health Organization, 2020. The top 10 causes of death. https://www.who.int/news-room/fact-sheets/detail/the-top-10-causes-of-death. (Accessed 23 May 2020).

Xia, Z., Jin, S., Ye, K., 2018. Tissue and organ 3D bioprinting. SLAS Technol. https://doi.org/10.1177/2472630318760515.

Xia, L., Wan, H., Hao, S., Li, D., Chen, G., Gao, C., Li, J., Yang, F., Wang, S., Liu, S., 2013. Co-transplantation of neural stem cells and Schwann cells within poly (L-lactic-co-glycolic acid) scaffolds facilitates axonal regeneration in hemisected rat spinal cord. Chin Med J (Engl) 126, 909–917. https://doi.org/10.3760/cma.j.issn.0366-6999.20120476.

Xu, M.M., Mei, F., Li, D., Yang, X.P., Sui, G., Deng, X.L., Hu, X.Y., 2007. Electrospun poly(L-lacticacid)/nano-hydroxyapatite hybrid nanofibers and their potential in dental tissue engineering. Key Eng. Mater. 330–332, 377–380. https://doi.org/10.4028/www.scientific.net/KEM.330-332.377.

Yang, Y., Chawla, A., Zhang, J., Esa, A., Jang, H.L., Khademhosseini, A., 2019. Chapter 29—applications of nanotechnology for regenerative medicine; healing tissues at the nanoscale. In: Atala, A., Lanza, R., Mikos, A.G., Nerem, R. (Eds.), Principles of Regenerative Medicine, Third ed. Academic Press, Boston, pp. 485–504, https://doi.org/10.1016/B978-0-12-809880-6.00029-1.

Yang, F., Murugan, R., Wang, S., Ramakrishna, S., 2005. Electrospinning of nano/micro scale poly(l-lactic acid) aligned fibers and their potential in neural tissue engineering. Biomaterials 26, 2603–2610. https://doi.org/10.1016/j.biomaterials.2004.06.051.

Yang, X., Yang, F., Walboomers, X.F., Bian, Z., Fan, M., Jansen, J.A., 2010. The performance of dental pulp stem cells on nanofibrous PCL/gelatin/nHA scaffolds. J. Biomed. Mater. Res. A 93, 247–257. https://doi.org/10.1002/jbm.a.32535.

Yeo, J.H., Lee, K.G., Kim, H.C., HYL, O., Kim, A.J., Kim, S.Y., 2000. The effects of Pva/chitosan/fibroin (PCF)-blended spongy sheets on wound healing in rats. Biol. Pharm. Bull. 23, 1220–1223. https://doi.org/10.1248/bpb.23.1220.

Yeong, W.Y., Sudarmadji, N., Yu, H.Y., Chua, C.K., Leong, K.F., Venkatraman, S.S., Boey, Y.C.F., Tan, L.P., 2010. Porous polycaprolactone scaffold for cardiac tissue engineering fabricated by selective laser sintering. Acta Biomater. 6, 2028–2034. https://doi.org/10.1016/j.actbio.2009.12.033.

Zamani, M., Prabhakaran, M.P., Thian, E.S., Ramakrishna, S., 2015. Controlled delivery of stromal derived factor-1α from poly lactic-co-glycolic acid core-shell particles to recruit mesenchymal stem cells for cardiac regeneration. J. Colloid Interface Sci. 451, 144–152. https://doi.org/10.1016/j.jcis.2015.04.005.

Zhai, P., Peng, X., Li, B., Liu, Y., Sun, H., Li, X., 2020. The application of hyaluronic acid in bone regeneration. Int. J. Biol. Macromol. 151, 1224–1239. https://doi.org/10.1016/j.ijbiomac.2019.10.169.

Zhang, S., 2003. Fabrication of novel biomaterials through molecular self-assembly. Nat. Biotechnol. 21, 1171–1178. https://doi.org/10.1038/nbt874.

Zhang, S., Holmes, T., Lockshin, C., Rich, A., 1993. Spontaneous assembly of a self-complementary oligopeptide to form a stable macroscopic membrane. Proc. Natl. Acad. Sci. U. S. A. 90, 3334–3338.

Zhang, J., Jiang, D., Zhang, J., Lin, Q., Huang, Z., 2010. Synthesis of dental enamel-like hydroxyapaptite through solution mediated solid-state conversion. Langmuir 26, 2989–2994. https://doi.org/10.1021/la9043649.

Zhang, H., Wang, K., Xing, Y., Yu, Q., 2015. Lysine-doped polypyrrole/spider silk protein/poly(l-lactic) acid containing nerve growth factor composite fibers for neural application. Mater. Sci. Eng. C 56, 564–573. https://doi.org/10.1016/j.msec.2015.06.024.

Zhang, W., Zhan, X., Gao, M., Hamilton, A.D., Liu, Z., Jiang, Y., Su, H., Dai, X., He, B., Kang, X., Zeng, Y., Wu, W., Guo, J., 2012. Self-assembling peptide nanofiber scaffold enhanced with RhoA inhibitor CT04 improves axonal regrowth in the transected spinal cord. J. Nanomater. 2012, 724857. https://doi.org/10.1155/2012/724857.

Zhao, X., Lang, Q., Yildirimer, L., Lin, Z.Y., Cui, W., Annabi, N., Ng, K.W., Dokmeci, M.R., Ghaemmaghami, A.M., Khademhosseini, A., 2016. Photocrosslinkable gelatin hydrogel for epidermal tissue engineering. Adv. Healthc. Mater. 5, 108–118. https://doi.org/10.1002/adhm.201500005.

Zhu, Y., Wang, A., Patel, S., Kurpinski, K., Diao, E., Bao, X., Kwong, G., Young, W.L., Li, S., 2011. Engineering bi-layer nanofibrous conduits for peripheral nerve regeneration. Tissue Eng. Part C Methods 17, 705–715. https://doi.org/10.1089/ten.tec.2010.0565.

Zhu, Z., Wang, Y.-M., Yang, J., Luo, X.-S., 2017. Hyaluronic acid: a versatile biomaterial in tissue engineering. Plast. Aesthet. Res. 4, 219–227. https://doi.org/10.20517/2347-9264.2017.71.

Zong, X., Bien, H., Chung, C.Y., Yin, L., Fang, D., Hsiao, B.S., Chu, B., Entcheva, E., 2005. Electrospun fine-textured scaffolds for heart tissue constructs. Biomaterials 26, 5330–5338. https://doi.org/10.1016/j.biomaterials.2005.01.052.

CHAPTER 7

Nanobiomaterials for bioimaging

Shamraja S. Nadar[a], Sadhana P. Patil[b], Radhika K. Kelkar[b], Neha P. Patil[b], Pradnya V. Pise[b], Manishkumar S. Tiwari[c], Ajay N. Phirke[d], and Pravin D. Patil[d]

[a]Department of Chemical Engineering, Institute of Chemical Technology, Mumbai, Maharashtra, India
[b]Department of Biotechnology Engineering, Kolhapur Institute of Technology's College of Engineering, Kolhapur, Maharashtra, India
[c]Department of Chemical Engineering, Mukesh Patel School of Technology Management and Engineering, SVKM's NMIMS University, Mumbai, Maharashtra, India
[d]Department of Basic Science and Humanities, Mukesh Patel School of Technology Management and Engineering, SVKM's NMIMS University, Mumbai, Maharashtra, India

7.1 Introduction

As the world advances in medical science, scientists seek to explore biological processes involved in several diseases without harming a living being. Bioimaging is an emerging process in medicine and diagnostics that utilizes digital technology in the real-time visualization of biological processes (Rostami et al., 2019). This novel imaging method shows images relating the anatomical structure connected to functional data where the camera captures the primary image of a biological object, and the sensors determine the characteristics such as shape, size, surface texture, and color. It is a nondestructive method that provides overall views of the human body progressively with minute details (Balas, 2009). In the past three decades, different advanced techniques have been developed for bioimaging, which includes three-dimensional (3D)/four-dimensional (4D) body images by computed tomography (CT) scans, X-ray/ultrasound (US) images, and magnetic resonance imaging (MRI) (Agnihotri et al., 2010). Bioimaging aims at minimum interference with biological samples in vivo employing nanoparticle (NP) architecture, which is used to diagnose cancer cells (Wolfbeis, 2015). Many considerable advancements exist in bioimaging, and it is preferred over any other technique (Xu et al., 2019). Nevertheless, certain drawbacks still exist in this technique that needs to be addressed. The image resolution is limited up to certain millimeters. Also, there is a hindrance to autofluorescence, which is not helpful for surgical guidance (Cheng et al., 2020). In this regard, researchers observed that using multiple microscopy techniques on

Nanotechnology in Medicine and Biology
https://doi.org/10.1016/B978-0-12-819469-0.00001-0

a single sample can eradicate such obstacles. However, this approach is practically inconvenient as the hardware and software used are highly expensive while having several biocompatibility issues (Ghamsari, 2018).

A superresolution image could be a solution for most of the existing limitations, which can be obtained possibly by employing nano-bioimaging. This approach uses nanomaterials, which enable the construction of high-resolution images of biological samples. Utilizing this method, various NPs have been synthesized as medicinal and clinical agents in the recent past (Li et al., 2020b). The superiority of nanomaterials in bioimaging is associated with its optical and physical properties that are easily modified and tuned through structural modulations. Additional magnetic properties, diverse surface chemistries, and chemical compositions make it a potential candidate (Saji et al., 2010). Also, some NPs consist of inherent therapeutic and optical properties that can add up to their efficiency. However, it is challenging to make favorable structural changes as many allied concerns emerge, such as biocompatibility, imaging capacity, toxicity, the complexity of the synthesis, and cost. Generally, a broad range of nanomaterials is used for bioimaging, including metals (Ag, Au, Pt, Pd, Cu, Mg, Fe, Ti, Zn, etc.), magnetic materials (metal oxides of Mn, Co, and Ni), organic carbon-based NPs (carbon nanotubes (CNTs), carbon-based quantum dots (QDs), graphene and its derivatives, fullerenes, and nanodiamonds (NDs)) (Wolfbeis, 2015). Fig. 7.1 depicts the general implementation of NPs in different bioimaging applications.

Even though nano-bio-optical imaging (nano-bioimaging) techniques offer higher resolution at the nanoscale, it can undergo strong attenuation of visible light by tissues (cellular components, such as lysosomes and mitochondria). Moreover, the image is restricted to the surface of the targeted tissue (Reineck and Gibson, 2017). To overcome such setbacks, either NPs should be developed that would not get hampered by the visible light or design such NPs that will operate at different wavelengths giving a well-resolved image while not disturbing the biological matters. In this regard, fluorescent NPs were developed to act in the near-infrared (NIR) region light, which can go deep inside the tissues at the molecular level, ultimately making it a viable alternative to the attenuation issue. Advanced research in this field can probably make its way to broader adoption for clinical purposes (Altınoğlu and Adair, 2010).

This chapter discusses the usage of different NPs (organic and inorganic nanomaterials) in bioimaging. Further, the properties of nanomaterials and their compatibility are comprehensively discussed. Finally, other bioimaging techniques and their potential applications in clinical fields are critiqued.

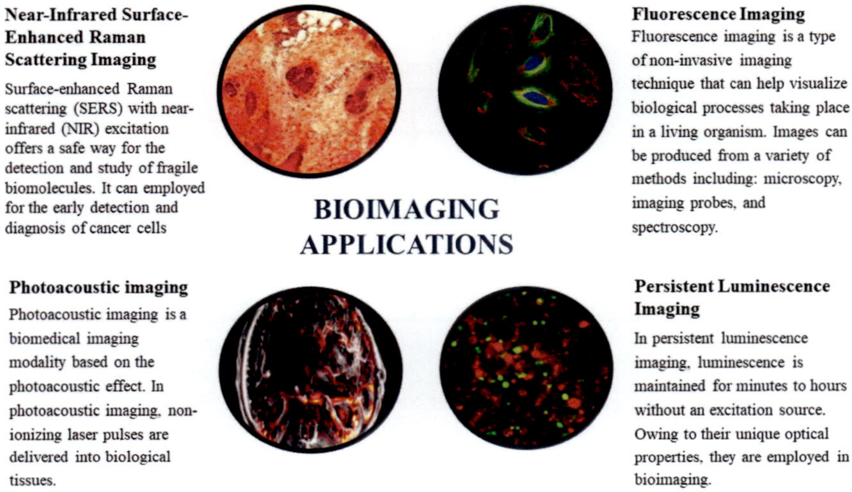

Fig. 7.1 Implementation of nanoparticles in different bioimaging applications.

7.2 Types of nanomaterials

The recent advancements in nanotechnology have resulted in the development of novel varieties of functional organic and inorganic nanomaterials with tunable morphology and well-defined characteristics that enable a wide variety of biomedical applications. Nanotechnology, along with biochemistry, makes up nanomedicine, which helps biomedical sciences diagnose and treat diseases at the molecular level. NPs offer unique physical and chemical properties such as electrochemical, thermodynamic, optical, catalytic, and magnetic (Mohanraj and Chen, 2006). The structure of NPs and their chemical compositions also affect their overall properties, and depending on such distinct properties, NPs have been employed in various bioimaging methods (Fig. 7.2).

7.2.1 Organic nanoparticles

Organic NPs are templated upon natural or synthetic organic molecules in bioimaging, depending on the target cells or organs. One of the most important features of organic NPs is that they offer relatively simple routes for encapsulating materials (Romero and Moya, 2012). This, together with the fact that the molecules used for the fabrication of the organic NPs can be biodegradable, makes organic NPs the most appealing biomedical applications system. Thus many different organic NPs have been synthesized for bioimaging in the recent past. They offer a variety of materials, such as graphene and its derivatives, graphene quantum dots (GQDs), carbon dots

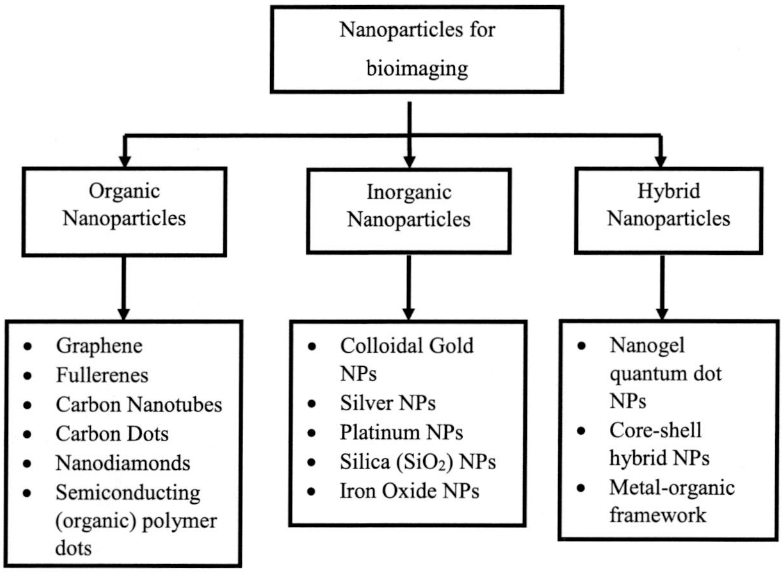

Fig. 7.2 Types of nanomaterials used in bioimaging applications.

(CDs), CNTs, and NDs, which are known for their exceptional contrasting properties, biocompatibility, high-resolution imaging properties, heat and chemical resistance, modifying/transporting capability, and optoelectronic properties. They can be tuned and employed against the dimension of biomaterials, such as proteins, DNA, and RNA (Wen et al., 2015). The luminescence, conductivity, magnetic permeability, and chemical reactivity of these particles are highly dependent on their size, which ultimately makes a small modification significant to its application (Saji et al., 2010). The following section covers several examples of organic NPs used in bioimaging.

7.2.1.1 Graphene

Graphene is the most putative nanomaterial for the fabrication of biomedical devices for bioimaging and biosensing purposes due to some of its stimulating qualities (Bhuyan et al., 2016; Dasari Shareena et al., 2018). There are different strategies for synthesizing graphene nanomaterials, summarized in Fig. 7.3. In 2004, Geim and co-workers first isolated graphene onto SiO_2 substrates and discovered its electrical properties while employing it in an application of graphene-based NPs (GBNs) in bioimaging (Blake et al., 2007). The stimulating qualities of graphene, such as excellent processability in aqueous medium and outstanding surface properties favoring light scattering and biocompatibility, makes it a favored NP for the design of

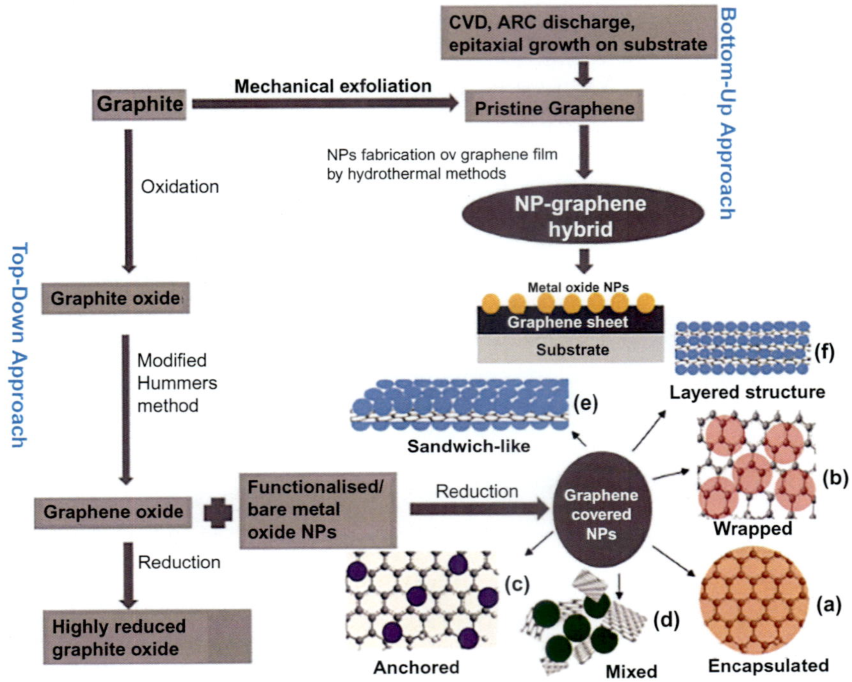

Fig. 7.3 The strategies to synthesize biocompatible graphene nanomaterials for bioimaging. *(From Jana, A., Scheer, E., Polarz, S., 2017. Synthesis of graphene–transition metal oxide hybrid nanoparticles and their application in various fields. Beilstein J. Nanotechnol. 8, 688–714. Creative Commons Attribution License © 2017 Jana et al.; licensee Beilstein-Institute.)*

biomedical sensors and can be applied for many different clinical applications such as therapeutics, bioimaging, and biosensing (Kumar et al., 2018). Graphene has found numerous applications in medicine and other fields due to its flexible nature to bind with a variety of functional groups in the form of chemically modified graphene, including graphene oxide (GO) and reduced graphene oxide (RGO), thus customizing its properties according to the application. The primary requirements of bioimaging materials are high specificity, nontoxicity, and sensitivity (Lin et al., 2018). While GBNs are capable of reducing the toxicity of designed probes, introducing the sensitivity and selectivity is still a hurdle in material synthesis. They are extensively explored in bioimaging methods, such as photoacoustic imaging (PAI), ultrasonography (USG), optical imaging (OI), MRI, radionuclide-based imaging (positron emission tomography (PET), single-photon emission computerized tomography (SPECT)), and CT, which facilitate observation while studying biological processes and organs at the cellular and subcellular levels (Dasari Shareena et al., 2018). The GQDs are mostly used GBNs and can be prepared from graphene sheets via simple hydrothermal cutting in the initial development stages. The fluorescence spectroscopy for the biological component imaging was the preferable technique developed due to the good photophysical properties of GQDs (Wang et al., 2015). Utilizing small polymers, NPs, dyes, biomolecules, etc., graphene and its derivatives can be easily modified and employed to serve different bioimaging techniques. Moreover, graphene can be used in bioimaging as an imaging contrast agent, carrier, fluorescence quencher, wrapping material, and building block. Therefore graphene has been gathering a huge interest due to its unique properties, which is crucial at nano levels. Nevertheless, several issues, such as nanotoxicity, the underlying mechanism, and signal pathway, still need to be addressed.

7.2.1.2 Fullerenes

Fullerenes are also known as the third allotrope of carbon after diamond and graphite. Fullerenes are hollow cage-like structures and have a hollow part of 1 nm diameter enclosed with atoms, molecules, etc. inside this cavity to make up endohedral fullerenes. In one such attempt, Lu et al. (2010) encapsulated metals inside fullerenes to form endohedral metallofullerenes (EMFs), where they obtained the first EMF called La@C_{60}. Fullerene, mainly C_{70}, is one of the nanosized carbon allotropes, being much smaller than CDs. The clinical applications of fullerene and its derivatives are mainly in drug delivery, cancer therapy, tissue engineering scaffolds, and radio imaging. Fullerenes, despite being color tunable, cannot be used for bioimaging because of their weak fluorescence. Fullerene, C_{60}, exhibits normal and late fluorescence, which is vigorously quenched by oxygen and significantly affected by temperature. To overcome the shortcomings of individual materials, chemical modifications and biconjugate reactions among several NPs can be introduced. The fullerene-like introduction of hydrophilic groups, such as polyhydroxy groups, carboxylic acids, and amino acids on the fullerenes' outer surfaces, produces derivatives with efficient water solubility and biocompatibility that can lead to targeted bioimaging (Biju, 2014). For instance, tumor sites (in vivo) can be easily imaged through higher resolution fluorescence imaging, which is possible by NIR fluorescence of hyaluronate fullerenes. Doubly targeting nanocrystals were procured by attaching 3-aminophenylboronic acid and hyaluronated fullerene to them. The two ligands assured specific targeting of cancer cells (Wolfbeis, 2015).

The two main categories of water-soluble fullerene derivatives, i.e., EMFs (e.g., fullerenols and carboxy fullerenes) and substituted fullerenes (e.g., malonic acid) have good significance in the biomedical field. These two groups of fullerene derivatives have shown excellent efficiency in bioimaging and cancer therapy. Moreover, their usefulness has led to their wide applications in different fields, including drug delivery, photodynamic therapy (PDT), and tumor cell nutrition supply reduction. Further, they can be employed as reactive oxygen species (ROS) and adjuvant in cancer medications (Zhang et al., 2019). The major advantage of fullerenes lies in its effective distribution in blood and appropriate localization at the target organ. Additionally, fullerenes are highly biocompatible and nontoxic, which cater to easy functionalization with biomolecules present in the human body while making the overall imaging process easier.

7.2.1.3 Carbon nanotubes

CNTs are one of the key carbon nanomaterials and can be classified as single-walled carbon nanotubes (SWNTs) and multiwalled carbon nanotubes (MWNTs; Cheung et al., 2002). Currently used processes for the synthesis of CNTs are chemical vapor deposition (CVD), arc discharge, and graphite laser ablation (Boskovic et al., 2002). CNTs offer a chief novel class of materials possessing unique mechanical, electrical, and physicochemical properties while offering large specific surface area and the ability to link with various biomolecules (such as protein and DNA) that can be employed for applications in biosensing, bioimaging, and drug delivery. The CNTs have a unique hollow monolithic structure with a distinct inner surface that can be occupied by several molecules and an outer surface, which can be modified by means of functionalization to get desired properties (Biju, 2014). A study showed that cell-specific imaging could be employed for targeting and imaging HeLa cells where they combined polystyrene and poly-(e-caprolactone) side chains containing a copolymer of poly(para-phenylene) with carboxyl-functionalized SWCNTs treated with folic acid (FA) (Ag et al., 2013). Further, Hashemzadeh and Raissi (2017) observed that loading CNTs with drugs did not hinder its chemiluminescence by using *Luciola cruciate* (luciferase)-labeled SWCNTs. Moreover, CNTs show good compatibility in the living body and can easily penetrate cellular membranes without any external transporter systems. CNTs, with their excellent properties, can emerge as a highly effective means of transporting cargos for therapeutic and diagnostic purposes in cancer nanotechnology and should be further explored in the bioimaging field.

7.2.1.4 Carbon dots

CDs are a zero-dimensional (0D) type of material with useful properties that make it an important carbon nanomaterial (Hola et al., 2014). For instance, the favorable properties of CDs such as permeability, ease of preparation photostability, low toxicity, biocompatibility, and low cost make them capable of using as agents for fluorescence labeling and imaging. Different synthetic methods such as arc discharge, electrolysis, hydrothermal, and laser ablation are employed in synthesizing CDs. They can be manifested in several forms, such as 0D spherical fullerenes or one-dimensional (1D) CDs, and many others. CDs are known for their excellent chemical as well as photostable properties while being rich in surface functional groups, such as hydroxyl, amino, and carboxyl, which is useful for tuning its optical properties (Wen et al., 2015). Their surface-state stability decides if their photoluminescence is excitation dependent (e.g., polyethyleneimine passivated CDs) or independent (e.g., N, S-CDs). On the other hand, their size is what decides their emission wavelength: ultraviolet (UV, 1.2 nm), bright visible (1.5–3 nm), and NIR (3.8 nm). These NPs also have low cost, excellent quantum yield, and very low cytotoxicity, making them a potential candidate for bioimaging analysis.

7.2.1.5 Nanodiamonds

With the emergence of technologies, such as high-pressure-high-temperature and CVD, the production of bulk diamonds and 2D diamond films have increased. Moreover, 1D diamond nanowires and 0D diamond NPs have diversified this material's use. Here, NDs refer to the diamond particles whose average diameter ranges from 1 to 100 nm. There are various methods for the preparation of NDs. Among many, oxidation is the most economically feasible and eco-friendly method, wherein they are prepared from explosives like 60 wt% trinitrotoluene ($C_6H_2(NO_2)_3CH_3$) and 40 wt% hexogen ($C_3H_6N_6O_6$), which are usually oxygen deficient. These are then detonated in a metallic tank, thus giving a product of NDs (4–5 nm diameter) along with some impurities that need to be separated (Dolmatov et al., 2004). A major advantage of NDs is that they undergo Brownian motion within cells like HeLa lines for more than 200 s, making them beneficial for long-term in vivo tracking (Prabhakar and Rosenholm, 2019). NDs are an excellent resource when it comes to the treatment of diseases like cancer. In one such study, the transforming growth factor (TGF) receptors (which are responsible for immunosuppression and metastasis in cancer cells) were coated with NDs and were successfully used to assess the trafficking process of TGF-beta receptors. The researchers obtained a localization accuracy of around 8 nm in the XY directions, and the accuracy was seen to be around 16 nm in the Z direction, which was far better than traditionally used dyes. This suggests that NDs can be beneficial for long-term monitoring of the intracellular protein delivery mechanism, which will help develop better therapeutic medicines. Another benefit of NDs for in vivo imaging is that they are chemically inert, unlike some NPs that use heavy metals. Moreover, it has also been reported that it can be tracked for a long time due to its high brightness. Due to their properties mentioned above, NDs can be employed in the superresolution microscopy using the stimulated emission depletion technique, and a remarkable resolution of 6–10 nm can be obtained in the process. Another factor that makes NDs a right candidate for bioimaging is its low exocytosis by cells, as seen in human cancer cell lines where the extent of exocytosis was seen to be around 15% after 6 days in multipotent stromal cells and HeLa cells (Perevedentseva et al., 2013). This property has also been used for tracking AS-B145-1R breast cancer cells. However, the higher concentration of these NDs can become toxic to cells, and therefore their nano-size forms tend to be helpful considering their easy internalization into cells. Moreover, the cells do not show cytotoxicity to these NDs at low concentrations because the cells tend to endocytose and exocytose the NDs continuously, thus regulating their amount in a cell at controlled levels, which makes NDs biocompatible along with being useful for long-term tracking. Additionally, they also have a fluorescence property that can be used as a good contrast agent against the background (Reineck and Gibson, 2017).

7.2.1.6 Semiconducting (organic) polymer dots

The polymer dots (PDs) have high brightness and small particle size of π-conjugated polymers and can be employed in a broad range of clinical applications. Semiconducting PDs are emerging as organic fluorescent NPs with high brightness, large Stokes shift, and intriguing energy-transfer properties (Wu and Chiu, 2013).These polymeric semiconductors were initially developed for optoelectronic devices and later used for highly sensitive chemical sensors. The PDs are commonly synthesized by nanoprecipitation or emulsion polymerization (Lee et al., 2007; Li Jia'En, 2011). The backbone of conjugated polymers acts like an array of light-harvesting units that manifest a broader optical cross section than small organic molecule dyes. However, their applications in bioimaging are less known to date. A blend of semiconducting PDs and fluorescent nanodots attached to the polypeptide is used for targeted imaging in clinical diagnosis. Nevertheless, more research is needed to make these NPs widely adaptable in bioimaging (Wolfbeis, 2015).

7.2.2 Inorganic NPs

In recent times, inorganic NPs have attracted much attention in the field of biomedical as organic NPs cannot be modified to a large extent, while some organic NPs cannot be modified at all. Moreover, synthesized inorganic NPs are mostly hydrophilic, and toxicity can be controlled, which makes them target specific while reducing unnecessary binding, whereas organic NPs in this regard are difficult to control (Paris et al., 2019). The inorganic NPs can be fabricated and incorporated in the living body and widely used in bioimaging for diagnosis purposes. Ease in the synthesis as well as modification in the size, shape, and surface properties have favored the synthesis of inorganic NPs (Lim et al., 2020). In recent times, researchers have designed and synthesized different types of inorganic NPs. They can be broadly classified into two categories: (i) noble metal NPs (gold, silver, platinum) and (ii) metal oxide NPs (silica, iron oxide, zinc oxide, etc.). Integral and multifunctional systems for bioimaging can be achieved by virtue of optical, electronic, and magnetic properties of various inorganic NPs. Inorganic NPs that are optically active can produce fluorescence or scattered light, which is used to develop an image and thus be employed in bioimaging (Kim et al., 2018). Some inorganic NPs have been studied thoroughly, and some yet need to be explored in terms of their application concerning biocompatibility and toxicity. Nevertheless, inorganic NPs can bring revolutionizing changes to the entire biomedical field.

7.2.2.1 Noble metal NPs

For decades noble metal NPs, predominantly of gold and silver, have been rigorously studied and applied in different sectors. They offer unique benefits, including retention of unusual optical, electronic, and thermal properties. Additionally, superficial synthesis and surface bioconjugation have made it feasible to become employed in the biomedical field (Yaqoob et al., 2020). The noble metal (platinum and palladium) NPs have relatively fewer clinical field applications and are under research scrutiny. A brief description of a few significant NPs is discussed here.

Colloidal gold NPs

The brilliant color, size, and shape of colloidal gold particles make them potential candidates to be applied in various areas, such as catalysis, biomedical, solar energy scavenging/power harvesting, sensing, and many others. The optical and electronic activity of gold NPs are easily tuned by modifying the size, shape, and surface chemistry, thus making it suitable for bioimaging. In bioimaging, gold NPs such as nanoshells, nanocubes, nanorods (NRs), nanospheres, nanostars, and nanocages have found rising interest in in vitro and in vivo imaging (Das et al., 2019). Many different methods are being employed for synthesizing gold NPs. Cheaper reagents and simple steps have made the Schiffrin-Brust biphasic synthesis process widely accepted back in 1994 (Biju, 2014). The properties of gold colloidal NPs include distinct surface chemistry, straight forward synthesis, nonhazardous nature, and large one/two-photon absorption cross sections, making them appropriate for applications in different bioimaging techniques (surface-enhanced Raman spectroscopy (SERS) of organic and biomolecules, SPR, optical coherence tomography, and photothermal/PA responses). According to reported applications, gold NPs are used in the detection of ovarian tumors by PAI (Wang et al., 2019). Moreover, in X-ray imaging, gold NPs are used as a potential agent for the accumulation of gold NPs in tumors causing attenuation of X-rays and thus differentiating tumor from healthy tissues. Therefore to intensify the gold NPs' therapeutic potency, a few pinpoint design factors such as toxicity and systemic interactions need to be considered (Mahan and Doiron, 2018).

Silver NPs

Silver NPs have been extensively explored in recent years. The photothermal ability and antimicrobial activity of silver NPs favor its use in bioimaging (Capanema et al., 2019). The various synthesis processes of silver NPs have been reported. Silver salts and surfactants in an aqueous solution, when irradiated with a laser, could synthesize suitable silver NPs with the desired shape and size (Sportelli et al., 2018). To improve the efficacy of the noble NPs, silver and gold NPs are used in a combination and reported in several biomedical studies. According to reports, both noble metals are combined into core-shell nanostructures. The shell is made up of gold, and the core is made up of silver NPs concerning its better NIR absorption. The synthesis of these structures is mostly fabricated by galvanic repulsion and seed-mediated growth. The nontoxic nature, optical activity, and easy fabrication are the properties that help in applying silver NPs in the bioimaging field (Austin et al., 2014). Furthermore, silver NPs are employed in SERS to detect critical proteins and biomolecules such as early cancer biomarkers or drug distribution in body fluids. Exploring more silver NPs while optimizing the characteristics and surface structures precisely can help increase bioconjugation and biocompatibility of silver NPs.

Platinum NPs

Platinum NPs are an appropriate biomedical field option due to its catalytic activity, antiinflammatory ability, and biocompatibility (Zhao et al., 2017). The synthesis of platinum NPs can be done by various means such as chemical, physical, and biologically assisted procedures. In chemical-based methods, galvanic displacement, wet chemical reduction (WCR), electrochemical reduction, and CVD have gained more attention (Pedone et al., 2017). In WCR, reducing agents are used to produce platinum NPs from platinum precursors, which controls the NPs' characteristics. Physically based methods are popular because they overcome the difficulties of chemical processes (e.g., toxic reagent and need for organic solvent). Physical methods follow flame synthesis, electron beam-induced reduction, laser ablation technique, and aerosol-assisted deposition. Though the synthesis of Pt NPs is relatively easy, there is a need to eradicate the cytotoxic effects and biocompatibility issues before they are employed in the bioimaging field (Pedone et al., 2017). Nevertheless, platinum could be considered as a potential NP agent for bioimaging similar to silver and gold.

7.2.2.2 Metal oxide NPs

The engineered metal oxide NPs are among the widest used NPs due to the unique features they possess. In bioimaging, many different NPs are currently synthesized from oxides of various metals such as iron, titanium, zirconia, hafnium, manganese, silica, and been explored in various imaging modalities.

Silica (SiO_2) NPs

Among various NPs, silica NPs have been widely investigated, and their properties are optimized for applying in different sectors. SiO_2 NPs have found applications in several fields such as bioimaging, catalysis in chemical industries, and drug and gene delivery applications due to their ease of synthesis, distinct surface chemistry, large surface area, and chemical and physical stabilities (Bagheri et al., 2018). The properties mentioned above for silica force them to design a protective shell that renders protection against biodegradation, toxic ions, and activation of the immune response. Many different procedures are described for synthesizing these silica NPs in the literature, with the sol-gel process being the most followed (Azlina et al., 2016). Although silica NPs have hydrophilic surfaces, assorted functional groups like amino acids, carboxyl, hydroxyl, or azide are necessary to be added on the surface or in pores for the higher conjugation of biomolecules for successful localization to target molecules or tissues or to protect against an immune response (Biju, 2014). Examples of bioimaging containing these silica NPs are comprehensive due to its ability to hold fluorescent MRI-PET contrast agents and medicine or genetic material molecules to their flexible exterior and pores. A combination of different bioimaging and drug delivery systems (DDSs) in single silica NPs are possible, which can be a promising aspect of biomedical science (Hu et al., 2018). The joint efforts of researchers in multidisciplinary fields can strengthen the application of silica in the biomedical field. Therefore to increase and explore the possibilities of silica NPs in the clinical field, targeted cell action and action on intracellular components should be rigorously studied.

Iron oxide NPs

Iron oxide NPs are composed of a hydrophilic polymer covering shell with the core as an iron oxide crystal. Superparamagnetic iron oxide NPs (SPIONs) and ultrasmall superparamagnetic iron oxides NPs (USPIONs) are two general classes of iron oxide NPs based on properties like size, shape, and other intrinsic characteristics. In comparison to SPIONs, USPIONs are considered favorable for biomedical purposes due to their reduced degree of opsonization (Al Zaki et al., 2017). In the recent past, different chemical methods are mentioned for the fabrication of iron oxide NPs, such as co-precipitation, thermal decomposition, and laser pyrolysis (Shaterabadi et al., 2017). Thermal decomposition is one such method that involves high-temperature disintegration of organometallic precursors, including iron pentacarbonyl and iron cupferronate using organic solvents/surfactants. The morphology of USPIONs can be modified or adjusted by controlling the process conditions and nature of solvents, precursors, and surfactants used (Zarschler et al., 2016). However, for the successful application of iron oxide NPs in bioimaging, the surface modification of iron oxide NPs is required to make them biocompatible and optically active. Also, conjugating them with any other species is necessary in some cases. Considering inherent properties (such as toxicity, optical activity, and compatibility of iron oxide NPs in the living body), the NPs can be employed in bioimaging.

7.2.3 Hybrid NPs

NPs synthesized by either organic or inorganic compounds are nowadays used on a large scale in the biomedical field due to its potential application in real-time biological imaging. The higher photostability, bright fluorescence, narrow emission, and broad excitation have attracted researchers to use it in the bioimaging field. However, cellular uptake efficacy is lower for these synthesized NPs (Li et al., 2020a). Hence, a compatible conjugate is required for making the NPs more compatible in the living body. Such types of conjugates are known as hybrid NPs. The hybrid NPs contain two or more distinct NPs assembled in a functional structure that itself is still of nanoscale dimensions. To date, various hybrid nanostructures are designed, such as core-shell, metal-organic framework (MOF), lipid-polymer, yolk-shell, heterodimer, dot-in-nanotube, dot-on-nanorod, and nanobranches. In a further section, a few hybrid NPs that can be potentially employed in the bioimaging field are briefly discussed.

7.2.3.1 Nanogel quantum dot hybrid NPs

QDs are used widely in the bioimaging field due to their inherent properties that support biological imaging; however, there is an issue regarding the uptake of NPs in living cells. Nevertheless, researchers have studied and found out that using a certain carrier with NPs can improve compatibility and uptake (Paysen et al., 2020). According to the reports, cationic liposomes were used as a carrier with NPs for imaging. However, the aggregation of these carriers in the cytoplasm was found, thereby demanding a novel approach to eradicating biocompatibility and aggregation. According to several other reports, the self-built structure of cholesterol-bearing pullulan gave rise to steady hydrogel NPs (nanogel). The nanogels make hydrophobic linkages with a range of drugs and proteins and deliver them upon encounter with specific cyclodextrin. The application of these hybrid nanogel QDs NPs was incorporated into human cervical cells, and real-time images were captured (Wang et al., 2018). To date, limited applications of nanogel NPs in bioimaging have been investigated; thus more research is needed for this hybrid NP to become employed in biological imaging.

7.2.3.2 Core-shell hybrid NPs

Typically, hybrid NPs are made up of a broad range of organic and inorganic nanomaterials (metals or polymers). One material acts as an inner layer core, while others act as an outer layer as a shell. These NPs are made up of a variety of nanomaterials, which make them unique by changing the properties (such as physicochemical, biological, and optical) of the core/shell layer. The classification of core-shell hybrid NPs are as follows: core-shell NPs (Pd@Pt), core-multishell NPs (NDCMS-NPs: Au nanodisks core with Ag outer layer), polyhedral core/shell NPs (Cu_2O@Ag), core-porous shell NPs (NPSNPs), and hollow-core-shell NPs (AgPt@Pt HNs). There are three approaches used to form core-shell NPs. In a one-pot approach, the simultaneous formation of the core and shell is carried out. In the two-pot approach, the core is formed at the initial stage, followed by the formation of a shell around the core surface. At the starting point, core formation takes place in the three-pot approach, and then the outer layers are formed (one by one), and the core is removed if hollow core-shell hybrid NPs are required. The core-shell hybrid NPs are easily internalized into the cell by interactions and are used in noninvasive imaging techniques. It also serves as a contrasting agent in MRI imaging (Hao et al., 2019).

7.2.3.3 Metal-organic framework

A type of hybrid material made up of metal ion/cluster connecting linkages and organic bridging ligands is called an MOFs. MOFs have found applications in biological imagining and sensing due to their useful properties such as manageable synthesis, pore size/wall alteration flexibility, and porosity (Nadar et al., 2018, 2019). MOFs possess good beneficial factors such as intrinsic decomposition and the capacity to use biocompatible building blocks that allow them to use in biological applications compared with inorganic nanomaterials (e.g., graphene and its derivative NPs, MoS_2) (Salgaonkar et al., 2018). Various synthesis methods are employed for making MOFs, including the traditional solvothermal method. Typically, a reaction vessel containing a solvent in which metal precursors and organic linkers are dissolved is used to form MOF crystals. Frequently used solvents for this purpose are ethanol, methanol, acetonitrile, etc.

Further, extensive research in MOFs has employed several advanced techniques, such as electrochemical, microwave-assisted, and mechanochemical synthesis (Bedia et al., 2019). These various methods allow the designing of large numbers of different MOFs. In virtue of these numerous advantages, scientists have recently used MOF as a contrasting agent for MRI and CT. Hence, the MOFs' attractive properties such as straightforward synthesis, predictable structures, and tunable optical features allow their interaction with various biological molecules and are easily incorporated in a living body in vivo for imaging (Luo et al., 2019). However, in bioimaging, MOFs are in the early stage, and MOF structures need to be scaled down at the nanoscale. Nevertheless, reducing the scale of MOFs is challenging (Wang, 2017). Therefore in the future, a suitable design of MOFs is necessary to create probes and carriers that are biocompatible, nontoxic, and have higher specificity to target molecules. Furthermore, the MOFs' precise activity should be evaluated to make them capable enough for use in in vivo for clinical diagnostic purposes. A successful investigation of this can make MOFs one of the potent NPs in the biomedical field (Wu and Yang, 2017).

7.3 Physicochemical properties

7.3.1 Photoluminescence

Bioimaging is a crucial part of a diagnostic study concerning its ability to observe biological component physical conditions, working under in vivo and in vitro conditions. Various techniques, such as US, OI, MRI, PET, single-photon emission CT (SPECT), and CT, and their variations have been introduced for this case with a progressing development in the field of electronics and information technology. NPs have various unique properties that make them a huge topic of interest, and photoluminescence is one of those properties. Photoluminescence is a type of luminescence in which the substance is exposed to photons of specified energy, which results in the excitation of its electrons to an upper energy state (S1, S2) (Wu et al., 2021). This transition needs to change to a higher energy state with equivalent vibrational and rotational energy. During this process, the electrons lose some energy in the form of radiation. This radiation has an energy equivalent to the Stokes shift, which basically refers to the difference between the wavelength necessary for excitation and the emitted luminosity (Jaque et al., 2016). The main requirements of any material that will be used in bioimaging are its sensitivity, biocompatibility, specificity, etc., and photoluminescence can be efficiently employed in this regard (Soufi and Iravani, 2020; Zhao et al., 2019a).

Recently, GBNs have been identified as a good agent in the biomedical sector employing the delivery of various drugs, combined cancer treatment, biomedical imaging, etc. (Dasari Shareena et al., 2018). It has been extensively experimented with in the bioimaging field because of its good photophysical properties. In one such investigation, nano GO-polyethylene glycol-Rituxan (nGO-PEG-Rituxan) was used to deliver therapeutic drugs for in vivo treatment. However, nGO-PEG-Rituxan was also used for fluorescence imaging that showed greater imaging depth, low autofluorescence, low photobleaching, as well as better phototoxicity (Sun et al., 2013). However, its emission gets mixed up with the autofluorescence of the body's natural components (Wei et al., 2016). The problem of autofluorescence was solved with the help of upconversion nanoparticles (UCNPs). UCNPs have the ability to tune lower energy source light into upper energy luminous emissions, which is crucial. The UCNPs have high fluorescence intensity under NIR irradiation as well as high uptake by cells and tissues, which results in good physical permanence while conferring low toxicity (Rostami et al., 2019). Another group demonstrated how UCNPs, with no modifications to the on/off emission, coated with amphiphilic biocompatible polymers, produced strong upconversion luminescence with low antistokes autofluorescence in the presence of a modest power continuous wave laser. Unfortunately, since the UCNPs are a new addition in the field of bioimaging, the required NIR sources for imaging are not designed or compatible with the usage of UCNPs and must be investigated further (Wu et al., 2015).

In terms of biocompatibility, silicon NPs (SiNPs) have shown easy biodegradability as they transformed into renal clearable molecules (i.e., silicic acid), which was next excreted out of the body without any toxicity evidence in vivo. This is a huge advantage over the other molecules in terms of cytotoxicity. They also have been approved by the Food and Drug Administration for first-in-human clinical trials, which resulted in the production of various forms of SiNPs (Reineck and Gibson, 2017). Among all the 0D fluorescent SiNPs, they showed various superior water-dispersibility properties, good fluorescence, and super low photobleaching. These properties are essential for the real-time tracking of live cells for the long term. Furthermore, the beneficial properties of the UCNPs and SiNPs were combined in the form of persistent luminescence (PL) imaging (Sun et al., 2018), where the luminescence can last for several seconds to days after turning off the source of excitation.

In this manner, various NPs were developed for utilization in bioimaging, where the GBNs had attractive photoluminescence properties. However, it cannot provide quantitative results concerning the interference occurring due to fluorescence quenching. Also, the critical factor that decides whether the material is usable in biology and medicine is the biocompatibility of that material, and this exact factor has prevented GBNs from going into clinical trials. On the other hand, UCNPs offered the ability of deep tissue penetration due to its upconversion abilities (González-Béjar et al., 2016). On the other hand, hybrid SiNPs offer various properties that made them suitable for real-time imaging. Nanoparticles of $ZnGa_{1.995}Cr_{0.005}O_4$ (n-ZGO) while lacking in deep tissue imaging, have shown great properties in terms of PL, broad excitation spectrum, etc. (Maldiney et al., 2014). This has led to a further search for photoluminescent NPs (PLNPs) that have better signal-to-noise ratios (SNRs) and emission in the NIR region, enabling deep tissue imaging. Moreover, attractive options have been offered by the Cr^{3+}-doped PLNPs, which have been reported to produce renewable PL under light-emitting diode (LED) light that can penetrate tissues. This helps eliminate the restriction of a light-emitting lifetime of nanoprobes while making the whole process efficient.

7.3.2 Absorbance

Absorbance, in terms of illumination, of any substance, is its ability to absorb the light incident on it and not let it transmit out of itself. Every substance absorbs light of a particular wavelength. The magnitude of absorbance (optical density) of any substance depends on the concentration of that substance, i.e., the higher the quantity of that substance per unit volume, the higher the amount of light absorbed. Hence, absorbance is of great importance in any quantitative analysis (Li et al., 2019). In bioimaging, absorbance plays a vital role. Plasmonic NPs show a great relationship between absorbance and fluorescence. The presence of plasmonic NPs around CDs has a significant influence on the CDs' absorption and coefficient. This effect greatly improves the fluorescence of these NPs (Emam et al., 2017). NPs possess a remarkable absorbance property; hence they are immensely explored in the DDSs, bioimaging, and in the overall biomedical field (Liang et al., 2014). However, traditional nanomaterials tend to get excited upon exposure to small amounts of UV or visible light while possessing autoluminescence. This, as a matter of fact, reduces the sensitivity of the diagnosis technique as well as causes damage to the surrounding cells and tissues. Therefore the synthesis of biocompatible NPs is of current interest. NPs can be attached to several biomarkers to aid in monitoring regular metabolic activity. In the case of abnormalities, particular biomarkers are synthesized. These NPs attach to the biomarkers, and the absorbance detected at that stage determines the biomarker producing cell concentration. The cells detected most of the time are cancer or tumor cells. Thus one major role of absorbance in biomedicine is that it helps in depicting the malignancy of cancer (Ye et al., 2018).

QDs are NPs that show astounding absorbance capacity (Huang et al., 2002). They belong to the semiconductor class and are close to or even smaller than the excitation Bohr radius. A high energy gap is generated due to the confinement of the electron-hole pair, thus demanding high energy (small wavelength) as well as absorbing a high amount of light.

Therefore a better output is gained when QDs are employed in bioimaging. Another justification regarding the huge interest in bioimaging using QDs is that some limitations are faced by fluorescent proteins (FPs) and fluorescent dyes, such as thin excitation spectra, low effective Stokes shifts, wide fluorescence bands, and their vulnerability to photobleaching (Martinić et al., 2017). Moreover, the lifetime of PL and autofluorescence are in the same time span window, i.e., a few nanoseconds. This property prevents them from the time-bound detection needed for improving the SNR; thus it does not help them in good differentiation among the various target molecules. However, disturbances in the crystal structures, most of the time on the surface of the QDs, may provide nonradiative fluorescence. Furthermore, the quantum confinement effect is also a consequence as in it causes size-dependent emission, and thus higher energy bandgap with a smaller size of the same material QDs and vice versa. This has resulted in the synthesis of hybrid NPs with varying sizes of QDs to develop a spectral range from UV to infrared. The PL of QDs yields a normal curve with a small full-width half-maximum of approximately 20–30 nm. They are also known to have quite negligible photobleaching. Their PL decay occurs in about 1–100 ns, which is often multiexponential (Dai et al., 2017). One of the most important properties to cater to bioimaging is high brightness. Brightness is a product of quantum yield (QY) (a ratio of the number of photons emitted to the number of those absorbed) and absorptivity. It is dependent upon QYs and molar extinction coefficients. Along with high brightness, QDs provide big two-photon cross sections. This is beneficial for the excitation of multiple photons. CdSe/CdS-quantum-dots-quantum-rods have recently been manufactured with two-photon cross sections of nearly 105 GM and quantum yields of 78%. A broad absorption spectrum provides for the efficient excitation of several dyes at a time. Excitation of multiple QDs using only one source of excitation (wavelength) along with the detection of simultaneous multiple QD PL opens up the possibility to multiplex the signals with around negligible noise of spectra. When weighing the advantages in terms of photostability, it has been witnessed that QDs are about 100 times more stable and 20 times brighter compared with Rhodamine 6G and some other superior organic dyes. Another advantage of QDs over traditional fluorophores is that it has around two orders larger two-photon cross section. This is a suitable property for the in vivo implementation using NIR excitation (Won et al., 2019). Despite the fantastic optical and photophysical properties of QDs, it has been reported that QDs cannot replace organic dyes or FPs in bioimaging due to their blinking, noncolloidal properties, and controversial toxicity issues. Moreover, a combination of many dyes with larger biomolecules, for example, antibodies, upsurge the overall brightness of the bioconjugate PL in addition to their biocompatibility. It displays an excellent opportunity for direct expression of the fluorophore in the targeted biological system, such that chemical coupling, which results in disrupted biological functionality, can be deliberately prevented (Wegner and Hildebrandt, 2015).

Thus absorbance plays a considerable part in any bioimaging process. The degree of absorbance is a direct implementation of the severity of the malignancy of cells. Several NPs have demonstrated remarkable photophysical properties, which could have been readily implemented in bioimaging. However, not all of them are biocompatible. Moreover, cytotoxicity is a major concern to be taken into account over the advantages of better absorbance of any material. Therefore one must see to it on a first priority basis while choosing any NP for bioimaging, whether that NP is biocompatible, among the set of favorable properties of any material.

7.3.3 Electrochemical properties

Bioimaging and biosensing are relatively a new addition to the field of nanotechnology. The field of bioimaging demands probes that have photoluminescence, but on the other hand, when the synthesized nanostructures retain the good electrochemical properties of their parent material(s), they can also be used for biosensing applications given that they are proven to have low cytotoxicity to cells (Pérez et al., 2019). Electrochemical biosensors are attracting much attention recently as they can be used efficiently for diagnosis in clinical applications and point-of-care devices.

The electrochemical properties that make certain NPs a good candidate in biosensing were assessed by Yu et al., where they tested graphene nanoplatelets (GNPs) GO, expanded graphite (EG), MWCNTs, and aminated graphene (NH_2-G) on various standards. Raman spectroscopy and Fourier-transform infrared analysis were performed to assess the existence of particular functional groups, such as carboxylic and carbonyl moieties, in some substances, which results in them having altered surface charges. This helps them have good water solubility and functionalization with biological, organic, inorganic, and polymeric species. It was also concluded that in the field of biosensing, electrochemical properties like small capacitance paired with large effective surface area is a much appreciated feature that was observed in composites of EG with nanocarbons. After investigating various other supporting tests, they employed EG and GNPs at a mass ratio of 2:1 for biosensing applications (Yu et al., 2018). Similarly, CDs are known for separating generated charges in the target interface and providing an electron transfer pathway to the electrode surface. So, in another attempt, a group used a CDs-based electrochemical DNA biosensor wherein they modified a disposable electrode using CDs that were nontoxic. The electrode was made for electrochemical transduction of signals when they found mutations in the human DNA from blood cells, and these CDs could efficiently enhance the transduction ability of those electrodes (García-Mendiola et al., 2018). However, CDs are essentially a semiconductor material, which means they inherently have low electronic conductivity. The CDs electrochemical features depended on activities between the carbon core, functional groups, and doped heteroatoms. CDs are trendy for their electrochemical signal transduction capabilities from the interface to the electrode. CDs capped with polyamidoamine (PAMAM) dendrimers were used along with a noble metal, which improved its intrinsic electrochemical properties to form polyamidoamine dendrimers capped-CDs (PAMAM-CDs)/Au nanocrystal nanocomposites. A nanostructure was prepared using a one-step process of microwave-assisted pyrolysis of citric acid and PAMAM. These structures were tested for their capabilities using a differential pulse voltammetry test and showed high stability and conductivity. These nanostructures are good materials for biosensors concerning their biocompatibility, high specific surface area, and available active sites that offer great functionalization (i.e., antibody immobilization) (Pirsaheb et al., 2019). On a different note, hybrid materials like MOF composites have also been used by integrating them with electrodes to make a DNA based on mimetic catalysis of MOFs and an allosteric switch of the hairpin DNA as shown in Fig. 7.4 (Wang, 2017). These NPs have good potential but need extensive research.

Carbon-based nanomaterials can be an excellent material for electrode surface modification. They have good electrochemical activity and an ability to provide a pathway to the electrons toward the electrode. Moreover, their greater specific surface area, hydrophilic edges, and hydrophobic planes increase the chances of analyte absorption on the electrode's surface. However, those being semiconductor means they inherently have low electronic conductivity. Therefore researchers have tried using other ways to improve the field of electrochemical sensing by using a combination of CDs with noble metal NPs as mentioned above or doped heteroatoms like ruthenium bipyridine sensitized MoO_3 multifunctional nanostructures. Even a graphene aerogel was employed to synthesize novel nanocomposites having superior electrochemical properties (Veerapandian et al., 2017).

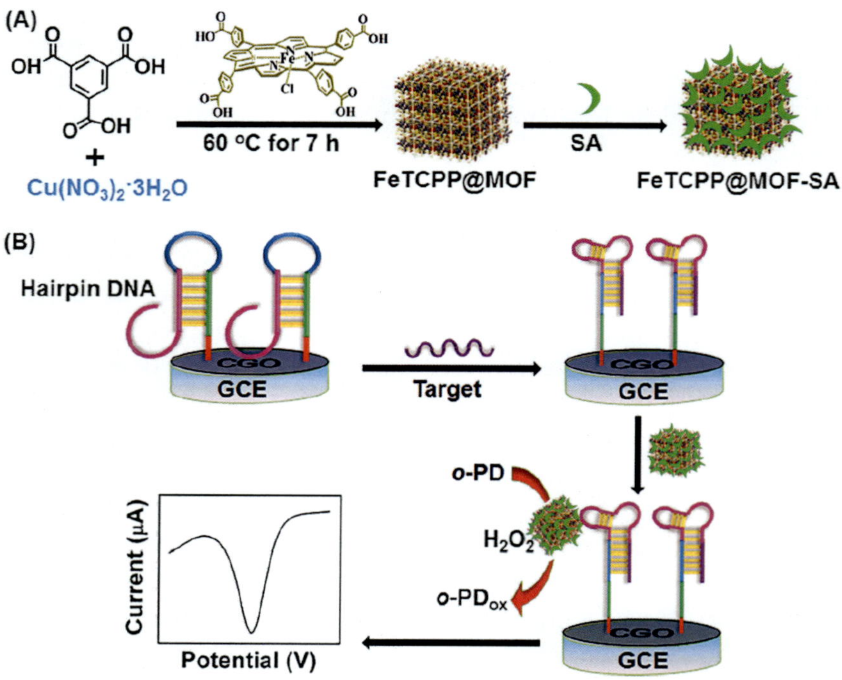

Fig. 7.4 A FeTCPP@MOF-SA composite for electrochemical DNA sensing. (A) Synthesis of the FeTCPP@MOF-SA composite and (B) electrochemical DNA sensing via the allosteric switch of the hairpin DNA. *(Reproduced with permission from Ling, P., Lei, J., Zhang, L., Ju, H., 2015. Porphyrin-encapsulated metal–organic frameworks as mimetic catalysts for electrochemical DNA sensing via allosteric switch of hairpin DNA. Anal. Chem. 87, 3957–3963. Copyright © 2015, American Chemical Society. All rights reserved.)*

7.3.4 Cytotoxicity

Cytotoxicity is a matter of major concern in bioimaging using NPs. The role of NPs in bioimaging is very intimate with the cells; hence, they must be least reactive to carry out only the desired function, which is bioimaging in this case. A NP journey in bioimaging follows from drug administration, distribution, metabolism (if any), and excretion (Ocampo-Nestor et al., 2017). Every process mentioned above takes place over a certain expected time interval, helping to prevent the accumulation of that nanomaterial in the human system and thus does not disturb its stability. Several organic NPs are known to be less toxic in comparison with inorganic NPs because of their natural origin. Nevertheless, not all organic nanomaterials are entirely free of toxicity.

Iron plays a vital role in oxygen transport across the body; however, the same iron, when taken in as a foreign material, in the form of nanomaterial, is highly reactive and, thus, may be toxic. Moreover, iron, in the form of Fe^0 and Fe_3O_4, is more ferocious than Fe_2O_3. Furthermore, iron NPs, rather any nanomaterial, is even more toxic because of their extremely small size. Since the nanomaterial is scaled down to nano-dimensions, more and more atoms start getting exposed to the particle's surface because of the increased surface area. These exposed atoms will have bonds dangling (vacancies and dislocations). This phenomenon gives the NPs high surface energy making them very reactive (Wagner et al., 2018). Thus the atoms' outer orbit electrons, which are usually found on the surface, will readily transfer themselves to the electron-acceptor groups, reducing them in the biological substances.

On the other hand, the surface vacancies can accept the electrons coming from the electron-donor group, in turn oxidize the molecules of biological substances. It ultimately leads to ROS production, and when it depends on the direct contact of a nanomaterial surface with the biomolecules, it is called the direct pathway of ROS generation. Opposite to that, ROS can be indirectly produced if the nanomaterial can disturb endogenous biochemical/physiological equilibria of the cells. All of these phenomena occur due to the nanomaterials' high surface energy that directs such activities to stabilize themselves by slowing down surface energy (Li et al., 2014).

To tackle such issues, surface coating and surface modifications to the NPs can be employed. Several materials, such as polyvinyl alcohol and dextran, have been experimented with to study numerous functional group comparative effects to seek better results. For example, iron oxide NPs when coated with different types of functional groups such as $-NH_2$, -OH, and -COOH showed differing cytotoxicity as well as genotoxicity using the L-929 fibroblasts. The NPs with a positive charge displayed dose-dependent genotoxicity upon testing with the cells, while the bare NPs and -OH group modified NPs caused no obvious genotoxicity at comparable concentrations (Mandal and Roy, 2020). In addition to that, iron oxide NPs having different coatings responded with a different kind of toxic effect on the primary cortical neurons. Additionally, the polydimethylamine-coated NPs had a damaging effect on the integrity of the membrane followed by induced death of cells, whereas aminosilane-coated NPs had much reduced toxicity comparatively and did not have any effects on the metabolic activity of cells at higher concentrations (Ung et al., 2017). Dextran-coated iron oxide NPs altered cell viability partially only at higher concentrations. However, considering the level of reactivity of iron oxide NPs, it is always more toxic when NPs are coated, as it mitigates the adverse reactions of NPs with the tissues. Moreover, the challenge of intactness of that coating throughout the bioimaging process still remains. The loss of coating from the nanomaterial in vivo may lead to absurd and uninvited ROS production and thus tissue damage (Li et al., 2014). Gold NPs, on the other hand, are more feasible for bioimaging because, unlike iron, gold has no background concentration in the biological system, which makes it appropriate to be measured at really low levels (Ning et al., 2017). However, they may be toxic on the basis of the organ distribution of gold NPs related to the particle size (Jia et al., 2017; Li Jia'En, 2011).

Thus for understanding the mechanism of toxicity and minimization/elimination of the toxicity of the NPs, it is really important to quantify and completely get rid of the excess reactants from the synthesis procedure of all the NPs. Every material possesses peculiar characteristics. Moreover, each material's properties changes with size; therefore a thorough study and valid experimentation are required to investigate the least toxic NPs along with superior bioimaging quality. Most importantly, it will be instructive to optimize the synthesis procedures for obtaining more safe NPs that can be used in biomedical applications accepted in the clinic.

7.4 Applications

7.4.1 Fluorescence imaging

NPs, whether they be organic, inorganic, or hybrid, have numerous applications in different imaging types such as fluorescence imaging, PAI, luminescence imaging, and many more. Depending on their properties and chemical nature, different NPs are employed in different applications of imaging. One such potential application of NPs is fluorescence imaging that uses the fluorescence properties of NPs. Fluorescence is the phenomenon that refers to the property of a material to absorb light of a shorter wavelength and emit out light at a certain wavelength. The advantage of fluorescence imaging over any other imaging technique is that it offers a unique property to visualize the morphological details of bio-species, from living cells to animals, without any harmful radioactive effects. The result and quality of the fluorescence imaging entirely depend on the fluorescent probes used to label the target biomolecules and amplify the fluorescence signals (Terai and Nagano, 2008). For several decades, small organic molecules and FPs have been used as probes; however, they have certain drawbacks, such as a small excitation spectrum, intrinsic susceptibility to proteolytic enzymes, and poor photostability. Therefore it is crucial to develop fluorescent probes that are photostable as well as biocompatible (Jensen, 2012). In recent studies, it was revealed that several NPs (such as QDs, organic and inorganic NPs, etc.) showed stability and a robust fluorescence.

One of the NPs with a strong potential application as a fluorescence probe is conjugated to conducting polymer (CP) NPs (CP NPs). Typically, CP NPs are prepared by initially dissolving CP in a specific organic solvent along with an amphiphilic polymeric encapsulation matrix. This organic solution is next added into a water phase (quickly), followed by sonication or stirring to facilitate stable NP dispersions. Further, the organic solvent is evaporated, and the polymer encapsulated CP NPs can be obtained. The optical properties, size, and shape of NPs can easily be manipulated or changed by using different polymer matrices (Li and Liu, 2012). A group used PEG-capped P8 NPs for performing nonspecific staining of HEp-2 cells. The internalization of NPs was recorded for 24 h. After 24 h of incubation, throughout the cytoplasm, intense NP fluorescence was detected clearly, while no specific toxicity was observed in cells over the course of the experiment (Howes et al., 2009).

GQDs are deemed good fluorescent probes due to the ease of functionalizing them using surface reagents (including biomolecules), narrow emission spectrum, superior photostability, and wide excitation wavelength (Chen et al., 2018). The intrinsic optical properties of GQDs form the basis for its applications in bioimaging. Different synthetic methods often lead to the formation of GQDs with edge defects, different functional groups, and sizes. These properties play an important part in the regulation of optical properties. The specially synthesized GQDs are used for in vitro and in vivo imaging. A group of researchers designed GQDs by a solvothermal method with strong green fluorescence properties; the synthesized NPs exhibited good biocompatibility, which could be used as labeling agents (Zhu et al., 2011). GQDs are also synthesized via a bottom-up approach using polycyclic aromatic hydrocarbons as the precursors. The internalization of the resultant GQDs by MCF-7 cells and their accumulation in the cytoplasm was investigated. For checking the efficiency of these synthesized probes, they were compared with Alexa Fluor 488 and fluorescein, which are the commonly used fluorescence probes for cellular imaging. It was observed that the higher photostability was exhibited by these GQDs (Wang et al., 2015).

In another study, a group used carboxylated GQDs for studying the biodistribution and OI in Balb/c nude mice with tumors. They first injected 5 and 10 mg/kg dosages of green GQDs in the mice, and they used a Kodak

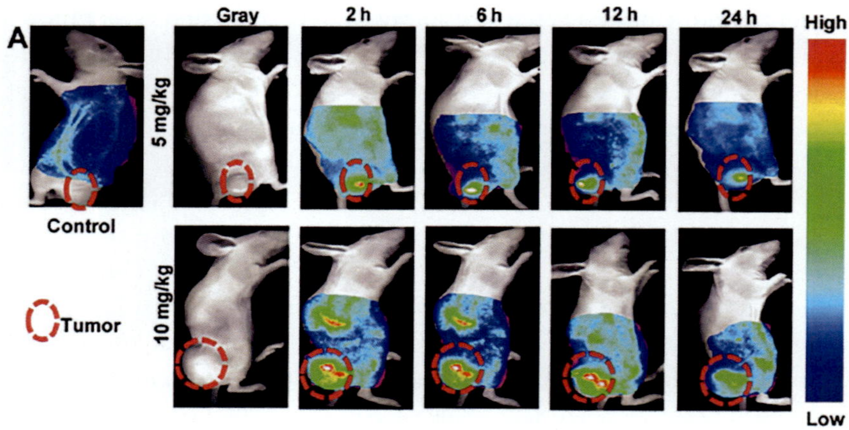

Fig. 7.5 Image showing time-dependent results for fluorescence imaging. *(Reproduced with permission from Nurunnabi, M., Khatun, Z., Huh, K.M., Park, S.Y., Lee, D.Y., Cho, K.J., Lee, Y., 2013. In vivo biodistribution and toxicology of carboxylated graphene quantum dots. ACS Nano 7, 6858–6867. Copyright © 2013 American Chemical Society.)*

Molecular Imaging System (4000MN PRO, Kodak, United States) for imaging the GQDs in a noninvasive manner. They saw that there were no signals from deep tissues in mice right after the injection at 505 nm in the emission wavelength. However, they received fluorescence signals from the tumor site 12 h after the injection. Fig. 7.5 illustrates the time-dependent images from the same study. The study evidently suggested that GQDs are competent enough to use as fluorescent probes in fluorescence imaging.

All the examples mentioned above have shown good fluorescence properties and can be employed in fluorescence imaging. As mentioned earlier, fluorescence imaging has emerged as a powerful platform compared to other imaging modalities due to its spatial-temporal imaging at the cellular level. It also helps to avoid issues of autofluorescence. Therefore fluorescence imaging can be efficiently employed in clinical fields for the real-time detection of the injured tissues or any other cells.

7.4.2 Persistent luminescence imaging

There are various types of luminescence, such as fluorescence, photoluminescence, phosphorescence, electro-chemiluminescence, PL, and chemiluminescence. The major difference in these luminescence techniques is the time in which the emission of energy takes place after absorbing the light (UV or visible) (Liu et al., 2019). PL is nearly the same as phosphorescence. It is an event in which luminescence is maintained for a few minutes to hours with no excitation source; due to the de-excitation between two electronic states, long emission is caused. It has been recognized that this phenomenon involves energy traps (such as electron or hole traps) in a material, which are filled during the excitation (Liang et al., 2019). After excitation, the stored energy is steadily released to emitter centers (which emit light), usually by a mechanism similar to that of fluorescence. Although it is said that PL is the same as phosphorescence, its entire mechanism is not understood. PLNPs show major growth in biomedical, data storage, phototherapy, bioimaging, and security techniques because of its unique properties, such as intensity, stability, and duration of PL (Wang et al., 2017). Rechargeable PLNPs with a great long afterglow life provide innovative methods for long-term phototherapy. Also, an enormous potential was observed concerning the elimination of external, optical rechargeable features, and multicolor PLNPs having higher decoding SNRs and high storage capability (Lecuyer et al., 2016).

Multidrug-resistance (MDR) bacterial strains that have evolved in the environment is a serious concern for human health. As a new drug is developed, after sometime, a specific bacterial strain may develop resistance toward that drug, which demands a new approach to combat MDR strains such as photothermal therapy (PTT) (Yan et al., 2020). Although PTT is an excellent move toward killing bacteria with physical heat, photothermal agents that are used in PPT cannot manage their circulation, which raises the temperature of regular cells present at the target site. To overcome this limitation, a group of researchers used pH-responsive nanoplatforms for PL imaging, which is a direct PTT technique to wipe out specific pathological cells. Core-shell nanomaterials were constructed for PL imaging, where PLNPs (NIR-emitting PLNP) were used as the core and covered with polyaniline (PANI). Furthermore, to add pH switchable properties, glycol chitosan (GCS, which is a water-soluble biopolymer with pH-dependent charge) was inserted on PLNP@PANI. When infected bacterial cells were detected in laboratory mice, PLNP@PANI-GCS NPs were introduced into the mice through injections. A normal cell inside the mice had a low affinity toward host cells (infected bacterial cells) due to a nearly high pH than infected cells (pH ~7.4); hence, they were not detected in PL imaging. Ultimately, the normal cells did not get killed in PTT. However, in the case of bacteria-infected cells, due to a low pH (pH <6.5), the affinity between the infected bacteria cells and PLNP@PANI-GCS NPs was found to be very high. Moreover, after exposing that particular mouse to LED light, a long-time luminescence was observed, which helped to guide the PTT to kill only infected cells while not harming the normal cells. An in vivo imaging system (IVIS) was used to capture the PL signal. Strong absorbance was observed due to the bending and stretching of various bonds with different wavelengths, such as PLNP@PANI, which gave strong absorption bands at 1580 and 1495 cm^{-1} for the C=C stretching vibration of the quinoid. In an acidic medium, conversion of charge took place that was observed by the Glasgow coma scale (GCS) modification in NPs. As the pH is lower (from pH 7.4 to 6.5), the charge on PLNP@PANI-GCS became more positive than negative concerning charge conversion that led to high affinity and ultimately led to an increase in the infected temperature cell and luminescent at the same time. Therefore in PTT, the infected cell can be specifically killed (Zhao et al., 2019b). Fig. 7.6 illustrates this study with a schematic for the preparation of PLNP@PANI-GCS.

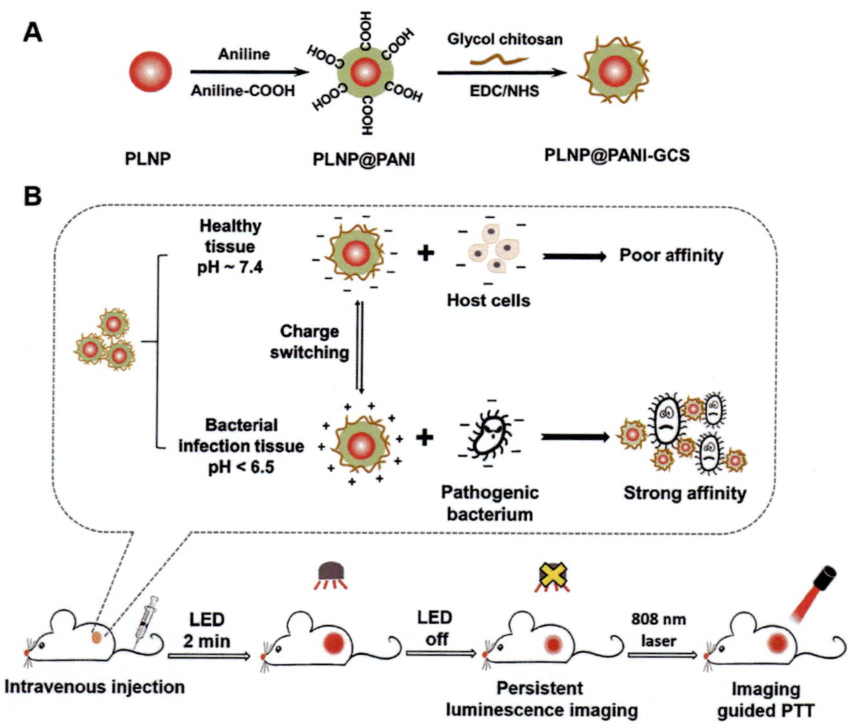

Fig. 7.6 (A) Schematic for the preparation of PLNP@PANI-GCS. (B) Illustration of PLNP@PANI-GCS for persistent luminescence imaging-guided photothermal therapy of bacterial infection. *(Reproduced with permission from Yan, L.X., Chen, L.J., Zhao, X., Yan, X.P., 2020. pH switchable nanoplatform for in vivo persistent luminescence imaging and precise photothermal therapy of bacterial infection. Adv. Funct. Mater. 30, 1–12. Copyright © 2020 WILEY-VCH Verlag GmbH & Co. KGaA, Weinheim. All rights reserved.)*

The latest techniques have been found to be very effective and less harmful than conventional ones. For instance, to locate the tumor, scientists have designed SWCNTs with NIR emission and silver sulfide nanoprobes to avoid autofluorescence, creating noise, and affecting the quality of the image. Even though designing such probes offers a few advantages, a needle imaging plate fails to penetrate more than 2 cm in tissue and cannot find a tumor located deep inside the tissue. Therefore the design of nano-size PL phosphors using solvothermal and silica-templating methods could result in the potential for deep tissue imaging.

Recent developments in the field revealed that X-rays can be helpful for imaging as well. They have a high penetration capacity, which is already used in clinical treatments and radiotherapies. Using this idea, a group worked on X-ray-induced PL, which provides ultrasensitive imaging (Xu and Tanabe, 2019). PLNs were firstly prepared with a silica-templating method in which metal ions doped with silicate formed typical spherical mesoporous zinc gallogermanates (with size 100.3 ± 10.6 nm). This could allow the NPs to create rechargeable X-ray-excited PL and inhibition of orthotopic tumors. For PL imaging, a human hepatocellular carcinoma (HepG2) cell line was used to introduce tumors inside the mice. NPs injected into the tumor were then exposed to X-ray, and the image was captured by IVIS. Along with this, cellular uptake, an in vivo X-ray PDT study, and cytotoxicity tests were also conducted. The results showed that PL lasted very long for a very low dose of X-ray irradiation. However, as doses of X-rays increased, the death rate of HepG2 also increased. Strong PL signals were observed after 24 h, indicating that NPs used in this study have high withholding properties in tumors. Moreover, no toxic effects were found in the major organs of mice (Shi et al., 2020). This shows that PL imaging can be coupled with various other technologies to eliminate tumor treatment limitations. This method is flexible and hence opens more opportunities for further studies.

Recently, nanoprobes possessing imaging as well as drug delivery capacities present a multifunctional appeal for diagnosing and treating tumors. Nanoprobes were prepared by combining the pH-low-insertion-peptide (pHLIP) to the surface of the core-shell structure of mesoporous silica-coated PLNPs (MSPLNPs) with the peptide GFLG and disulfide bond as bridges, which are responsible for drug release in chemotherapy and PL imaging of tumors. The pHLIP is used since it allows a high uptake rate in adenocarcinomic human alveolar basal epithelial (A549) and HepG2 cells at very low pH (pH < 6.5). The probe was prepared employing a hydrothermal method. Further, PL imaging of HepG2 cells was acquired using an IVIS (irradiated with a 254 nm UV light for 5 min). Along with this, cytotoxicity assays and chemotherapy were also conducted. The outcome showed that the synthesis of pHLIP-SS-GFLG-MSPLNPs@DOX improved the nanoprobe bioavailability while providing drug loading channels. In a 48-h interval, the probe maintained significant PL characteristics after UV excitation and LED lamp repeated excitation. Confocal laser scanning microscopic images unveiled that pHLIP-SS-GFLG-MSPLNPs@DOX imaged tumor cells under acidic conditions. The research evidently showed that the pHLIP-SS-GFLG-MSPLNPs@DOX could conduct in vivo targeting PL imaging of tumors. Thus PL imaging can be used for complex tumor conditions and should be extensively explored (Zhang et al., 2020).

Although the PL imaging method has had several limitations in the past, such as autofluorescence by using nanoprobes, the need for various light sources, and varying experimental conditions (e.g., pH), it will be helpful for various diseases while not harming nontargeted cells.

7.4.3 Near-infrared surface-enhanced Raman scattering imaging

When light is incident upon some object, basically, many photons are thrown on that object, which has a particular frequency. Most of these photons, upon striking the object, bounce off with the same frequency; this phenomenon is called the Rayleigh effect. On the other hand, the photons coming back with lower or higher frequency than its initial value are said to follow the Raman effect. However, a major concern with the Raman effect is that it gives off very weak signals. Nevertheless, this limitation is overcome by the SERS technique, in which a metal with increased surface area employed with nanoscale roughness is used to adsorb the material to be studied. This results in Raman signal enhancement of around 10^{14-15} times. SERS technology has been largely developed in the last few decades for tissue and cell imaging. Silver NPs exhibited more sensitive SERS signals as compared to gold. Researchers tend to make bimetallic nanostructures that incorporate both of the elements. To demonstrate the increase of an analytical enhancement factor (AEF) in the presence of silver, a research group made Au-Ag NRs and deposited them on a substrate, which in turn gave out 10 times higher SERS signal of AEF as compared to Au NRs (Khlebtsov et al., 2013). Such composite NPs can also be applied for targeted cancer imaging, where they prepared chitosan encapsulated Au-Ag nanoflowers that gave out stable and strong SERS signals compared to Au-NPs when they were coupled with tumor cell-specific targeting ligands like

FA (Zhang et al., 2015). In other studies, it was observed that better reproducibility, as well as AEF, was offered by silicon nanohybrids (Au/Ag NPs-decorated silicon wafer or SiNWs arrays) (Ji et al., 2018). Therefore SERS imaging is an advantageous technique and must be explored in the field of bioimaging. However, it still is not a regularly used clinical technique due to the requirement of hi-end equipment that adds costs making it expensive. Another challenge to this technique is the development of nanomaterials that can improve the SERS signals given off by target cells by cutting off the interference from nonspecific molecules, i.e., autofluorescence (Zhang et al., 2018). While technology simplification will take time, imaging in the NIR window can prevent autofluorescence and tissue scattering of signals. This also helps in the excitation of light that penetrates deeper into the tissues giving better outputs for the field of in vivo imaging. The NIR part of the electromagnetic spectrum has two parts NIR-I (700–900 nm) and NIR-II (1000–1700 nm). Another review highlighted that the NIR-II window is preferably chosen for bioimaging applications instead of the NIR-I window. In contrast, the NIR-II window has very low autofluorescence, a high SNR, and reduced photon scattering, which provides better resolution images (He et al., 2018).

Therefore most of the research was focused on making NPs that have an emission spectrum in response to NIR excitation. Typically, such NPs have to be synthesized in multiple steps that include linking of noble metal particles, Raman reporters (dye molecules that have emission in the NIR region), and coating with a biocompatible materials (such as PEG, GO). A study reported GO-wrapped gold nanorods (GNRs) with an IR-780 dye (GO@GNRs/IR-780). These were synthesized by first preparing GO-wrapped GNRs (GO@AuNRs) and further analyzed by UV-Vis-NIR spectroscopy. Later, it was tagged with six NIR emission dye molecules named IR-780, IR-820, MB, MG, CV, and 2-ATP. The IR-780 had an absorption peak around 780 nm, which is why it exhibited the surface-enhanced resonance Raman scattering (SERRS) effect and improvised the SERS signal, and possessed in vitro stability for more than an hour. They used these GO@GNRs/IR-780 nanocomposites as labels in the imaging of 143B cells and obtained distinguishable good Raman signals from the cytoplasmic area, mainly when overlaid with bright-field images, showing good potential in bioimaging. The Raman signals from these nanocomposites were heterogeneously distributed according to the probe distribution. Additionally, they observed that due to the SERS, graphene-enhanced Raman scattering (GERS) and dye molecule enrichment on a GO sheet resulted in a faster image formation than other Raman probes images where integration took as less as ~0.04 s per pixel. This method, upon further tests, proved to be constructible using other cell lines as well as NIR dyes (Qiu et al., 2017). Thus this method could be easily applied for versatile, high-clarity, multicolor, superfast NIR-SERS imaging. Moreover, it can also be used for real-time monitoring of the photothermal cancer cell abscission using SERS and the imaging-guided photothermal treatment of cancerous cells. A group of scholars produced a nanocomposite made up of the Ag shell-Au satellite (Ag-Au SS) structure and excited them for in vivo imaging at 532, 647, and 785 nm, where these wavelengths rendered an AEF of 4.1-, 3.1-, and 2.5-fold, respectively, when compared with that of Ag shells. Moreover, they observed that upon photoexcitation at 785 nm, these nanocomposites gave out uniform and intense SERS signals where the SERS enhancement factor was $\sim 1.4 \times 10^6$, which was the highest compared with the other two laser lines along with an 11% relative standard deviation. The detectability of single particles under laboratory conditions was also observed to be 100%, which is an excellent feature for the production of good quality images. The study also unveiled that the AEF values from these nanocomposites were highly uniform and were attributed to its reproducibility to the shell-satellite structure of these nanocomposites, which gave rise to multiple hot spots. These nanocomposites were highly stable under laser irradiation, indicating that these were good choices for NIR-SERS imaging concerning their reproducibility, sturdiness, and signal uniformity, irrespective of incident laser polarization. As a proof-of-concept, they studied these nanocomposites in vivo using nude mice, where they witnessed that the injected area gave stronger SERS signals that matched well to the injected probe spectrum, whereas the other skin regions exhibited no Raman signals (Chang et al., 2014). Therefore these Ag-Au SS probes can be used in vivo for sensitive bioimaging. All the NIR-SERS imaging attempts were related to probes that had to be delivered on-site. However, applying an innovative approach, a group produced nanocomposites that selectively detect cancerous cells. They targeted the human epidermal growth factor receptor 2 (HER2) signaling pathway, which in most cases, is upregulated in breast cancer and prepared nanotags that could detect the HER2 receptors expressed by specified cancerous cells. It was obtained by conjugating nanocomposites with two HER2-recognition motifs: a full anti-HER2 monoclonal antibody (170 kDa) and an scFv anti-HER2 (26 kDa) antibody. Researchers also checked that these motifs had high selectivity toward HER2-positive cells so that they would not bind to nontargeted cells. On performing

NIR-SERS imaging, they obtained intense SERS signals from the particles located on the surface of HER2-positive cells, while no signals were obtained from their other regions or HER2-negative cells (MDAMB231 cells). NIR-SERS has a major issue associated with the development of high-sensitivity probes, as most of them are available in the UV/Vis range. 3,3′-Diethylthiatricarbocyanine (DTTC) is a cyanine derivative that is used as a standard in NIR-SERS imaging; however, it has moderate intensity. Therefore for making high-sensitivity probes, researchers prepared a library of structurally varying tricarbocyanines with the hope of finding a molecule with sensitivity higher than DTTC. It was observed that CyNAMLA-381 was selected as the best Raman reporter since it was good in terms of both signal intensity and stability. It also exhibited nearly a 12-fold higher sensitivity compared to the standard DTTC (Samanta et al., 2011). Thus these CyNAMLA-381-AuNPs were considered to be a good candidate for targeted in vivo cancer cells in bioimaging using NIR-SERS imaging.

Nevertheless, there are still several shortcomings, including dye molecules bound electrostatically to the noble metals while having poor stability in the physiological environment. Moreover, the chemical attachment process of metals to dyes is a costly process and thus cannot be emulated efficiently on commercial levels. Cytotoxicity of the dye molecules is another disadvantage. To make these nanocomposites biocompatible, most of the time, they are coated with biocompatible hydrophilic polymers. However, even these coatings get deformed morphologically (melting) when exposed to high-power NIR irradiation. These disadvantages must be taken into account. A dye-free technology, where a conducting polymer, can be employed as a biocompatible polymer as well as an NIR Raman reporter molecule. GNRs were investigated as the noble metal particle and coated with polypyrrole (PPy) and PANI to form GNR-PPy and GNR-PANI, respectively. It was employed in studying A549 cells employing a confocal Raman microspectrometer with 785 nm excitation. It obtained distinguishable images, which upon overlapping with bright-field microscopic images, showed that these probes were usually located in the cytoplasm of the cells. It was also demonstrated that the multiplex imaging could be obtained by incubating GNR-PANI and GNR-PPy together in cells while obtaining noninterfering signals from these probes at the same wavelength concerning the narrow spectral features of Raman peaks (Liu et al., 2015). Fig. 7.7 illustrates the NIR-SERS imaging of A549 cells using GNR-CPs as novel probes. This is an effective economical method that can be scaled up for applications in bioimaging as well as PTT of cancerous cells.

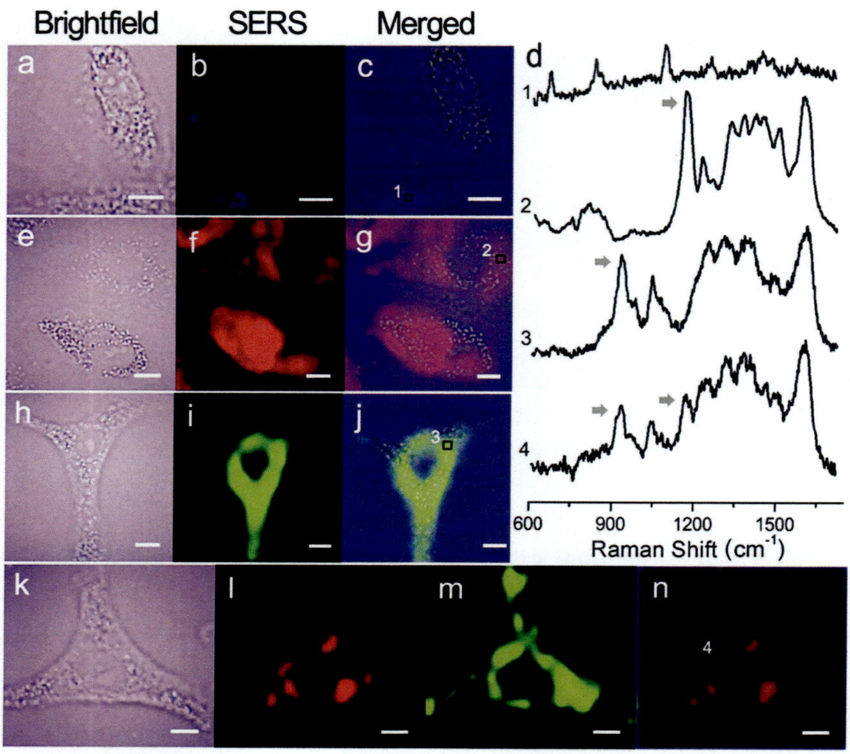

Fig. 7.7 NIR-SERS imaging of A549 cells using GNR-CPs as novel probes. *(Reproduced with permission from Liu, Z., Ye, B., Jin, M., Chen, H., Zhong, H., Wang, X., Guo, Z., 2015. Dye-free near-infrared surface-enhanced Raman scattering nanoprobes for bioimaging and high-performance photothermal cancer therapy. Nanoscale 7, 6754–6761. Copyright © 2015 The Royal Society of Chemistry, UK. All rights reserved.)*

Therefore the development and quest of finer, deep penetration, and low autofluorescence nanomaterial-based imaging methods have concluded that the NIR-SERS was an excellent method that has various additional properties (ability to produce multicolor imaging by multiplexing different NPs for imaging at the same time, superfast imaging, etc.). Various studies focused on the comparison of various Raman probes to get a better Raman reporter while others discovered new high-sensitivity NIR-Raman probes. Targeted cancer cell imaging using NIR-SERS was also investigated. Moreover, the cytotoxicity of these nanocomposites was also considered and taken care of by the introduction of dye-free NIR-Raman probes, which resulted in giving an economical and up-scalable imaging method that could produce high-resolution in vitro as well as in vivo images. With advancements in the current technology and wider availability of the same, this technology could be used for noninvasive, high-speed, and colorful imaging of targeted cells, tissues, and organs.

7.4.4 Photoacoustic imaging

PAI, as the name suggests, is a bioimaging technique in which the end image obtained is the result of the formation of ultrasonic waves after light waves are incident on the tissue (Attia et al., 2019). As stated above, the principle underlying PAI is the absorption of light leading to the emergence of sound waves. The resulting image is, therefore, the plot of the assembled sound waves thus produced. When compared with conventional methods, such as fluorescence imaging, PAI leads to deeper tissue imaging penetration and higher spatial resolution (Upputuri and Pramanik, 2019). Further, PAI yields exceedingly weaker optical signals in biological tissues (as a result of scattering of ultrasonic signals), possesses elevated spatial resolution, and much gaping tissue penetration (Brunker et al., 2017). Moreover, due to the comparison between optical properties of tissues or contrast agents and ultrasonic imaging (which is limited to the tissues' mechanical properties), PAI offers superior contrast (Talekar et al., 2017). Therefore all these advantages of PAI give rise to multiple applications (designed for varying imaging types ranging from an organ to a perfect animal) in the field of biomedical imaging, such as PA computer tomography, PA endoscopy, and PA microscopy. To reduce the interference of imaging (which commonly occurs due to the biological compound optical absorption), PAI agents with strong absorption in the range of NIR region and excessive absorption coefficients are of great importance (Salgaonkar et al., 2019). To yield a target-specific bioimage, absorption of light by specific contrast agents is desired. Numerous contrast agents, such as carbon materials, inorganic NPs, FPs, 2D materials, and NIR dyes, have been specially devised for PA imaging. Among all other contrast agents, NPs have an astounding role to play and thus invite several applications of NPs in PAI (Beard, 2011).

Graphene, for example, possessing intrinsic physical and especially optical characteristics, can be used as biosensors and employed in bioimaging. The outstanding optical properties of graphene and its derivatives, such as PA and photothermal responses, characteristic Raman bands, and visible and NIR photoluminescence, make them inviting for bioimaging, primarily in live cells (Wen et al., 2015). Polymer dots (PDs) exhibit the benefits of reduced biotoxicity, superficial surface functionalization of fluorescence, fine photostability, and elevated brightness, which makes it a suitable candidate in bioimaging.

However, the absence of the use of other optical techniques, along with stimulated Raman scattering, is questionable. Despite their unusual optical properties, such as nonradiative heat generation, high extinction coefficient, and NIR absorption, PDs have been broadly employed as PAI agents. Moreover, as versatile agents for PAI-guided PTT, conjugated PDs serve more potential applications. As reported by Chang et al., the novel 4,8-*bis*(5-(2-ethylhexyl)thiophen-2-yl)-2,6-*bis*(trimethylstannyl)benzo(1,2-*b*,4,5-*b*′)dithiophene-6-6′-dibromo-*N*,*N*′-(2-ethylhexyl)isoindigo (BDT-IID) PDs can be readily fabricated through nano reprecipitation and their absorption can vary between 650 and 700 nm in the spectrum. Furthermore, BDT-IID PDs possess a stable nanostructure and significantly decrease bio-toxicity. More essentially, in vivo results showed that the BDT-IID PDs are able to concurrently improve PA contrast and sufficient photothermal effect. The BDT-IID PDs can be used for PAI-guided PTT of tumors as distinctive theranostics nanoplatforms, holding high assurance for their restarting clinical development. The PDs hold impressive biocompatibility attributes and a remarkable photothermal conversion efficiency of up to 45%. Eventually, the BDT-IID PDs for succeeding clinical employment in PAI-guided PTT of various tumor species display great biosafety as well, making them a likely choice (Solhi and Hasanzadeh, 2019).

In addition to NP conjugation with peculiar molecules, a combination of PAI with fluorescence imaging offers dual-modality with the synthesized PEGylated RGO nanocomplex (RNGO) with indocyanine green (ICG) as a novel imaging agent. The speciality of the RNGO-PEG/ICG nanocomposite is that it has a durable circulation time, more intense imaging signals, reduced toxicity, better passive selecting capacity, and enhanced stability with obscure accumulation, displaying a promising future of image-guided diagnosis and therapy (Chen et al., 2016). Similarly, Qu et al. (2018) have synthesized a novel nanocomposite, i.e., GO/bismuth selenide/polyvinylpyrrolidone (PVP) by depositing Bi_2Se_3 NPs on GO in the presence of PVP, which could serve as a good bimodal contrast agent to concurrently improve X-ray, CT imaging, and PAI imaging in vivo.

An interesting application of CNTs along with their conjugates could be a favorable contrast agent for PAI of tumors, as it provides an extraordinary photothermal-acoustic response and photo-to-acoustic conversion efficiency. Recently, Wang et al. reported for the first time that Arginine-Glycine-Aspartic Acid (RGD)-conjugated silica-coated gold NRs on the surface of MWCNTs were well incorporated in targeted PAI of gastric cancer cells in vivo. The prepared probe exhibited favorable water solubility and low cellular toxicity and could target gastric cancer cells in vivo while providing excellent PAI in a nude animal model (Wang et al., 2014). Another group demonstrated a family of novel PA contrast agents based on small optical dye binding to SWCNTs (SWCNT-dye). They noted that SWCNTs were coated with either QSY21 (succinimidyl ester), i.e., SWCNT-QSY, or ICG (SWCNT-ICG) displayed over a hundred times better PA contrast in living animals with enhanced sensitivity compared to plain SWCNTs. Further, conjugation of SWCNT-dye with cyclic RGD peptides was done to target $\alpha v\beta 3$ integrins (which is associated with tumor angiogenesis) at the molecular level. When these tumor-targeted imaging agents were administered to tumor-bearing mice intravenously, a remarkably stronger PA signal in the tumor was observed, compared to mice injected with an untargeted contrast agent. Moreover, spectral separation of the PA signals of SWCNT-QSY and SWCNT-ICG in living animals (injected subcutaneously with both particles in the same location) was also obtained, thus assuring the possibility of in vivo multiplexing studies (de la Zerda et al., 2012). Similarly, Li et al. (2019) synthesized a smart nanoprobe, c(RGDyK)-MHDA/LSC@AuNPs, for PA detection and tumor imaging. These nanoprobes possess the properties of precise and targeted cancer cell PAI. Additionally, they yield signals only upon exposure to acidic microenvironments, which is a peculiar characteristic of solid tumors (regardless of their type). The latter characteristics of these smart nanoprobes proved to be practically helpful as it serves advantages of targeted and selective bioimaging as well as superintended drug release in vivo. This smart property of the Ph-sensitive PAI nanoprobes is governed by the meticulous control of the ratio of two thiol ligands on the surface of gold NPs. Upon exposure to overexpressed $\alpha v\beta 3$ integrins, these nanoprobes transfer the citraconic amides to primary amines (positive charge). Hence, they lead to NP aggregation and yield output in the form of an NIR signal (Fig. 7.8).

Further, CDs are also employed as contrast agents in PAI, as CDs cause evident acoustic waves after laser irradiation while offering a remarkable spatial resolution that can offer immoderate information even in the smallest areas. For instance, CDs are useful in detecting axillary lymph nodes where cancer cells can be spread in breast cancer and soon be excreted from the body while manifesting low toxicity during definitive optical signal production. The application of CDs in PA visualization of the sentinel lymph nodes and vessels was reported by a team, in which CDs exhibited vigorous signal enhancement upon injecting and were removed comparatively faster from the vessels. Furthermore, CDs have also been utilized as PA contrast agents as photosensitizers for PDT and PTT (Hola et al., 2014).

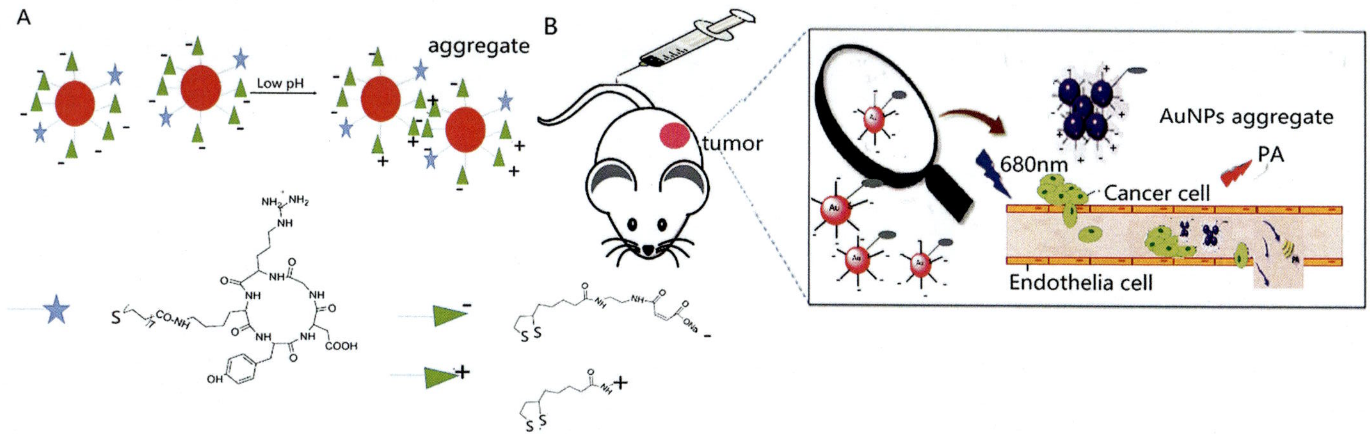

Fig. 7.8 Aggregation of nanoprobes in an acidic environment results in a near-infrared signal to give a photoacoustic image. *(From Li, S., Lui, K.H., Tsoi, T.H., Lo, W.S., Li, X., Hu, X., Chi-Shing Tai, W., Hiu-Ling Hung, C., Gu, Y.J., Wong, W.T., 2019. PH-responsive targeted gold nanoparticles for: in vivo photoacoustic imaging of tumor microenvironments. Nanoscale Adv. 1, 554–564. Creative Commons Attribution License @ 2019, Royal Society of Chemistry.)*

Thus nanomaterials possess major functionality in applications of PAI concerning their compatible characteristics. They exhibit high spatial resolution at extraordinary depths as PA waves and are much less scattered (2–3 orders of magnitude) than optical waves in biological tissue, and at the same time, PAI does the least harm to the cells, unlike conventional imaging techniques. NPs, when conjugated with peculiar biomolecules, enhance their applicability by assisting in PTT and PDT along with bioimaging. With the mentioned nanomaterial applications in PAI, there are several other NPs and their conjugates to be explored and to be applied in PAI.

7.5 Conclusion and future perspectives

In summary, the comprehensive investigation of the application of NPs has offered new insights into interesting developments in the field of biological imaging for real-time detection. Among many, fluorescence imaging has appeared as a powerful platform compared to other imaging techniques concerning its extraordinary spatial-temporal imaging ability at the cellular level while avoiding autofluorescence issues. The research also suggests that PL imaging can be employed in complex tumor conditions and be extensively explored. It is to be noted that PL imaging techniques suffer a few setbacks due to several limitations, such as autofluorescence, requirements of various light sources, and varying experimental conditions. NIR-SERS is an excellent method of producing superfast imaging, which serves a demand for finer and low autofluorescence-producing nanomaterial-based imaging methods that can efficiently penetrate deep in tissue. PAI has several applications concerning their compatible features. They exhibit high spatial resolution at extraordinary depths in biological tissue while not being harmful to nontargeted cells. Given the number of potential applications of NPs in the vast medical field (such as cancer diagnosis, therapy, and bioanalysis), it is difficult to make a general recommendation. However, the authors anticipate that this chapter will help readers understand the fundamentals behind applying distinct NPs for bioimaging purposes.

References

Ag, D., Seleci, M., Bongartz, R., Can, M., Yurteri, S., Cianga, I., Stahl, F., Timur, S., Scheper, T., Yagci, Y., 2013. From invisible structures of SWCNTs toward fluorescent and targeting architectures for cell imaging. Biomacromolecules 14, 3532–3541.

Agnihotri, P., Fazel-Rezai, R., Kaabouch, N., 2010. Comparative analysis of various brain imaging techniques. In: 2010 Annual International Conference of the IEEE Engineering in Medicine and Biology. IEEE, pp. 3029–3032.

Al Zaki, A., Cormode, D., Tsourkas, A., Dorsey, J.F., 2017. Increasing the therapeutic efficacy of radiotherapy using nanoparticles. In: Increasing the Therapeutic Ratio of Radiotherapy. Springer, pp. 241–265.

Altınoğlu, E.İ., Adair, J.H., 2010. Near infrared imaging with nanoparticles. Wiley Interdiscip. Rev. Nanomed. Nanobiotechnol. 2, 461–477.

Attia, A.B.E., Balasundaram, G., Moothanchery, M., Dinish, U.S., Bi, R., Ntziachristos, V., Olivo, M., 2019. A review of clinical photoacoustic imaging: Current and future trends. Photoacoustics 16, 100144.

Austin, L.A., Mackey, M.A., Dreaden, E.C., El-Sayed, M.A., 2014. The optical, photothermal, and facile surface chemical properties of gold and silver nanoparticles in biodiagnostics, therapy, and drug delivery. Arch. Toxicol. 88, 1391–1417.

Azlina, H.N., Hasnidawani, J.N., Norita, H., Surip, S.N., 2016. Synthesis of SiO_2 nanostructures using sol-gel method. Acta Phys. Pol. A 129, 842–844.

Bagheri, E., Ansari, L., Abnous, K., Taghdisi, S.M., Charbgoo, F., Ramezani, M., Alibolandi, M., 2018. Silica based hybrid materials for drug delivery and bioimaging. J. Control. Release 277, 57–76.

Balas, C., 2009. Review of biomedical optical imaging—a powerful, non-invasive, non-ionizing technology for improving in vivo diagnosis. Meas. Sci. Technol. 20, 104020.

Beard, P., 2011. Biomedical photoacoustic imaging. Interface Focus 1, 602–631.

Bedia, J., Muelas-Ramos, V., Peñas-Garzón, M., Gómez-Avilés, A., Rodríguez, J.J., Belver, C., 2019. A review on the synthesis and characterization of metal organic frameworks for photocatalytic water purification. Catalysts 9, 52.

Bhuyan, M.S.A., Uddin, M.N., Islam, M.M., Bipasha, F.A., Hossain, S.S., 2016. Synthesis of graphene. Int. Nano Lett. 6, 65–83.

Biju, V., 2014. Chemical modifications and bioconjugate reactions of nanomaterials for sensing, imaging, drug delivery and therapy. Chem. Soc. Rev. 43, 744–764.

Blake, P., Hill, E.W., Castro Neto, A.H., Novoselov, K.S., Jiang, D., Yang, R., Booth, T.J., Geim, A.K., 2007. Making graphene visible. Appl. Phys. Lett. 91, 63124.

Boskovic, B.O., Stolojan, V., Khan, R.U.A., Haq, S., Silva, S.R.P., 2002. Large-area synthesis of carbon nanofibres at room temperature. Nat. Mater. 1, 165–168.

Brunker, J., Yao, J., Laufer, J., Bohndiek, S.E., 2017. Photoacoustic imaging using genetically encoded reporters: a review. J. Biomed. Opt. 22, 70901.

Capanema, N.S.V., Carvalho, I.C., Mansur, A.A.P., Carvalho, S.M., Lage, A.P., Mansur, H.S., 2019. Hybrid hydrogel composed of carboxymethylcellulose–silver nanoparticles–doxorubicin for anticancer and antibacterial therapies against melanoma skin cancer cells. ACS Appl. Nano Mater. 2, 7393–7408.

Chang, H., Kang, H., Yang, J.K., Jo, A., Lee, H.Y., Lee, Y.S., Jeong, D.H., 2014. Ag shell–Au satellite hetero-nanostructure for ultra-sensitive, reproducible, and homogeneous NIR SERS activity. ACS Appl. Mater. Interfaces 6 (15), 11859–11863.

Chen, J., Liu, C., Zeng, G., You, Y., Wang, H., Gong, X., Zheng, R., Kim, J., Kim, C., Song, L., 2016. Indocyanine green loaded reduced graphene oxide for in vivo photoacoustic/fluorescence dual-modality tumor imaging. Nanoscale Res. Lett. 11, 1–11.

Chen, W., Lv, G., Hu, W., Li, D., Chen, S., Dai, Z., 2018. Synthesis and applications of graphene quantum dots: a review. Nanotechnol. Rev. 7, 157–185.

Cheng, H.-B., Li, Y., Tang, B.Z., Yoon, J., 2020. Assembly strategies of organic-based imaging agents for fluorescence and photoacoustic bioimaging applications. Chem. Soc. Rev. 49, 21–31.

Cheung, C.L., Kurtz, A., Park, H., Lieber, C.M., 2002. Diameter-controlled synthesis of carbon nanotubes. J. Phys. Chem. B 106, 2429–2433.

Dai, X., Deng, Y., Peng, X., Jin, Y., 2017. Quantum-dot light-emitting diodes for large-area displays: towards the dawn of commercialization. Adv. Mater. 29, 1607022.

Das, P., Fatehbasharzad, P., Colombo, M., Fiandra, L., Prosperi, D., 2019. Multifunctional magnetic gold nanomaterials for cancer. Trends Biotechnol. 37, 995–1010.

Dasari Shareena, T.P., McShan, D., Dasmahapatra, A.K., Tchounwou, P.B., 2018. A review on graphene-based nanomaterials in biomedical applications and risks in environment and health. Nano-Micro Lett. 10, 1–34.

de la Zerda, A., Bodapati, S., Teed, R., May, S.Y., Tabakman, S.M., Liu, Z., Khuri-Yakub, B.T., Chen, X., Dai, H., Gambhir, S.S., 2012. Family of enhanced photoacoustic imaging agents for high-sensitivity and multiplexing studies in living mice. ACS Nano 6, 4694–4701.

Dolmatov, V.Y., Veretennikova, M.V., Marchukov, V.A., Sushchev, V.G., 2004. Currently available methods of industrial nanodiamond synthesis. Phys. Solid State 46, 611–615.

Emam, A.N., Loutfy, S.A., Mostafa, A.A., Awad, H., Mohamed, M.B., 2017. Cyto-toxicity, biocompatibility and cellular response of carbon dots-plasmonic based nano-hybrids for bioimaging. RSC Adv. 7, 23502–23514.

García-Mendiola, T., Bravo, I., López-Moreno, J.M., Pariente, F., Wannemacher, R., Weber, K., Popp, J., Lorenzo, E., 2018. Carbon nanodots based biosensors for gene mutation detection. Sensors Actuators B Chem. 256, 226–233.

Ghamsari, M.S., 2018. Introductory Chapter: Nano-bioimaging—Past, Present, and Future. IntechOpen, Rijeka (Chapter 1).

González-Béjar, M., Francés-Soriano, L., Pérez-Prieto, J., 2016. Upconversion nanoparticles for bioimaging and regenerative medicine. Front. Bioeng. Biotechnol. 4, 1–9.

Hao, C., Wu, X., Sun, M., Zhang, H., Yuan, A., Xu, L., Xu, C., Kuang, H., 2019. Chiral core–shell upconversion nanoparticle@ MOF nanoassemblies for quantification and bioimaging of reactive oxygen species in vivo. J. Am. Chem. Soc. 141, 19373–19378.

Hashemzadeh, H., Raissi, H., 2017. The functionalization of carbon nanotubes to enhance the efficacy of the anticancer drug paclitaxel: a molecular dynamics simulation study. J. Mol. Model. 23, 222.

He, S., Song, J., Qu, J., Cheng, Z., 2018. Crucial breakthrough of second near-infrared biological window fluorophores: design and synthesis toward multimodal imaging and theranostics. Chem. Soc. Rev. 47, 4258–4278.

Hola, K., Zhang, Y., Wang, Y., Giannelis, E.P., Zboril, R., Rogach, A.L., 2014. Carbon dots—emerging light emitters for bioimaging, cancer therapy and optoelectronics. Nano Today 9, 590–603.

Howes, P., Thorogate, R., Green, M., Jickells, S., Daniel, B., 2009. Synthesis, characterisation and intracellular imaging of PEG capped BEHP-PPV nanospheres. Chem. Commun., 2490–2492.

Hu, Q., Li, H., Wang, L., Gu, H., Fan, C., 2018. DNA nanotechnology-enabled drug delivery systems. Chem. Rev. 119, 6459–6506.

Huang, D., Ou, B., Hampsch-Woodill, M., Flanagan, J.A., Deemer, E.K., 2002. Development and validation of oxygen radical absorbance capacity assay for lipophilic antioxidants using randomly methylated β-cyclodextrin as the solubility enhancer. J. Agric. Food Chem. 50, 1815–1821.

Jaque, D., Richard, C., Viana, B., Soga, K., Liu, X., García Solé, J., 2016. Inorganic nanoparticles for optical bioimaging. Adv. Opt. Photon. 8, 1.

Jensen, E.C., 2012. Use of fluorescent probes: their effect on cell biology and limitations. Anat. Rec. Adv. Integr. Anat. Evol. Biol. 295, 2031–2036.

Ji, X., Wang, H., Song, B., Chu, B., He, Y., 2018. Silicon nanomaterials for biosensing and bioimaging analysis. Front. Chem. 6, 38.

Jia, Y.-P., Ma, B.-Y., Wei, X.-W., Qian, Z.-Y., 2017. The in vitro and in vivo toxicity of gold nanoparticles. Chin. Chem. Lett. 28, 691–702.

Khlebtsov, B.N., Khanadeev, V.A., Tsvetkov, M.Y., Bagratashvili, V.N., Khlebtsov, N.G., 2013. Surface-enhanced Raman scattering substrates based on self-assembled PEGylated gold and gold–silver core–shell nanorods. J. Phys. Chem. C 117, 23162–23171.

Kim, D., Kim, J., Park, Y.I., Lee, N., Hyeon, T., 2018. Recent development of inorganic nanoparticles for biomedical imaging. ACS Cent. Sci. 4, 324–336.

Kumar, R., Singh, R., Hui, D., Feo, L., Fraternali, F., 2018. Graphene as biomedical sensing element: state of art review and potential engineering applications. Compos. Part B Eng. 134, 193–206.

Lecuyer, T., Teston, E., Ramirez-Garcia, G., Maldiney, T., Viana, B., Seguin, J., Mignet, N., Scherman, D., Richard, C., 2016. Chemically engineered persistent luminescence nanoprobes for bioimaging. Theranostics 6, 2488.

Lee, B.H., Kwon, K.-W., Shim, M., 2007. Semiconductor–polymer hybrid colloidal nanoparticles. J. Mater. Chem. 17 (13), 1284–1291.

Li Jia'En, J., 2011. Cytotoxicity of Gold Nanoparticles in vitro.

Li, K., Liu, B., 2012. Polymer encapsulated conjugated polymer nanoparticles for fluorescence bioimaging. J. Mater. Chem. 22, 1257–1264.

Li, J., Chang, X., Chen, X., Gu, Z., Zhao, F., Chai, Z., Zhao, Y., 2014. Toxicity of inorganic nanomaterials in biomedical imaging. Biotechnol. Adv. 32, 727–743.

Li, J.-B., Liu, H.-W., Fu, T., Wang, R., Zhang, X.-B., Tan, W., 2019. Recent progress in small-molecule near-IR probes for bioimaging. Trends Chem. 1, 224–234.

Li, J., Wang, J., Yao, Q., Li, T., Yan, Y., Li, Z., Zhang, J., 2020a. Why synthetic virus-like nanoparticles can achieve higher cellular uptake efficiency? Nanoscale 12, 14911–14918.

Li, Y., Wang, X., Zhang, Y., Nie, G., 2020b. Recent advances in nanomaterials with inherent optical and magnetic properties for bioimaging and imaging-guided nucleic acid therapy. Bioconjug. Chem. 31, 1234–1246.

Liang, R., Wei, M., Evans, D.G., Duan, X., 2014. Inorganic nanomaterials for bioimaging, targeted drug delivery and therapeutics. Chem. Commun. 50, 14071–14081.

Liang, L., Chen, N., Jia, Y., Ma, Q., Wang, J., Yuan, Q., Tan, W., 2019. Recent progress in engineering near-infrared persistent luminescence nanoprobes for time-resolved biosensing/bioimaging. Nano Res. 12, 1279–1292.

Lim, J.Y.C., Yu, Y., Jin, G., Li, K., Lu, Y., Xie, J., Tan, Y.N., 2020. Establishing empirical design rules of nucleic acid templates for the synthesis of silver nanoclusters with tunable photoluminescence and functionalities towards targeted bioimaging applications. Nanoscale Adv. 2, 3921–3932.

Lin, J., Huang, Y., Huang, P., 2018. Graphene-Based Nanomaterials in Bioimaging, Biomedical Applications of Functionalized Nanomaterials: Concepts, Development and Clinical Translation. Elsevier Inc.

Liu, Z., Ye, B., Jin, M., Chen, H., Zhong, H., Wang, X., Guo, Z., 2015. Dye-free near-infrared surface-enhanced Raman scattering nanoprobes for bioimaging and high-performance photothermal cancer therapy. Nanoscale 7, 6754–6761.

Liu, J., Lécuyer, T., Seguin, J., Mignet, N., Scherman, D., Viana, B., Richard, C., 2019. Imaging and therapeutic applications of persistent luminescence nanomaterials. Adv. Drug Deliv. Rev. 138, 193–210.

Lu, X., Akasaka, T., Nagase, S., 2010. Rare earth metals trapped inside fullerenes–endohedral metallofullerenes (EMFs). In: Rare Earth Coordination Chemistry: Fundamentals and Applications, pp. 273–307.

Luo, Z., Fan, S., Gu, C., Liu, W., Chen, J., Li, B., Liu, J., 2019. Metal–organic framework (MOF)-based nanomaterials for biomedical applications. Curr. Med. Chem. 26, 3341–3369.

Mahan, M.M., Doiron, A.L., 2018. Gold nanoparticles as X-ray, CT, and multimodal imaging contrast agents: formulation, targeting, and methodology. J. Nanomater. 2018.

Maldiney, T., Bessière, A., Seguin, J., Teston, E., Sharma, S.K., Viana, B., Bos, A.J.J., Dorenbos, P., Bessodes, M., Gourier, D., Scherman, D., Richard, C., 2014. The in vivo activation of persistent nanophosphors for optical imaging of vascularization, tumours and grafted cells. Nat. Mater. 13, 418–426.

Mandal, T.K., Roy, D.B., 2020. A review on fabrication methods, characterization and applications of nanomaterials, magnetic iron oxide. Iran. J. Mater. Sci. Eng. 17.

Martinić, I., Eliseeva, S.V., Petoud, S., 2017. Near-infrared emitting probes for biological imaging: organic fluorophores, quantum dots, fluorescent proteins, lanthanide (III) complexes and nanomaterials. J. Lumin. 189, 19–43.

Mohanraj, V.J., Chen, Y., 2006. Nanoparticles-a review. Trop. J. Pharm. Res. 5, 561–573.

Nadar, S.S., Varadan, N., Suresh, S., Rao, P., Ahirrao, D.J., Adsare, S., 2018. Recent progress in nanostructured magnetic framework composites (MFCs): synthesis and applications. J. Taiwan Inst. Chem. Eng. 91, 653–677.

Nadar, S.S., Vaidya, L., Maurya, S., Rathod, V.K., 2019. Polysaccharide based metal organic frameworks (polysaccharide–MOF): a review. Coord. Chem. Rev. 396, 1–21.

Ning, L., Zhu, B., Gao, T., 2017. Gold nanoparticles: promising agent to improve the diagnosis and therapy of cancer. Curr. Drug Metab. 18, 1055–1067.

Ocampo-Nestor, A.L., Trujillo-Ferrara, J.G., Abad-Garcia, A., Reyes-Lopez, C., Geninatti-Crich, S., Soriano-Ursua, M.A., 2017. Boron's journey: advances in the study and application of pharmacokinetics. Expert Opin. Ther. Pat. 27, 203–215.

Paris, J.L., Baeza, A., Vallet-Regí, M., 2019. Overcoming the stability, toxicity, and biodegradation challenges of tumor stimuli-responsive inorganic nanoparticles for delivery of cancer therapeutics. Expert Opin. Drug Deliv. 16, 1095–1112.

Paysen, H., Loewa, N., Stach, A., Wells, J., Kosch, O., Twamley, S., Makowski, M.R., Schaeffter, T., Ludwig, A., Wiekhorst, F., 2020. Cellular uptake of magnetic nanoparticles imaged and quantified by magnetic particle imaging. Sci. Rep. 10, 1–8.

Pedone, D., Moglianetti, M., De Luca, E., Bardi, G., Pompa, P.P., 2017. Platinum nanoparticles in nanobiomedicine. Chem. Soc. Rev. 46, 4951–4975.

Perevedentseva, E., Lin, Y.-C., Jani, M., Cheng, C.-L., 2013. Biomedical applications of nanodiamonds in imaging and therapy. Nanomedicine 8, 2041–2060.

Pérez, J.A.C., Sosa-Hernández, J.E., Hussain, S.M., Bilal, M., Parra-Saldivar, R., Iqbal, H.M.N., 2019. Bioinspired biomaterials and enzyme-based biosensors for point-of-care applications with reference to cancer and bio-imaging. Biocatal. Agric. Biotechnol. 17, 168–176.

Pirsaheb, M., Mohammadi, S., Salimi, A., 2019. Current advances of carbon dots based biosensors for tumor marker detection, cancer cells analysis and bioimaging. TrAC Trends Anal. Chem. 115, 83–99.

Prabhakar, N., Rosenholm, J.M., 2019. Nanodiamonds for advanced optical bioimaging and beyond. Curr. Opin. Colloid Interface Sci. 39, 220–231.

Qiu, X., You, X., Chen, X., Chen, H., Dhinakar, A., Liu, S., Guo, Z., Wu, J., Liu, Z., 2017. Development of graphene oxide-wrapped gold nanorods as robust nanoplatform for ultrafast near-infrared SERS bioimaging. Int. J. Nanomedicine 12, 4349.

Qu, Y., He, F., Yu, C., Liang, X., Liang, D., Ma, L., Zhang, Q., Lv, J., Wu, J., 2018. Advances on graphene-based nanomaterials for biomedical applications. Mater. Sci. Eng. C 90, 764–780.

Reineck, P., Gibson, B.C., 2017. Near-infrared fluorescent nanomaterials for bioimaging and sensing. Adv. Opt. Mater. 5 (2), 1600446.

Romero, G., Moya, S.E., 2012. Synthesis of organic nanoparticles. In: Frontiers of Nanoscience. Elsevier, pp. 115–141.

Rostami, I., Alanagh, H.R., Hu, Z., Shahmoradian, S.H., 2019. Breakthroughs in medicine and bioimaging with up-conversion nanoparticles. Int. J. Nanomedicine 14, 7759–7780.

Saji, V.S., Choe, H.C., Yeung, K.W.K., 2010. Nanotechnology in biomedical applications: a review. Int. J. Nano Biomater. 3, 119–139.

Salgaonkar, M., Nadar, S.S., Rathod, V.K., 2018. Combi-metal organic framework (Combi-MOF) of α-amylase and glucoamylase for one pot starch hydrolysis. Int. J. Biol. Macromol. 113, 464–475.

Salgaonkar, M., Nadar, S.S., Rathod, V.K., 2019. Biomineralization of orange peel peroxidase within metal organic frameworks (OPP–MOFs) for dye degradation. J. Environ. Chem. Eng. 7, 102969.

Samanta, A., Maiti, K.K., Soh, K., Liao, X., Vendrell, M., Dinish, U.S., Yun, S., Bhuvaneswari, R., Kim, H., Rautela, S., Chung, J., Olivo, M., Chang, Y., 2011. Ultrasensitive near-infrared raman reporters for SERS-based in vivo cancer detection. Angewandte Chemie. Zuschrift., 6213–6216.

Shaterabadi, Z., Nabiyouni, G., Soleymani, M., 2017. High impact of in situ dextran coating on biocompatibility, stability and magnetic properties of iron oxide nanoparticles. Mater. Sci. Eng. C 75, 947–956.

Shi, T., Sun, W., Qin, R., Li, D., Feng, Y., Chen, L., Liu, G., Chen, X., Chen, H., 2020. X-ray-induced persistent luminescence promotes ultrasensitive imaging and effective inhibition of orthotopic hepatic tumors. Adv. Funct. Mater. 30, 1–9.

Solhi, E., Hasanzadeh, M., 2019. Recent advances on the biosensing and bioimaging based on polymer dots as advanced nanomaterial: analytical approaches. TrAC Trends Anal. Chem. 118, 840–852.

Soufi, G.J., Iravani, S., 2020. Eco-friendly and sustainable synthesis of biocompatible nanomaterials for diagnostic imaging: current challenges and future perspectives. Green Chem. 22, 2662–2687.

Sportelli, M.C., Izzi, M., Volpe, A., Clemente, M., Picca, R.A., Ancona, A., Lugarà, P.M., Palazzo, G., Cioffi, N., 2018. The pros and cons of the use of laser ablation synthesis for the production of silver nano-antimicrobials. Antibiotics 7, 67.

Sun, Z., Huang, P., Tong, G., Lin, J., Jin, A., Rong, P., Zhu, L., Nie, L., Niu, G., Cao, F., Chen, X., 2013. VEGF-loaded graphene oxide as theranostics for multi-modality imaging-monitored targeting therapeutic angiogenesis of ischemic muscle. Nanoscale 5, 6857–6866.

Sun, S.-K., Wang, H.-F., Yan, X.-P., 2018. Engineering persistent luminescence nanoparticles for biological applications: from biosensing/bioimaging to theranostics. Acc. Chem. Res. 51, 1131–1143.

Talekar, S., Joshi, A., Kambale, S., Jadhav, S., Nadar, S., Ladole, M., 2017. A tri-enzyme magnetic nanobiocatalyst with one pot starch hydrolytic activity. Chem. Eng. J. 325.

Terai, T., Nagano, T., 2008. Fluorescent probes for bioimaging applications. Curr. Opin. Chem. Biol. 12, 515–521.

Ung, L., Pattamatta, U., Carnt, N., Wilkinson-Berka, J.L., Liew, G., White, A.J.R., 2017. Oxidative stress and reactive oxygen species: a review of their role in ocular disease. Clin. Sci. 131, 2865–2883.

Upputuri, P.K., Pramanik, M., 2019. Photoacoustic imaging in the second near-infrared window: a review. J. Biomed. Opt. 24, 40901.

Veerapandian, M., Avti, P.K., Ravichandiran, V., 2017. Ruthenium bipyridine sensitized MoO_3 multifunctional nanostructures: study of opto-electrochemical properties, biocompatibility and bioimaging. Colloids Surf. B: Biointerfaces 154, 315–320.

Wagner, H., Cheng, J.W., Ko, E.Y., 2018. Role of reactive oxygen species in male infertility: an updated review of literature. Arab J. Urol. 16, 35–43.

Wang, H.S., 2017. Metal–organic frameworks for biosensing and bioimaging applications. Coord. Chem. Rev. 349, 139–155.

Wang, C., Bao, C., Liang, S., Fu, H., Wang, K., Deng, M., Liao, Q., Cui, D., 2014. RGD-conjugated silica-coated gold nanorods on the surface of carbon nanotubes for targeted photoacoustic imaging of gastric cancer. Nanoscale Res. Lett. 9, 1–10.

Wang, D., Chen, J.F., Dai, L., 2015. Recent advances in graphene quantum dots for fluorescence bioimaging from cells through tissues to animals. Part. Part. Syst. Charact. 32, 515–523.

Wang, J., Ma, Q., Wang, Y., Shen, H., Yuan, Q., 2017. Recent progress in biomedical applications of persistent luminescence nanoparticles. Nanoscale 9, 6204–6218.

Wang, H., Chen, Q., Zhou, S., 2018. Carbon-based hybrid nanogels: a synergistic nanoplatform for combined biosensing, bioimaging, and responsive drug delivery. Chem. Soc. Rev. 47, 4198–4232.

Wang, J., Hsu, S., Gonzalez-Pech, N., Jhunjhunwala, A., Chen, F., Hariri, A., Grassian, V., Tao, A., Jokerst, J.V., 2019. Copper sulfide nanodisks and nanoprisms for photoacoustic ovarian tumor imaging. Part. Part. Syst. Charact. 36, 1900171.

Wegner, K.D., Hildebrandt, N., 2015. Quantum dots: bright and versatile in vitro and in vivo fluorescence imaging biosensors. Chem. Soc. Rev. 44, 4792–4834.

Wei, Y., Yang, X., Ma, Y., Wang, S., Yuan, Q., 2016. Lanthanide-doped nanoparticles with near-infrared-to-near-infrared luminescence for bioimaging. Chin. J. Chem. 34, 558–569.

Wen, J., Xu, Y., Li, H., Lu, A., Sun, S., 2015. Recent applications of carbon nanomaterials in fluorescence biosensing and bioimaging. Chem. Commun. 51, 11346–11358.

Wolfbeis, O.S., 2015. An overview of nanoparticles commonly used in fluorescent bioimaging. Chem. Soc. Rev. 44, 4743–4768.

Won, Y.-H., Cho, O., Kim, T., Chung, D.-Y., Kim, T., Chung, H., Jang, H., Lee, J., Kim, D., Jang, E., 2019. Highly efficient and stable InP/ZnSe/ZnS quantum dot light-emitting diodes. Nature 575, 634–638.

Wu, C., Chiu, D.T., 2013. Highly fluorescent semiconducting polymer dots for biology and medicine. Angew. Chem. Int. Ed. 52, 3086–3109.

Wu, M.-X., Yang, Y.-W., 2017. Metal-organic framework (MOF)-based drug/cargo delivery and cancer therapy. Adv. Mater. 29, 1606134.

Wu, X., Chen, G., Shen, J., Li, Z., Zhang, Y., Han, G., 2015. Upconversion nanoparticles: a versatile solution to multiscale biological imaging. Bioconjug. Chem. 26, 166–175.

Wu, S., Zhou, B., Yan, D., 2021. Recent advances on molecular crystalline luminescent materials for optical waveguides. Adv. Opt. Mater. 3, 768.

Xu, J., Tanabe, S., 2019. Persistent luminescence instead of phosphorescence: history, mechanism, and perspective. J. Lumin. 205, 581–620.

Xu, X., Zhong, J., Su, Y., Zou, Z., He, Y., Hou, X., 2019. A brief review on mass/optical spectrometry for imaging analysis of biological samples. Appl. Spectrosc. Rev. 54, 57–85.

Yan, L.X., Chen, L.J., Zhao, X., Yan, X.P., 2020. pH switchable nanoplatform for in vivo persistent luminescence imaging and precise photothermal therapy of bacterial infection. Adv. Funct. Mater. 30, 1–12.

Yaqoob, S.B., Adnan, R., Khan, R.M.R., Rashid, M., 2020. Gold, silver, and palladium nanoparticles: a chemical tool for biomedical applications. Front. Chem. 8.

Ye, F., Zhao, Y., El-Sayed, R., Muhammed, M., Hassan, M., 2018. Advances in nanotechnology for cancer biomarkers. Nano Today 18, 103–123.

Yu, J., Zhang, Y., Li, H., Wan, Q., Li, Y., Yang, N., 2018. Electrochemical properties and sensing applications of nanocarbons: a comparative study. Carbon N.Y. 129, 301–309.

Zarschler, K., Rocks, L., Licciardello, N., Boselli, L., Polo, E., Garcia, K.P., De Cola, L., Stephan, H., Dawson, K.A., 2016. Ultrasmall inorganic nanoparticles: state-of-the-art and perspectives for biomedical applications. Nanomedicine 12, 1663–1701.

Zhang, G., Li, J., Shen, A., Hu, J., 2015. Synthesis of size-tunable chitosan encapsulated gold–silver nanoflowers and their application in SERS imaging of living cells. Phys. Chem. Chem. Phys. 17, 21261–21267.

Zhang, Y., Wang, G., Yang, L., Wang, F., Liu, A., 2018. Recent advances in gold nanostructures based biosensing and bioimaging. Coord. Chem. Rev. 370, 1–21.

Zhang, X., Cong, H., Yu, B., Chen, Q., 2019. Recent advances of water-soluble fullerene derivatives in biomedical applications. Mini. Rev. Org. Chem. 16, 92–99.

Zhang, H.J., Zhao, X., Chen, L.J., Yang, C.X., Yan, X.P., 2020. pH-driven targeting nanoprobe with dual-responsive drug release for persistent luminescence imaging and chemotherapy of tumor. Anal. Chem. 92, 1179–1188.

Zhao, L., Ge, X., Yan, G., Wang, X., Hu, P., Shi, L., Wolfbeis, O.S., Zhang, H., Sun, L., 2017. Double-mesoporous core–shell nanosystems based on platinum nanoparticles functionalized with lanthanide complexes for in vivo magnetic resonance imaging and photothermal therapy. Nanoscale 9, 16012–16023.

Zhao, M., Liao, H., Molokeev, M.S., Zhou, Y., Zhang, Q., Liu, Q., Xia, Z., 2019a. Emerging ultra-narrow-band cyan-emitting phosphor for white LEDs with enhanced color rendition. Light Sci. Appl. 8, 1–9.

Zhao, X., Chen, L.-J., Zhao, K.-C., Liu, Y.-S., Liu, J., Yan, X.-P., 2019b. Autofluorescence-free chemo/biosensing in complex matrixes based on persistent luminescence nanoparticles. TrAC Trends Anal. Chem. 118, 65–72.

Zhu, S., Zhang, J., Qiao, C., Tang, S., Li, Y., Yuan, W., Li, B., Tian, L., Liu, F., Hu, R., Gao, H., Wei, H., Zhang, H., Sun, H., Yang, B., 2011. Strongly green-photoluminescent graphene quantum dots for bioimaging applications. Chem. Commun. 47, 6858–6860.

CHAPTER 8

Nanobiomaterials for medical devices and implants

Ankit A. Agrawal, Kaustubh A. Pawar, Vaibhav N. Ghegade, Archana A. Kapse, and Vandana B. Patravale
Department of Pharmaceutical Sciences and Technology, Institute of Chemical Technology, Mumbai, Maharashtra, India

8.1 Introduction

Medical devices and implants have been employed for several years. Over the last few decades, the use of medical devices and implants has dramatically increased in response to high demand for various reasons. Advances in metal, ceramic, and polymer science have also opened up new horizons in developing new technologies for the generation of nanobiomaterials.

Nanoscale materials that are biocompatible or biodegradable and which can positively interact with human biological systems are being increasingly developed to diagnose and treat human diseases. Medical devices and implants are an indispensable part of today's medical world, and applications of nanobiomaterials to these devices and implants can significantly improve their functionality and biocompatibility. The global market of medical devices and implants is expected to grow to more than $110 billion by 2022. The demand for novel and safe nanobiomaterials is increasing to circumvent existing issues associated with these devices. Apart from disease treatment, nanobiomaterials are also explored extensively in the prevention of biofilms and implant-associated infection.

Nanobiomaterials used for the manufacturing of these devices can be categorized into metals, polymers, composites, bio-ceramics, carbon-based materials, etc. The vast range of materials and interdisciplinary approaches to modify the material properties have created tremendous opportunities in the manufacturing of sophisticated and novel medical devices and implants having unique functionalities. Novel fabrication technologies for the development of such devices are being developed, such as additive manufacturing along with other prevailing technologies. As nanobiomaterials interact

Nanotechnology in Medicine and Biology
https://doi.org/10.1016/B978-0-12-819469-0.00008-3

at the cellular level, safety and toxicity measures are of critical importance in the development of such products. Novel nanobiomaterial-based medical devices and implants aim to provide improved functionality, real-time diagnosis and the occurrence of fewer adverse events than currently used devices. Such novel devices have the potential to emerge as "multifunctional therapeutics" that can deliver therapeutics as well as monitor its effective delivery.

8.2 Types of nanobiomaterials used in medical devices and implants

8.2.1 Metallic nanobiomaterials

Metals are used as nanobiomaterials, principally because of their good mechanical strength and corrosion resistance property. They have been extensively employed to manufacture different types of implants. About 70% of implants are used for orthopedic and cardiovascular applications (Niinomi et al. 2012). Pure metals are generally used, but alloys can enhance strength and corrosion resistance. The main properties required are biocompatibility, optimal mechanical properties, corrosion resistance in the presence of body fluids, durability, and cost-effectiveness. These properties depend on the chemical composition of the material. For instance, Ti-6Al-4V alloy has more tensile strength as compared to only titanium (Ti) because of the addition of aluminum and vanadium into it. The metallurgical state decides its mechanical properties; for instance, the annealing enhances ductility as compared to that of cold-worked metals. Further, metal treatments also determine their microstructure and physical properties. For example, the forging process generally gives higher strength than cast metal implants. The most widely used metals for implants are stainless steel (316L type), cobalt-chromium (Co-Cr), and Ti alloys. To fix the fractured bone segments together during healing, metal plates and screws are used. Depending on the recovery of bone and the extent of the injury, the plates and screws or rods may be removed (Schindhelm and Milthorpe 2003) (Table 8.1).

(A) Stainless steel:

Stainless steel AISI 316L has wide applications in orthopedic implants as compared to other metallic materials. It has several advantages such as better mechanical properties, low cost, ease of processing, good corrosion resistance, and abundant in supply (Talha et al. 2012). The typical stainless steel used is austenitic stainless steel (AISI 316L, ASTM F-55, and F-138), with 17%–20% Cr, 12%–15% nickel, 2%–3%

Table 8.1 General applications of metal nanobiomaterials used in implants and medical devices.

Metal type	Applications
Stainless steel	Orthopedic: bone fixation, joint replacements, bone plates, hip nails, shoulder prosthesis Dental: dental root implant, tooth fixation Cardiovascular: artificial heart valves, pacer, catheters, coronary stents Neural: spinal implant, screws, fracture plates
Co-Cr alloys	Orthopedic: joint replacement, fixation screws, orthopedic prosthesis Dental: dental root implant Cardiovascular: stents, pacer Surgical instruments, suture
Ti and Ti alloys	Orthopedic: total hip and knee joint replacement, bone plate, screws, orthopedic prosthesis Dental: implants, tooth fixation, and parts for orthodontic surgery Cardiovascular: artificial heart valves, pacemakers, stents Miscellaneous: cochlear implants
Cobalt-chromium alloys	Joint replacements, bone fracture fixation
Silver	Dental implants
Platinum	Cochlear implants

molybdenum, and small amounts of other elements. After implantation of stainless steel containing implants, nickel ions release into the body and hence, it is necessary to make nickel-free steel for making implants, which are used for long-term application (Talha et al. 2013).

(B) Co-Cr alloys:

Cobalt-based alloys have been broadly used as implant components, principally in orthopedic implants, due to their excellent corrosion resistance and wear properties (Yan et al. 2007). The Co-Cr alloys, including wrought and cast alloys, are widely used in clinical applications. For instance, wrought alloys containing 33–37 wt% Ni (ASTM F562, MP35N) are utilized extensively in orthopedic devices. A Co-Cr-Mo alloy (ASTM F75, Vitallium) has been used in the hip prostheses (Arden et al. 1970).

(C) Titanium and its alloy:

Ti and its alloys are the most attractive implant nanobiomaterials owing to their high strength-to-weight ratios, excellent corrosion resistance, and biocompatibility as compared to other metallic materials (Niinomi 2011). Commercial pure Ti (CP-Ti) was used commercially because of its high biocompatibility among various metals. As compared to other metallic biomaterials, they are commonly used due to high biocompatibility and greater strength to weight ratios. The widely used Ti alloy, Ti-6Al-4V, has high tensile strength and less pitting corrosion. Nitinol, an alloy of Ni and Ti, has a shape memory effect. This property of Nitinol is used in dental restoration wiring (Rack and Qazi 2006) and coronary stents. CP-Ti is used for cardiovascular stents, lead wires, and spinal fixation devices. When it contains low Fe, it has a low possibility of adverse effects. CP-Ti is used for hard tissue regeneration (Li et al., 2014). Ti-based alloys are also employed for load-bearing applications in orthopedic and dental devices (Hayashi et al. 1991). These nanobiomaterials are used for artificial valves in the heart, stents, replacement implants in shoulders, knees, hips, elbows, ears, and dental structures (Alves 2017; Gepreel and Niinomi 2013). They are also used as a cardiac simulator and for urinary tract reconstruction. Ti and its alloys are widely used for spinal, hip, and knee replacement implants. Ti-based alloys are used as implant devices for dental applications and replacing failed hard tissues such as artificial hip joints, artificial knee joints, bone plates, dental implants, crowns, dentures, artificial tooth roots, and screws, etc. They are also used to fix soft tissue like blood vessels (Li et al., 2014).

8.2.2 Ceramic nanobiomaterials

Ceramics are generally defined as inorganic nonmetallic materials. Ceramics are widely used in orthopedics, mainly in total hip and knee replacements. The bio-ceramic materials prevent the release and reduce wear rates of bearing components. The major drawback of ceramics is their intrinsic brittleness and high fracture rate (Campbell et al. 2004). Bio-ceramics are inert (e.g., alumina and zirconia) and biodegradable [tricalcium phosphate (TCP)]. They are an ideal material for the artificial bone because they are replaced by autologous bone. Bioactive materials, such as hydroxyapatite (HA), are major inorganic materials for artificial bone replacement. HA is not absorbed by the body and thus remains permanently in the body. Instead of metallic and polymeric components, ceramic has been used in the artificial hip joint to increase the toughness of joint replacement. The ceramic femoral head and acetabular cup are some examples of this design (LINEAGE of Wright Medical Technology, Inc. has a ceramic-ceramic acetabular cup system).

(A) Zirconia:

Zirconia exhibits highly favorable physical and mechanical properties, which include desirable hardness, elastic modulus, and thermal conductivity. It is also highly biocompatible and has similar color with the tooth (Depprich et al. 2008), which permits its use in dental implants. In dentistry, zirconia is also widely employed in applications like root posts and orthodontic brackets.

(B) Alumina:

For over 20 years, alumina has been used in orthopedic surgery because it is extremely biocompatible and forms a very thin capsule, which permits cementless fixation of prostheses with exceptionally lower coefficients of friction and wear rate (Hench 1995). Alumina has more chemical-physical stability. However, it is not used for complex shapes and thin ceramic components because of poor toughness. On the other hand, zirconia is tough and durable but less stable. Hence, an alumina matrix composite material is a mixed material that has positive characteristics of both materials called as Biolox Delta (CeramTec AG, Plochingen, Germany) (Dalla Pria 2007), but it has a major concern about ceramic fracture and squeaking. The fourth-generation ceramic Biolox forte is a composite made of 82% alumina and 17% zirconia. Although mechanical properties greatly increased, it is not plastically deformable and has brittle characteristics due to which the risk of fracture remains (Lee et al. 2017) (Table 8.2).

8.2.3 Polymeric nanobiomaterials

Polymeric nanobiomaterials are the most widely used materials in developing medical implants and devices. Polymers are so versatile in nature that it is difficult to be matched by metals and ceramics. The broad range of physicochemical and mechanical properties of polymers has substantially boosted the research and development of polymeric nanobiomaterials. They are highly recommended for developing any implant or device because of

Table 8.2 General applications of ceramic nanobiomaterials used in implants and medical devices.

Ceramics types	General applications
Aluminum oxides	Dental crown, hip implants, dental implants, cochlear replacement
Zirconia	Hip implants, dental implants
Calcium phosphate	Used as bone graft substituent, surface coating on joint replacement

their flexibility, high tensile strength, easy fabrication, biocompatibility, and biostable nature.

Biological as well as synthetic biopolymers are used in the development of polymeric nanobiomaterials. The following are a few examples of biopolymers: polysaccharides such as starch, alginate, chitin/chitosan, hyaluronic acid derivatives and proteins such as collagen, fibrin gel, and silk. Whereas synthetic polymers include poly(lactic acid) (PLA), poly(glycolic acid) (PGA), poly(ε-caprolactone) (PCL), poly(lactic glycolic acid) (PLGA), polyhydroxybutyrate (PHB), etc. (Avti et al. 2011). Biological polymers help in cell adhesion and tissue regeneration; however, synthetic polymers have better mechanical strength but lower biocompatibility and biodegradability.

Any material that is going to be used to manufacture implants and medical devices should not directly or indirectly produce adverse effects. The selection of a polymeric material is challenging, and thus, to choose a sustainable polymer, one has to consider chemical composition, pH, and other mechanical parameters. Hence, the nanobiomaterial used for a device in one region of the body may not be suitable for another device, even in a different region of the body. Polysaccharides, proteins, PLGA, PLA, PGA, PCL, epoxies, silicones, polyurethanes, polyimides, silicon-polyimides, parylenes, polycyclic-olefins, silicon-carbons, liquid crystal polymers, and benzocyclobutenes are a few examples of biocompatible polymers of high interest (Joung 2013).

Apart from biocompatibility, another advantage of polymeric materials over ceramics and metals is that it can be easily fabricated into shapes and structures of various complexity. This is attributed to their high mechanical strength as well as flexibility. Most of the time, polymer composites are utilized to make implants and devices. When different polymers are used in cohesion in one thin layer, polymer composites are formed. Thus, the properties of composites differ from their parent materials. They usually have low elastic modulus and high strength with possibly better structural biocompatibility compared to the parent materials. Additional advantages of these materials are that they are nonmagnetic and radiotransparent making them compatible for X-ray radiography and magnetic resonance imaging MRI scans (Teo et al. 2016).

An essential class of polymeric nanobiomaterials is polymeric nanofibers. Extensive research work has been carried out to develop and understand the properties of nano-fibers. Nano-fibers have a size less than 100 nm, which imparts a high surface area to volume ratio. Nanocomposites are currently being explored for dental implants, controlled drug delivery, medical devices and implants, and biosensors (Hasirci 2006).

Despite having numerous advantages, implants made of polymeric nanobiomaterials have to face the staggering challenge of sterilization. Conventional sterilization processes could inadvertently damage the polymeric implant. For instance, gaseous sterilization may lead to the exudation of toxic ethylene oxide from the polymeric material, which is not desirable. High temperatures created during dry heat sterilization would cause deformation owing to differences in transition and melting temperature of each material, or even reduce the ductility, or else cause chalking and color change. Therefore the industry is working on low heat sterilization techniques for polymeric implants like microwave sterilization and pulsed high-intensity light (McDonnell 2012).

Polymeric nanobiomaterials have been widely studied to prepare cardiovascular system, central nervous system, ophthalmic, dental, orthopedic, obstetric, and gynaecologic implants. Neurological applications are one of the most prominent research activities in the field. A device was studied to record and stimulate the neural signals occurring in the case of neural damage (Buchko et al. 2001). This neural prosthetic device was developed from biodegradable porous protein polymeric films. It was made by coating silicon substrates with a thin nanofibrous polymer film, which acted as an interphase and also decreased the chances of the implant failure.

Electrospun polymeric nanobiomaterials are also used in the production of orthodontic implants. Here, the mechanical properties were highly improved (Price et al. 2003). Traditional resin matrix materials for dental application are also being replaced by polymeric composites. The polymeric materials help in the prolonged service lives than inorganic fillers (generally more than 18 months). Polymers like nylon-6 nano-fibers were used to make composite resins in the formulation of dental implants (Fong 2004). Addition of very small amount of nano-fibers resulted in a significant improvement in elastic modulus and flexural strength. Nano-fiber composites of nylon-6 increased the resistance of a material and was able to deflect the cracks and thus showed fewer fractures than a normal resin composite. This reflects the importance of nanobiomaterials in the preparation of such implants.

As polymeric nano-fibers have a large surface area to weight ratio, they are extensively being utilized in biosensor medical device applications. This characteristic enhances material sensitivity; thus, it is possible to detect substances with very low concentrations. Glucose biosensors were developed from a composite of gold nanoparticles (NPs) and conductive polyaniline nano-fibers. This device used nano-fibers having immobilized glucose oxidase for detection of glucose. The device exhibited high reproducibility (less than 5% relative standard deviation) and good operational stability (over 2 weeks, Xian et al. 2006). Along with polyaniline nano-fibers, other polymers like poly(vinylpyrrolidone) are being studied to develop medical devices (Sawicka et al. 2005).

As we all know, medical devices are objects that require either chemical or electrical form of energy to produce a reaction to either remedy certain bodily functions or to obtain information from the body. Therefore attempts have been made to use polymeric nanobiomaterials along with other materials to form composites which would generate the bioenergy needed to run the medical device. This bioenergy will be generated from the heartbeat by converting the mechanical energy into electric power that can charge or even power implanted devices such as a pacemaker. In a study, it has been demonstrated that the combination of polyvinylidene difluoride (PVDF) nano-fibers and a graphene composite can harvest energy from the expansion and contraction of blood vessels in the human body (Fadhil et al. 2014). The assembly constituted dual layers of PVDF nano-fibers and graphene composites that are embedded into a self-curling biocompatible silicone. The device is performed by converting mechanical actions of a blood artery (pulsated pressure of expansion and contraction) into a corresponding voltage. Hence, using novel nanobiomaterials, self-powering implantable devices can be developed.

Bio-based hyperbranched polyurethane and iron oxide nanocomposites were tested as smart antibacterial biomaterials for the manufacturing of medical devices and implants (Das et al. 2013). These nanocomposites (average diameter of 7.65 nm) of biomaterial polyurethane also displayed magnetic behavior with enhanced biocompatibility, biodegradation, antimicrobial properties, and shape recovery. Thus, such materials may be used as a thermally and magnetically controlled smart biomaterial.

Nanocomposites of biomaterials have been intensely researched for hard tissue implants. These materials have both desired fracture toughness and elasticity to mimic the mechanical properties of bone. HA is widely used material for this purpose due to its high chemical and physical resemblance to the mineral part of the bone (Kim et al. 2006). It is an osteoconductive material, i.e., shows good osteoblast cell adherence and proliferation necessary for bone repair and growth. Nanobiocomposites of HA along with other materials like PLA and chitosan have been used as bone implants

(Kokubo et al. 2003). The DePuy Orthopedics, Inc. (Warsaw, IN, USA) developed a nanobiomaterial-based implant, Healos, which is made up of cross-linked collagen fibers coated with HA for bone implant substitutes in spinal fusions (Avti et al. 2011).

However, the majority of top pharmaceutical companies are still not majorly involved in nanobiomaterial-based product development owing to uncertainties in the Food and Drug Administration (FDA) approval process (Boyd 2006). This is the prime reason for the low number of nanobiomaterial commercialized medical devices and implants. Polymeric nanobiomaterials will have a great influence on the medical device and implant industry due to its biocompatibility, mechanical strength, and wide array of applicability. Currently, there are numerous polymeric biomaterials used for the same, but a few have a nanoscale version of it.

8.2.4 Carbon-based nanobiomaterials

The nano-sized structures created by using organic materials like carbon-based nanobiomaterials have attracted attention in the biomedical field. Carbon-based nanobiomaterials have great potential due to their small size and high contact surface area. Some of the well-known carbon-based nanobiomaterials are carbon nanotubes (CNTs), graphene quantum dots (QDs), graphene oxide, and fullerenes (Maiti et al., 2019). These nanobiomaterials have been investigated as building blocks for complex and miniaturized medical devices and implants. Various allotropes of carbon nanobiomaterials are shown in Fig. 8.1.

The large aspect ratio of carbon nanobiomaterials, their excellent electrical conductivity, and mechanical robustness have made them a prime choice for molecular electronic and bioelectronic applications. Its unique photophysical and photochemical properties have been used to prepare various medical devices such as biochips, bio-nanoelectromechanical systems (BioNEMs), biosensors, and bioimaging (Avti et al. 2011).

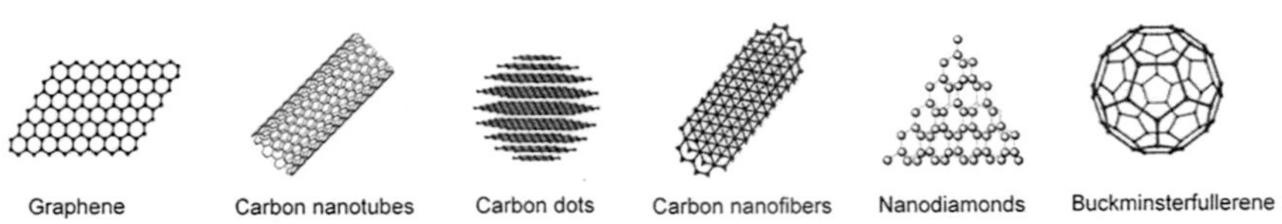

Fig. 8.1 Different allotropes of carbon nanobiomaterials. *Reproduced from Wang, Z., Dai, Z., 2015. Carbon nanomaterial-based electrochemical biosensors: an overview, Nanoscale 7(15):6420–6431, 2015 with permission from Royal Society of Chemistry.*

CNTs are the most widely studied carbon-based nanobiomaterial. They have tubular shapes made up of carbon hexagons with the diameter ranging from 0.4 nm to 3 nm and the length varying from a few nanometres to several microns. Some applications are the miniaturization of medical devices, the development of electronic systems, and biosensors that interact with the human body to monitor complex interactions (Colvin 2003). Biosensors made up of CNTs can detect the electrical signal and chemical interactions within the body in a few seconds with ultra-high sensitivity (Sotiropoulou and Chaniotakis 2003). In this category, CNT composites, the strongest materials with high tensile strength, elastic modulus, high surface area, and flexibility (Jensen et al. 2007) are being utilized for implants.

From the structural point of view, CNTs are usually described as an arrangement of carbon hexagons that form tiny tubes and is a true macromolecular system with the architecture of ideal graphene sheets. A single-walled CNT (SWCNTs) is a tubular form of carbon with the diameter ranging from 0.4 nm to 2–3 nm and the length varying from a few nanometres to several microns. The electrical properties of CNTs aid in acting as semiconductors, and they are dependent on diameters and chirality. This behavior helps in the construction of a new generation of the biosensor (Popov 2004). The mechanical properties of CNTs are way better than these previously known materials. It is characterized by strong covalent bonding and chemical inertness as it lacks functional groups (Niyogi et al. 2002). Reactivity and stability are absolutely decisive for biomaterial functions. The inertness of CNTs greatly contributes to their biocompatibility and stability when in contact with the living body. However, the fabrication process and modification approaches may cause alterations in chemical stability. As CNTs are hydrophobic, various surface modification methods have been adopted to utilize it for biomedical applications.

Toxicity is one of the major limitations of carbon-based nanobiomaterials. The metal impurities generated during CNT synthesis cause toxicity to the cells. Moreover, higher diameter and longer length also affect cellular internalization and toxicity. Graphene also has limitations in biomedical applications due to its toxicity. Along with dimension and impurities, other parameters such as functional groups and surface property should also be considered for toxicity evaluation (Maiti et al., 2019). Despite these limitations, numerous applications for carbon-based nanobiomaterials are being explored in the field of medical devices and implants. Some of the medical devices and implants that are being developed using carbon-based nanobiomaterials are discussed below.

Neural prostheses are used to apply and monitor electrical signals in neural tissues to restore nerve function. CNT fibers possess excellent electrical properties and high surface energy, which have been proven useful in the area of neural implants. Nanotubes function as a support for nerve cell growth. This was proven by growing embryonic rat brain neurons on CNTs of a diameter similar to nerve fibers (Mattson et al. 2000). The conductivity of nanotubes makes them a valuable candidate for electrophysiological analysis of neuronal microcircuitry. The carbon nano-fibers can limit astrocyte functions, leading to decreased glial scar tissue formation (McKenzie et al. 2004). These characteristics promote the development of CNT miniaturized devices that help in the formation of a nerve cell network, which restores damaged neuronal circuit. Hence, carbon-based nanobiomaterials can be used to develop implant devices for the central nervous system.

CNT composites are also useful as high load-bearing orthopedic implants and can promote the precipitation and materialization of HA in such implants (Li et al. 2011). The advantage of CNT orthopedic implants over other material implants is that it offers favorable conditions to induce cellular functions, possess excellent packing density without any macroscopic porosity, have good bonding strength between them and the metal substrates, and reinforce the composite coatings that help in high load bearing. Apart from the orthopedic applications, it can be used in dental implants and three-dimensional (3D) scaffolds for tissue engineering (TE). CNTs can attach to the surfaces of dentin and thus could be explored as dental implants.

Medical devices like biosensors are one of the most prominently researched fields in the case of carbon-based nanobiomaterials. Especially, CNTs are considered as appropriate nanobiomaterials for biosensing devices (Lin et al. 2004; Zhao et al. 2002). Biomolecules are immobilized on the surface of the biosensor that leads to enhanced recognition and signal transduction process. These medical devices are used for the detection of DNA, oligonucleotides, enzymes, receptors, antibodies, intact cells, toxic substances, as well as for therapeutic drug monitoring. Several biological events, such as genotoxicity, immunotoxicity, biotoxins, and endocrine effects, are measured using biosensors (Nakamura and Karube 2003; Stradiotto et al. 2003). These devices were even studied for in vivo and in vitro evaluation. One such instance is the construction of a nanotube-electrode for neurotransmitters involving dopamine, using bromoform as a binder for in vitro and in vivo investigation (Britto et al. 1996). Moreover, these biosensors are utilized for the clinical detection of biomolecules, such as antibodies, associated with human autoimmune diseases. The clinical detection of medical devices acts on two principal applications: selective detection of serum proteins after vaccination or therapeutic intervention and detection of different proteins without labeling via electrical transducers. Another application includes CNT glucose biosensors (Gaitán et al. 2017). Those are designed based on the conjugation of glucose oxidase with CNTs. One such example is a device made up of CNT nonwoven fabrics in conjugation with glucose oxidase impregnated with a polyvinyl alcohol solution (Zhu et al. 2014). Along with CNTs, Graphene QDs-based biosensor devices have largely been developed and used for practical applications such as detection of biomacromolecules with better selectivity and sensitivity (Kumawat et al. 2017).

Biochips are novel medical devices fabricated using carbon-based nanobiomaterials. This device could be used for the analysis of different DNA or proteins simultaneously as well as single-nucleotide polymorphism, mutation, genetic disease, protein-DNA interactions. Graphene oxide nanobiomaterials are being used in selective electrochemical sensing of single- and double-stranded DNA biochips (Liu et al. 2017; Tang et al. 2015). The electrochemical properties of graphene are attributed to the high sensitivity of biochips. Numerous biochips have been developed using graphene oxide; a few of them are: graphene nanowire biosensors by Akhavan et al. (2012) for detection of DNA bases, carboxyl-functionalized graphene oxide, and polyaniline-modified graphene oxide DNA biochips (Cheng et al. 2017); DNA biochips by Ping et al. (2016), a single-layer graphene-based field-effect transistor biosensor capable of detecting 10 fM concentrations of DNA (Zheng et al. 2015), a biochip composed of silicon nanowires modified with graphene for detecting oligonucleotides with sensitivity and selectivity (Kim et al. 2016); and medical devices for the detection of tuberculosis via analyzing DNA of *Mycobacterium tuberculosis* using graphene-based surface plasmon resonance-sensing chip (Prabowo et al. 2016).

Nanoelectromechanical systems are novel medical devices fabricated with carbon-based nanobiomaterials and can be biofunctionalized for biological and clinical applications (BioNEMs). Their length is less than 100 nm and are referred as intelligent nanodevices that can sense analyte-induced changes, which measurably alter dynamical device properties. These devices have the ability for sensing, processing, and/or actuating functions. For example, single-molecule manipulations such as DNA and proteins are feasible using these devices to provide information about the molecular conformation, chromatin organization, and biomolecular interaction dynamics (Avti et al. 2011).

Medical nanorobots are futuristic medical nanodevices, designed for maintaining the human body and protecting it against pathogenic agents. They will also be helpful for indirect in vivo surgery on individual human cells (Polizu et al. 2006). These medical devices could assist the immune system by finding and disabling unwanted bacteria or viruses. Predetermined search patterns could be useful in identifying invaders and destroying them by mechanical or chemical phagocytosis (Cavalcanti et al. 2004). Such devices could also be explored for targeted cancer drug delivery, as it enables one to distinguish every cell type by checking their surface antigen through chemotactic sensors keyed to specific antigens target cells. To a further extent, these could replace stents by clearing arteriosclerotic deposits and widening the diseased blood vessels (Menezes et al. 2001). It is a challenge to develop such sophisticated medical devices but can be possible by manipulating CNTs at both the atomic and molecular scale and integrating it with biological entities like DNA and proteins (Polizu et al. 2006).

Carbon-based nanobiomaterials thus have a huge potential in the development of medical devices and implants. However, regulatory challenges and industrial mass production are prime hurdles limiting their real-life implementation.

8.2.5 Miscellaneous nanobiomaterials

Collagen and modified collagen are used in periodontal and implant therapy due to their cell-occlusiveness, biocompatibility, and regenerative capacity. Collagen-based implants are naturally degraded by the collagenase enzyme, which attacks the helical region in collagen (Patino et al. 2002). Inorganic core and organic shell NPs like SiO_2/TiO_2 are used as dental brace materials and fillers. They can be used according to their physical properties like elasticity and thermal expansion (Yoshida and Prasad 1996). Composites are a mixture of two or more types of materials. Bioresorbable internal fixation devices made of poly-L-lactic acid (PLLA) with HA showed ultra-high strength, good processability. PLLA also has a very similar elastic modulus to natural bone (Shikinami and Okuno 2001). A femoral stem made up of a composite layer of epoxy resin reinforced with carbon and glass fibers has been used (Dalla Pria 2007). A biodegradable composite made of TCP particles and gelatin has been used for cranial bone repair. It showed good in vivo results such as more biocompatibility and biodegradability (Migliaresi and Nicolais 1980). A PLA composite made up of 15%–25%

bioglass particles was used to heal a bone fracture in internal fixation devices (Kellomäki et al. 2000). Polymeric acrylic or methacrylic matrix reinforced with ceramic particles were used as a dental composite (Ensaff et al. 2001).

8.3 Fabrication techniques for nanobiomaterials-based medical devices and implants

A wide range of nanobiomaterials has been used for the manufacturing of medical devices and implants. As dealt with earlier, such materials include metals, polymers, composites, bio-ceramics, carbon-based materials, etc. These medical devices and implants include invasive external communicating medical devices like catheters with coatings of nano-silver for bladder drainage, hemodialysis, and local administering of anesthesia; polymer-based dental composite filler materials and dental cement containing NPs; layer-on-layer coated electrodes to improve the electrode-tissue interface, nano-porous micro-electrodes for an improved brain-machine interface, as well as surgical and dental instruments like scalpels, needles, catheters, burs for cutting bone or teeth, etc. with nanostructures used to enhance the cutting behavior and wear resistance (Ferracane 2011). They may also include invasive implantable medical devices like CNT-based bone cements for implants (van der Zande et al. 2010), bone fillers with HA and TCP NPs, cardiovascular stents, and stent-grafts with various functional nanocoatings like aluminum oxide, glycoproteins, platinum or Ti dioxide (TiO_2) (Puranik et al. 2013), joint replacement and fracture implants, sutures (Ho et al. 2013), joint prosthetics (hip, knee) with nano-HA coating, surface nanocoatings for antibacterial action, e.g., silver nanocoating for various catheters, contact lenses, endotracheal tubes, etc.

The manufacturing of such devices is an interdisciplinary approach. Novel fabrication technologies for developing such devices are being developed, such as additive manufacturing and prevailing technologies. In the following section, we briefly explore the various methods reported for the fabrication of such devices. Given below is a summary of the various techniques known currently for the fabrication of nano-bio material-based medical devices and implants.

8.3.1 Additive manufacturing

Additive manufacturing, popularly known as 3D printing, has been one of the most important recent developments in science and technology. As per the US FDA, additive manufacturing or 3D printing is "a process that

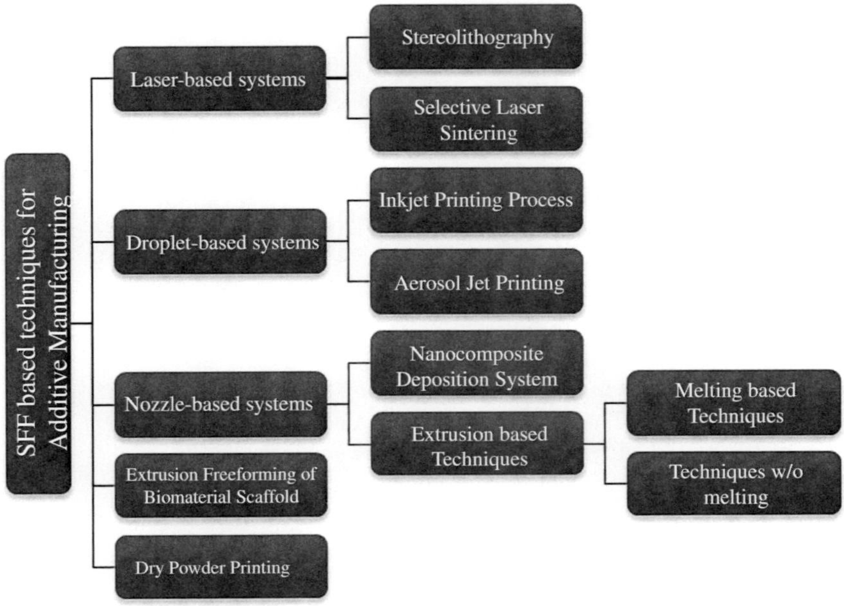

Fig. 8.2 Solid freedom fabrication (SFF) techniques for additive manufacturing.

creates a 3D object by building successive layers of raw material." "Each new layer is attached to the previous one until the object is complete." "Objects are produced from a digital 3D file, such as a computer-aided design (CAD) drawing or a MRI." This has made it possible to create devices and implants that were previously impossible to make and are personalized to suit individual patients' needs (US FDA, 2020).

Among the various methods available for additive manufacturing, the solid freeform fabrication (SFF) processes based on layer-by-layer manufacturing have shown immense promise (Fig. 8.2). SFF is a fabrication technique used to build 3D components, one layer after another, with the help of CAD data (Vaezi and Yang 2014). Schematic of various rapid prototyping-based fabrication methods is presented in Fig. 8.3.

Worldwide, upwards of 30 different SFF methods are currently being explored, of which almost 20 methods have the capability to process biomaterials. These could have potential applications in the biomedical industry (Chua et al. 2004). SFF techniques can also indirectly produce molds or 3D negatives that can then be used to produce the final product (Dong-Woo et al. 2007).

1. Additive manufacturing
   - i) Laser-based systems:
     - i. Stereolithography
     - ii. Selective laser sintering
   - ii) Droplet-based systems:
     - i. Inkjet printing process
     - ii. Aerosol jet printing
   - iii) Nozzle-based systems:
     - i. Nanocomposite deposition system
     - ii. SFF by extrusion
       - Techniques based on melting:
         1. Fused deposition modeling
         2. Three-dimensional (3D) fiber deposition
         3. Precision extrusion deposition
         4. Precision extrusion manufacturing
         5. Multiphase jet solidification
       - Techniques without melting:
         1. Pressure-assisted microsyringe
         2. Low-temperature deposition modeling
         3. 3D bioplotting
         4. Robocasting
         5. Solvent-based extrusion free-forming
         6. Direct-write assembly
   - iv) Extrusion free forming of biomaterials scaffold (fabrication of scaffolds for TE)
   - v) Dry powder printing
2. Nanopatterning
   - i) Nano biopatterning
   - ii) Chemical patterning
   - iii) Topographical patterning
   - iv) Combinatorial patterning
   - v) 3D patterning
3. Electro-spraying and electrospinning
   - i) Coaxial electrospinning
   - ii) Multi-needle electrospinning
   - iii) Needleless electrospinning
   - iv) Electronetting
   - v) Near-field electrospinning
   - vi) Centrifugal spinning
   - vii) Melt electrospinning

4. Molecular self-assembly
    i) Self-assembled architecture of bone tissue
    ii) Self-assembled block copolymers
    iii) Self-assembly of nanocrystals
    iv) Template assisted the growth of carbon nanotube
    v) Self-assembly of quantum dots
    vi) Self-assembly of nano-thin films
    vii) Self-assembly of crystalline liquid nanostructures
5. Surface modification techniques
    i) Anodization of implant surface (Ti implants): nanotopography
    ii) Fluorine-electrolyte nanotopography
    iii) Nanostructured carbon coatings
        - Nanocrystalline diamond (NCD), ultra-NCD, and nanostructured diamond coatings (load-bearing implants)
        - Chemical vapor deposition (CVD) method (thermal CVD, photo-assisted CVD, plasma-enhanced CVD)
        - Thermal-sprayed nanostructured bioactive coatings

8.3.1.1 Stereolithography (SL) process

Stereolithography (SL) is a technique that utilizes an ultraviolet (UV) light-based approach for layer-by-layer polymerization of photosensitive resin. This process was first developed on a commercial scale by a USA-based company called 3D Systems Inc. There are two main SL techniques based on the type of beam delivery system used—scanning SL and projection SL. Scanning-type SL solidifies the photopolymer (including UV photoinitiator, monomer, and other additives) either in a point-by-point or a line-by-line fashion in each layer. In projection SL, the whole photopolymer layer is cured at once via controlled exposure with a photomask. The dynamic mask used in this process is usually a digital micro-mirror device embedded in digital light processing projectors (Vaezi and Yang 2014). Bionanofillers can be incorporated in a photosensitive polymer resin matrix to manufacture 3D nanocomposite parts using the SL process. This process is mostly used to reinforce the final nanocomposite part.

Different parts have been fabricated from water or acrylate-based, photocurable resins by incorporating nano/micron-sized ceramic particles such as alumina (Greco et al. 2001; Hinczewski et al. 1998), HA (Griffith et al. 1995), silica, silicon nitride (Griffith and Halloran 1996), etc. The matrix used for these alumina or HA NPs is usually made from acrylate

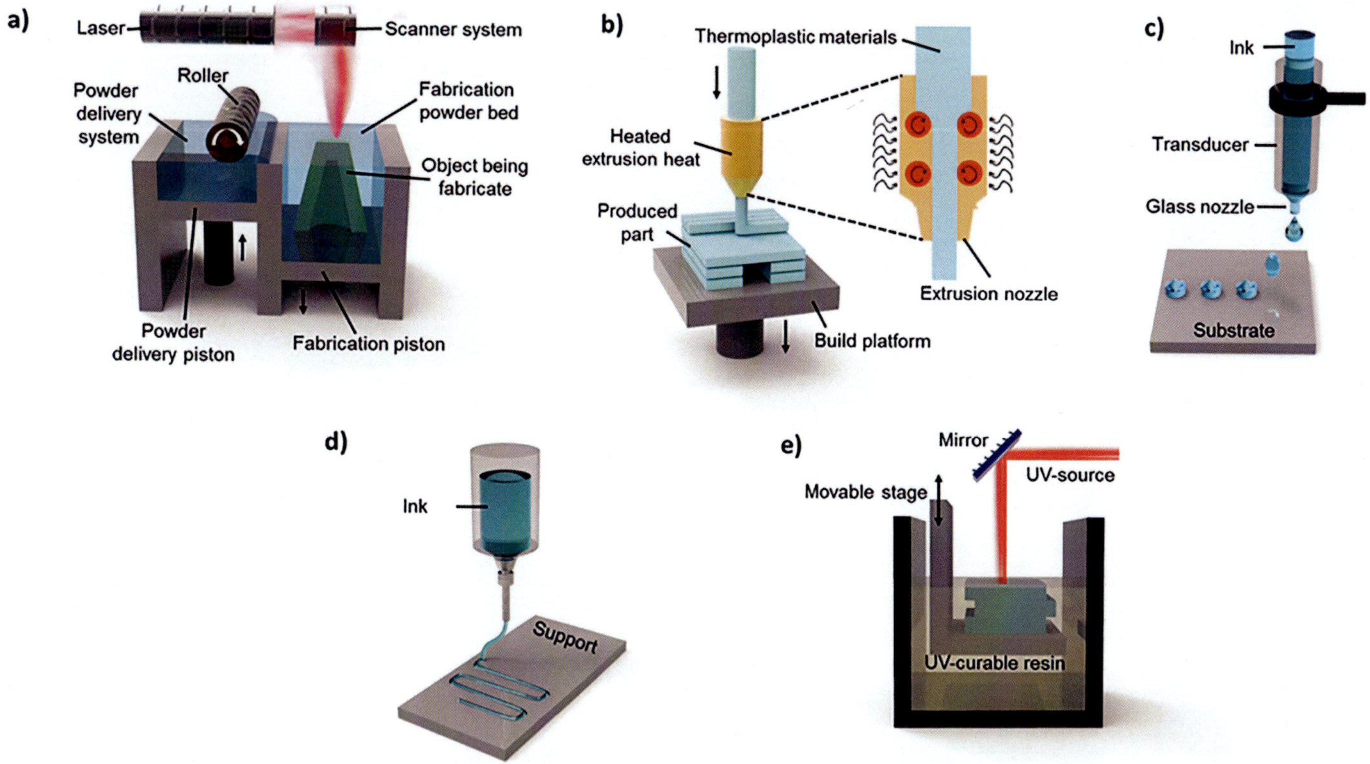

Fig. 8.3 Schematic illustration showing various rapid prototyping-based fabrication methods. (A) Selective laser sintering process, (B) fused deposition modelling, (C) inkjet printing/multijet modelling, (D) extrusion-based printing, and (E) laser-based stereolithography. *Reproduced from Kankala, R.K., Zhu, K., Li, J., Wang, C.S., Wang, S.B., Chen, A.Z., 2017. Fabrication of arbitrary 3D components in cardiac surgery: from macro-, micro- to nanoscale. Biofabrication 9(3):032002, under Creative Commons Attribution 3.0 Licence (https://creativecommons.org/licenses/by/3.0/).*

prepolymers. To prevent aggregation of these NPs and to reduce the viscosity of the prepolymer, a suitable dispersing agent must be included in the formulation. Along with NPs, CNTs have also been explored as nanofillers to enhance the mechanical strength of the nanocomposites (Sandoval et al. 2007).

8.3.1.2 Selective laser sintering process

In this process, 3D structures are built by sintering polymer layers or powdered polymer composites by using a CO_2 laser beam. Different biomaterials including biopolymers, bio-ceramics, and biocomposites having possible medical applications have been produced by this method (Yang et al. 2002).

The selective laser sintering (SLS) process has been used to fabricate bone implants from calcium phosphate that has been coated with a polymer, poly(methyl methacrylate) (Lee and Barlow 2003). Reinforced polyethylene composites for bone implants are also produced by this process (Hao et al. 2006). Using the SLS process, the biological or mechanical properties of biopolymers can be drastically modified using a small number of nanofillers. Certain properties of these nanofillers (NPs or nanofibers) like their high surface area to volume ratios can be used to control the biodegradability and bioactivity properties of biomaterials. Apart from these, optical and mechanical properties, thermal conductivity, and resistance can also be improved. Mechanical properties of nanocomposites can be enhanced by using nano-silica and nano-alumina (Chung and Das 2008). Similarly, CNTs have been used with much success as nanofillers by various researchers.

8.3.1.3 Inkjet printing process

Inkjet printing is a noncontact 3D printing technology that has its origins in normal ink-based paper printing. Today, it has evolved as a high-resolution, high-throughput, and reproducible additive manufacturing technology. In this method, the liquid ink which is dispensed in a droplet form is solidified by cooling (which may occur either by vitrification or crystallization), chemical alteration, or simply by solvent evaporation (Hon et al. 2008).

This method can be optimized either for speed or for accuracy, namely by using either the drop on demand (DOD) mode or the continuous inkjet (CIJ) mode. CIJ systems have been optimized for speed. They use lower viscosity fluids and higher drop velocity as compared to DOD. In contrast, DOD systems typically use thermally or piezoelectrically induced acoustic pulses to dispense smaller drops, which have been optimized for accuracy. Owing to the principles behind their operation, a number of different solvents can be used with piezoelectric DOD in contrast to thermal DOD in which only water is used as a solvent (De Gans and Schubert 2003).

The physical properties of the ink chosen influence the quality of the inkjet printing, and they remain the single most important parameter in inkjet printing. These physical properties include surface tension, viscosity, and inertia of the ink. The ink should have an adequately low viscosity to prevent overloading with a low-power piezoelectric diaphragm, while at the same time must have a sufficiently high surface tension to prevent leakage of ink from the nozzle. These physical properties of ink can also be analyzed by using certain dimensionless variables such as Reynolds' number (Re), Weber's number (We), and Ohnesorge's number (Oh) (Vaezi and Yang 2014).

To date, inkjet printing has successfully been able to handle a number of different bioinks. Inkjet printing has also been carried out using nanobioceramic inks containing nano-TiO_2 (Hosseini Zori and Soleimani-Gorgani 2012) and nano-inks containing SWCNTs and multiwalled CNTs (MWCNTs) and grapheme (Chen et al. 2010). Ink containing gold NPs for producing true 3D parts have also been explored (Ko et al. 2010). Lastly, inkjet printing of antibiotics and calcium-eluting two-dimensional micropatterns was also explored. This facilitated the development of osteogenic cells on orthopedic Ti implant surfaces and prevented the biofilm formation on the surface of the implant (Gu et al. 2012).

8.3.1.4 Aerosol jet printing

Aerosol jet process is a direct writing process that uses a focused aerosol stream instead of liquid ink to deposit various materials in a 3D arrangement. It is a low temperature process utilizing low kinetic energy, femtoliter-scale droplets which do not damage living cells and holds much promise as a suitable technique for biomanufacturing. Although initially developed for flat surface printing, recent advances in aerosol jet printing have enabled it produce true 3D nanobiomaterials (Hon et al. 2008). This process was pioneered by OPTOMEC under the trademark M3D (maskless mesoscale material deposition) (Vaezi and Yang 2014; Fig. 8.4). Today, aerosol jets include materials like polymers such as PLGA, metals, ceramics, and biomaterials in the form of suspension, NPs, protein, and antibody solutions (Hon et al. 2008).

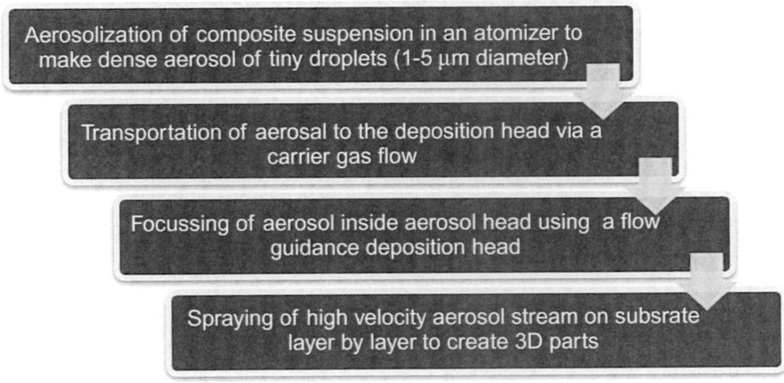

Fig. 8.4 Aerosol jet printing process.

8.3.1.5 Nanocomposite deposition system

Although many rapid prototyping or additive manufacturing technologies have been described, many still face the problem of the stair-step effect, which leads to poor surface quality. In response to this and to the problem of recoating faced during the production of nanofiller-loaded resin by the SL process, the nanocomposite deposition system (NCDS) process was developed by Won-Shik et al. (2007).

NCDS is a hybrid SFF technique in which biodegradable resins containing NPs are deposited and cured layer after layer. Usually, biocompatible bionanofiller containing UV-curable resins are used as the matrix. After deposition and curing, the excess material is removed using micromachining. It is a hybrid process because while, on the one hand, it uses the deposition principles from rapid prototyping, it uses the material removal process of "mechanical micromachining" on the other.

The hardware system deposits the nanoparticulate matter containing polymer mixture with the help of a PMAC board controlled the 3D stage with a linear encoder for each axis. It then cures the resin with UV light of a wavelength of 365 nm. Following this, the extra deposited material is removed by micromachining. This setup achieves a resolution of 1 μm. Using this technique, the authors successfully fabricated multiwalled CNTs (MWCNTs) composites and HA composites, which could have potential applications in the development of functional medical devices and implants (Kim et al. 2007). Nanocomposite deposition system developed by Kim et al. (2007) is illustrated in the Fig. 8.5. To cite another example, Chu et al. (2007) fabricated the smallest human bone, the stapes using HA and the error in geometry was only 0.26%. Further, they also found that the

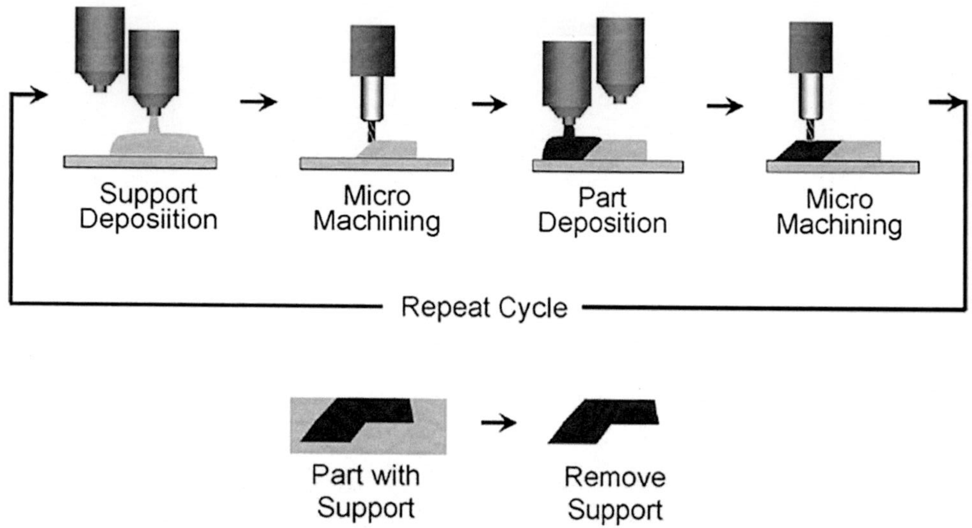

Fig. 8.5 A typical fabrication sequence of the nanocomposite deposition system. These processes repeat to fabricate a 3D part. developed by Kim et al. (2007). *Reproduced with permission from Kim, S.G., Chu, W.S., Jung, W.K., Ahn, S.H., 2007. Evaluation of mechanical and electrical properties of nanocomposite parts fabricated by nanocomposite deposition system (NCDS), J. Mater. Process Technol., 3rd International Conference on Advanced Forming and Die Manufacturing Technology 187–188:331–334.*

addition of NPs improved the mechanical properties of the implant (Chu et al. 2007).

8.3.1.6 Extrusion-based techniques

Extrusion-based techniques and droplet-based techniques were classically grouped together as direct ink writing techniques. Being much more mechanically simple than other SFF process, extrusion-based techniques have received widespread recognition for being able to process a variety of biomaterials. Briefly, extrusion-based techniques use a pneumatic or mechanically (piston or screw type) controlled robotic device to extrude continuous filaments (15–300 nm diameter) of material to fabricate the component. This technique can handle biomaterials from low to high viscosity hydrogels melt polymers as well as ceramics and can produce 3D products with a resolution of 200 μm.

Extrusion-based techniques can be briefly classified as follows:

- Techniques based on melting
  - (i) Fused deposition modeling (FDM)
  - (ii) 3D fiber deposition
  - (iii) Precision extrusion deposition (PED)
  - (iv) Precision extrusion manufacturing (PEM)
  - (v) Multiphase jet solidification
- Techniques without melting
  - (i) Pressure-assisted microsyringe (PAM)
  - (ii) Low-temperature deposition modeling (LDM)
  - (iii) 3D bioplotting
  - (iv) Robocasting
  - (v) Solvent-based extrusion free forming
  - (vi) Direct-write assembly

To improve mechanical properties and the bioactivity of the implant/medical device, various types of nanofillers have been employed. Nanofiber-reinforced biopolymers can also be fabricated by FDM which results in bionanocomposites without any porosity. The pressure-assisted microsyringe technique has been employed to fabricate nano-HA/PCL bionanocomposite bone TE scaffolds (Heo et al. 2009). The 3D bioprinting of a novel photo-cross-linkable bioink made of gelatin methacrylate and decellularized extracellular matrix (ECM) for hepatocytes (from the porcine liver) and cardiomyocytes (from the porcine heart left ventricle) was also done (Yu et al. 2019).

8.3.1.7 Extrusion free-forming of biomaterial scaffolds

A scaffold is a porous structure that permits cell growth in favored orientations and also facilitates cell adhesion, proliferation, and differentiation by acting as a synthetic ECM (Sachlos and Czernuszka 2003). Scaffolds have a lot of importance in TE as they give a structure onto which the cells can be grown as per the required 3D geometry. Currently, various techniques like solvent casting/leaching, foaming, phase separation, and textile meshes are being used to fabricate TE scaffolds. However, they all have certain shortcomings, which include issues like the inability to control pore size, geometry, or the pore distribution pattern on the scaffold. These shortcomings can easily be addressed by additive manufacturing techniques like extrusion free forming, which allow precise control over the internal and external structure of the fabricated scaffold, and can help in overcoming the limitations of conventional methods like shape restrictions and inconsistent and inflexible fabrication procedures.

Extrusion free-forming of biomaterial scaffolds is an extension of the extrusion-based direct ink writing technique. Therefore extrusion free-forming of scaffolds is also divided into two techniques: extrusion free-forming with material melting and extrusion free-forming without melting.

Material melting techniques like FDM have been employed to fabricate 3D scaffolds having pores and filaments of micron size. FDM has been used to make scaffolds with a resolution of 250 μm using polymers like PCL, polypropylene/TCP, PCL/HA, and PCL/TCP. Along these lines, highly porous PLGA scaffolds modified by type II collagen for cartilage TE were developed by Hung-Jen et al. (2009) using an FDM process. Biomimetic polybutylene terephthalate trabecular scaffolds were also fabricated by Tellis et al. (2008) using the FDM process involving micro-computed tomography.

PEM is another process that can be used to fabricate TE scaffolds. Various porous PLLA and PLLA/TCP bone TE scaffolds with various properties were fabricated using this technique (Xiong et al. 2001). The PED process is another material melting extrusion-based process (Wang et al. 2004). It is based on a similar principle as FDM except for the fact that material pellets or granules are deposited and liquefied in a chamber and extruded by a rotating screw through the nozzle. PCL and PCL/HA 3D scaffolds having a uniform pore size of 250 μm have been made using PED material (Shor et al. 2007).

However, higher temperatures and melting are often seen as problematic, especially when working with biological/bioactive materials. Therefore attempts have been made to develop new configurations. The PAM process is a technique developed by Vozzi et al. (2003), which resembles FDM except that there is no need for heating. PAM uses a pneumatic-driven microsyringe to deposit a biomaterial on a substrate and have been employed to fabricate scaffolds using different polymer compositions such as PCL, PLLA, PLGA, PCL/PLLA, gelatin, and alginate hydrogel scaffolds with three different geometries—square grids, hexagonal grids, and octagonal grids (Vozzi et al. 2004; Vozzi and Ahluwalia 2007). All other non-melting techniques like LDM, 3D bioplotting, robocasting, solvent-based extrusion free-forming, and direct-write assembly have been widely utilized for developing and fabricating a large variety of TE scaffolds.

8.3.1.8 Dry powder printing

Dry powder printing technology was developed specifically with the aim of being able to precisely meter, dispense, and deposit dry powder particles for the purposes of solid free-forming and additive manufacturing. This technology has also been incorporated with powder-based additive manufacturing technologies like SLS and 3D printing to improve product quality and functionality.

In this process, acoustic energy produced from a piezoelectric disc is applied to control the dispensing of dry powder from a system, which contains a glass capillary as a funnel and a computer control system. The vibrations from a piezoelectric disc are used to initiate and stop the powder flow from the nozzle. The powder keeps flowing while the disc remains on, while the flow is arrested as soon as the disc is switched off. The frequency and amplitude of the vibration can be modified to adjust the flow rate of the powder (Yang and Evans, 2004, 2005). Some other processing parameters include nozzle size and time of vibration (T_v). Careful attention must be paid to the selection of nozzle size as it has a significant impact on the dispensing of the nanobiomaterial powders. Powder-related factors like particle size, shape, and powder flowability must also be taken into account while selecting the nozzle size. The other processing parameter, T_v, is the most effective way to control powder dosage (Vaezi and Yang 2014). Multi-material 3D parts can be built using powder-based systems, and currently, research focusing on incorporating dry powder printing with SLS is ongoing in multi-material and micromanufacturing areas (Vaezi and Yang 2014).

8.3.2 Nanopatterning

Nanopatterning refers to the process of fabricating a nanoscale pattern having at least one dimension below 100 nm. This is being increasingly used for the generation of novel nanobiomaterials for applications in medical devices and implants with superior surface properties. Various forms of nanopatterns have been described in the literature, which includes, but are not limited to, columns, pits, islands, protrusions or nodes, anisotropic structure, and isotropic nano-islands distributed uniformly over the surface of the implant. These nanoscale patterns facilitate various functions like cell growth and are also thought to play an essential role in a range of metabolic cellular events. Some well-known techniques of nanopatterning include chemical patterning, topographical patterning, combinatorial patterning, 3D patterning, and nano-biopatterning.

In chemical patterning, different nanoscale patterns are created by chemical modification process of a biomaterial substrate. An example of this technology is self-assembled monolayers (SAMs), which are molecular assemblies used to impart enhanced surface functionalities to the nanobiomaterial. The conventional photolithography technique also uses the basics of chemical patterning to control cell growth and functions. These techniques can be used in applications that require sustainable cellular growth and in biomedical microdevices for sustaining long-term cell-biomaterial interactions (Manickam et al. 2017).

Topographical patterning is a process in which the shape of the substrate is modified with textured patterns of dimensions of a few microns to nanometres. For this purpose, lithographic techniques have been employed to create the desired topography on the substrate surface. One such lithographic process is nanoimprint lithography. It is a relatively simple and straight-forward technique that requires neither expensive instruments nor elaborate cleanroom facilities. Another method is colloidal lithography—which has been used to produce periodic nanotopographical patterns across large surfaces (Dalby et al. 2004).

Combinatorial patterning is another technique by which chemical and topographical cues can be incorporated on biomaterials as in the case of cell-based biosensors and TE (Charest et al. 2005) to support growth, cell orientation, and overcome other functional challenges.

One of the latest techniques in nanopatterning is 3D patterning. It has been made possible due to the development of 3D bioprinting. Recently, high-content graphene scaffolds for use in electronic and biomedical applications were fabricated using 3D patterning. It was found that this material had a unique set of properties and could be fabricated with ease. These results point to the fact that this technique could be used in the fabrication of a wide range of functional electronic, biological, and bioelectronic medical and nonmedical devices and implants (Jakus et al. 2015). Lastly, in nano-biopatterning, biological materials such as biomolecules, cells are patterned precisely at a nanometer scale. Nano-biopatterning is especially useful in applications like TE and molecular diagnostic devices/implants and nano-biosensors (Cui et al. 2001; Demidov 2004; Shekhawat et al. 2006; Zheng et al. 2005).

8.3.3 Electrospraying and electrospinning

Electrospraying (ES) is a versatile technique for fabricating different nanomaterials of various compositions, morphologies, shapes, textures, and sizes. ES involves the dispersion of a bulk liquid into very fine liquid droplets by applying a high voltage (few kilovolts; Boda et al. 2018). Owing to its advantages, ES technology finds applications for the fabrication of numerous materials like nano/microparticles and thin films for pharmaceutical and biomedical applications. It can be used to successfully control the surface texture of polymer coatings, which are applied on implant surfaces. In 2015 Guo and coworkers were able to successfully achieve different surface textures and microtopographies of the polymer coating on the surface of 316L stainless steel coronary stents (implant devices) by varying various parameters of the coating process. They electrosprayed a 0.5 wt% solution of polyhedral oligosilsesquioxane thermoplastic polyurethane in tetrahydrofuran onto the metallic stents connected to a rotating device, separated by a distance of 3.5 cm. As they increased the electric field from 1.5 kV/cm to 1.61 kV/cm to 1.8 kV/cm, the sprayed droplets underwent progressively greater elongation in their morphology in the increasing electric fields. This resulted in the variation of the coating surface from smooth to roughened to a fibrous coating topography (Guo et al. 2015). It is thought that such control of ES coating topography on implant devices enables regulation of their integration with the surrounding tissue (Boda et al. 2018). ES has also been used in fabricating dental/orthopedic implants and in TE. Commercial Ti alloy discs (Ti-6Al-4V) were coated with nanoscale calcium phosphate and collagen composite coatings through ES (de Jonge et al., 2009).

The electrospinning technique is used for the fabrication of porous nanofibers. In this, charged threads of a polymer solution or melt in the nano- or micro-sized diameters are drawn by using electric fields. A wide range of materials can be handled using this technique, which produces submicron assemblies having many functional properties (Chronakis 2005). Various styles of electrospinning are currently known, which include coaxial electrospinning, multi-needle electrospinning, needleless electrospinning, electronetting, near-field electrospinning, centrifugal spinning, and melt electrospinning (Ding et al. 2019). The fibers produced from the various electrospinning techniques have a porous structure that is conducive to cell culture, as it acts as a supporting structure with the appropriate rigidity. Consequently, these fibers find application in various biomedical and TE applications (Aznar-Cervantes et al. 2012; Kai et al. 2011). Polymers like collagen, chitosan, hyaluronic acid, and gelatin have all been used specifically for such TE applications. A lot of work has been reported in relation to cardiac tissue. Electrospinning has also been used to replicate the anisotropic nature of cardiac cells. In another instance, a combination of electrospun polyurethane with a polyethylene glycol-based hydrogel was used to fabricate a model of the heart valve tissue (Puperi et al. 2016). Attempts have also been made to use a core-shell nanofibrous cardiac patch to stimulate the regeneration of cardiac tissue after an episode of myocardial infarction (Ravichandran et al., 2015).

8.3.4 Molecular self-assembly

Self-assembly is the spontaneous assembly of constituents to form a complex nanostructure without any significant external intervention. There are two types of self-assembly: intermolecular and intramolecular self-assembly. Self-assembly is a useful technique because it provides a means for very small atoms, molecules, particles, monomers, and biological components to organize themselves into organized patterns that have various utilities, including the fabrication and coating of medical devices and implants. Naturally, this technique holds great promise for the fabrication of nanostructured materials. Various self-assembled materials like block copolymers, nanocrystals, CNTs, QDs, and thin nanofilms have been reported (Joshi et al. 2016). Self-assembled block copolymers like polyacrylic acid, poly(methyl acrylate), polystyrene-polyethylene oxide, polybutadiene, poly-*N*-isopropyl acrylamide, etc. find very wide applications in a number of medical devices and implants. They are basically amphiphilic molecules that contain two or more polymers quantitatively in the form of blocks.

SAMs is another such concept which has its origins in the concept of molecular self-assembly. In this, molecules like surfactants spontaneously orient themselves in the form of a monolayer on the surface of a substrate. These SAMs are stable, well-defined, and well-organized organic structures that have the ability to produce surface modifications at the nanoscale level, which can be utilized in the fabrication of various medical devices and implants. SAMs can be produced in two ways—solution deposition or aerosol spraying/vapor deposition. In solution deposition, the substrate is immersed into a solution of the coating surfactant. The surface of the substrate is first cleaned thoroughly and is immersed for 12–48h in a dilute 1–10mm solution of the coating surfactant, which has been prepared in a high-purity solvent. Following this, the substrate is withdrawn, rinsed with solvent, and nitrogen-dried. In aerosol spraying/vapor deposition, the aerosol or vapors of the coating surfactant is simply deposited on the substrate surface. Work has been reported using SAMs as a nanoscale surface modification technique for Ti implants for use in dental implants (Freitas et al. 2018).

A number of biomimetic materials have also been developed using self-assembly techniques. These have many potential biomedical applications, such as fabricating synthetic bone tissue for replacement, support frames for implant devices, and biological sensors. Nanoscale CNTs and QD probes have also been developed using principles of self-assembly for the detection and measurement of biological macromolecules like DNA and proteins in a time-efficient and cost-effective manner (Joshi et al. 2016).

8.3.5 Surface modification techniques

Surface modification techniques involve the alteration of surface features of the nanobiomaterial like surface composition, structure, and topography to improve the performance of the biomaterial implant/device. They are broadly classified into two categories: (i) physical/chemical surface modification and (ii) surface coating with biocompatible/bioactive agents (Manickam et al. 2017).

One example of chemical surface modification is that of anodization. Anodization is an electrochemical process that is used to render the metal surface more resistant to corrosion by increasing the thickness of the natural oxide layer on its surface. This process has been used to improve the surface features of Ti implants (Webster 2006). In anodization, the surface is first activated with the use of a combination of mineral acids (e.g., nitric and hydrofluoric acids). Subsequently, a constant voltage or current is applied between the anode and cathode to initiate electrode reactions and field-driven ion diffusion. Fluorine electrolytes are also used to obtain a nanostructured topography through a process called self-ordered nanotubular structure formation. However, care must be taken to ensure that the voltage is below the dielectric breakdown point. Many researchers have developed self-ordered nanotubular Ti oxide films using HF/H_2SO_4, CH_3COOH/NH_4F (Boehm et al. 2011).

HA coatings have been recently accomplished on implants to overcome the bio-inert nature of Ti implants. This has been achieved with techniques like plasma spraying. They are most successful as they induce a bidirectional growth of bones (Porter et al. 2002). In fact, the US FDA has recently approved a HA coating on orthopedic implants by plasma spraying for use in the United States (Magesh et al. 2018). Coatings composed of carbon-based nanostructures have also been applied, most notably on load-bearing implants. For instance, nanocrystalline coatings have been applied to metallic implants. The particle size of such coatings is below 100 nm and generally lies between 50 and 100 nm. Ultra-nanocrystalline diamond films have also been described, which are about 3–5 nm in thickness and contain diamond grains with size below 10 nm. Various fabrication technologies have been utilized to fabricate nanostructured carbon coatings on metal implants, one of them being chemical vapor deposition (CVD). This process involves the diffusion-based deposition of thin solid films on the substrate, produced by gaseous-phase homogeneous/heterogeneous chemical reactions. Precursor gases like methane and hydrogen gas are activated inside the CVD chamber by using heat (thermal CVD), high-frequency radiation (photo-assisted CVD), or plasma (plasma-enhanced CVD). CVD is a versatile process that has the capability to deposit a uniform diamond coating over a large surface area of components having irregular/complex shapes and is uniquely positioned to produce wear-resistant coating for orthopedic implants (Magesh et al. 2018).

8.4 Conclusion and future perspectives of Nanobiomaterials-based medical devices and implants

Nanobiomaterials have made a profound commercial impact on the medical device and implant sector. Devices and implants that are currently in clinical practice have their own limitations. Device or implant-acquired infections result in serious illness, physical, and psychological trauma to the patient necessitating the removal of the device. Ti implants are widely used in orthopedic surgeries. Many times, the implant fails due to poor adherence of the Ti surface to biological tissue. Nanobiomaterials, such as Ti oxide-based ceramic nanowires, have shown to improve Ti adhesion to the biological tissue (Dong et al. 2007). Nanobiomaterials are also being explored to improve the surface characteristics of coronary stents to address the lingering problem of restenosis. Such a variety of unmet medical needs can be addressed by specially engineered nanobiomaterials.

New applications of these novel materials also come with safety concerns such as toxicity and environmental issues. The toxicity level of nanomaterials can be affected by the type of material, metal impurities, size of the particles, type of dispersing agents used, the formation of aggregates, functionalization, and surface modification. The nanobiomaterials also present new challenges in fabrication, biostability, biocompatibility, and biodistribution. The characterization of nanobiomaterial interactions at the cellular level is essential to understand the mechanism of toxicity as well as to explore and develop unique nanobiomaterials that can interact with the biological system in a controlled way. The possible exposure to nanomaterials should be considered in all cases, including fixed nanomaterials forming a coating on implants or embedded nanomaterials as an integral part of the implant. Additionally, nano-sized particles may generate by wear-and-tear of medical devices. For the risk assessment of nanobiomaterials used in medical devices and implants, a phased approach is recommended (SCENIHR (Scientific Committee on Emerging and Newly Identified Health Risks), 2015). Phase 1 includes exposure assessment through particle release. Phase 2 deals with particle distribution and persistence. Phase 3 includes hazard assessment by toxicological evaluations. In phase 4, risk assessment is categorized based on the possibility of exposure.

Nanobiomaterials can be tuned to explore specific applications and bypass current limitations pertaining to medical devices and implants. As discussed in this chapter, a wide range of biomaterials can be processed, and the desired properties can be achieved by manipulation of manufacturing conditions. Also, with the advancement in new technologies and the increasing need to address clinical demands, extensive research is being undertaken to develop better and safe nanobiomaterials to improve the quality of life. The clinical translation of the developed nanobiomaterials-based medical devices and implants can be successful only after thoroughly evaluating in vivo safety and efficacy. However, the application of nanobiomaterials for the development of novel medical devices and implants seems a potentially rewarding opportunity.

References

Akhavan, O., Ghaderi, E., Rahighi, R., 2012. Toward single-DNA electrochemical biosensing by graphene nanowalls. ACS Nano 6, 2904–2916.

Alves, G., 2017. The importance of metallic materials as biomaterials. Adv. Tissue. Eng. Regen. Med. Open Access 3, 300–302. https://doi.org/10.15406/atroa.2017.03.00054.

Arden, G.P., Taylor, A.R., Ansell, B.M., 1970. Total hip replacement using the McKee-Farrar prosthesis. In rheumatoid arthritis, Still's disease, and ankylosing spondylitis. Ann. Rheum. Dis. 29, 1–5. https://doi.org/10.1136/ard.29.1.1.

Avti, P.K., Patel, S.C., Sitharaman, B., 2011. Nanobiomaterials: current status and future prospects. In: Nanobiomaterials Handbook. CRC Press, Boca Raton, pp. 1-1–1-15.

Aznar-Cervantes, S., Roca, M.I., Martinez, J.G., Meseguer-Olmo, L., Cenis, J.L., Moraleda, J.M., Otero, T.F., 2012. Fabrication of conductive electrospun silk fibroin scaffolds by coating with polypyrrole for biomedical applications. Bioelectrochemistry 85, 36–43. https://doi.org/10.1016/j.bioelechem.2011.11.008.

Boda, S.K., Li, X., Xie, J., 2018. Electrospraying an enabling technology for pharmaceutical and biomedical applications: a review. J. Aerosol Sci. 125, 164–181. https://doi.org/10.1016/j.jaerosci.2018.04.002. From Electro-Hydro-Dynamics of liquids for the production of charged droplets by Electro-Spray to applications for tailored Materials (aerosols, powders, coatings) and Environment.

Boehm, R.D., Jin, C., Narayan, R.J., 2011. Carbon and diamond. In: Ducheyne, P. (Ed.), Comprehensive Biomaterials. University of North Carolina and North Carolina State University, Raleigh, NC, pp. 109–126.

Boyd, R.S., 2006. Scientists Race to Create Bionic Arm: Federal Government Wants Better Prostheses for Wounded Soldiers. Charlotte Observer.

Britto, P.J., Santhanam, K.S.V., Ajayan, P.M., 1996. Carbon nanotube electrode for oxidation of dopamine. Bioelectrochem. Bioenerg. 41, 121–125. https://doi.org/10.1016/0302-4598(96)05078-7.

Buchko, C.J., Kozlo, K.M., Martin, D.C., 2001. Surface characterization of porous, biocompatible protein polymer thin films. Biomaterials 22, 1289–1300.

Campbell, P., Shen, F., Mckellop, H., 2004. Biologic and tribologic considerations of alternative bearing surfaces. Clin. Orthop. Relat. Res. 90007, 98–111.

Cavalcanti, L.R., Kretly, L.C., Rosenfeld, M., Einav, S., 2004. Proceedings of the IEEE INT'l Conference on Electronics, Circuits and Systems. 447.

Charest, J.L., Eliason, M.T., García, A.J., King, W.P., Talin, A., Simmons, B., 2005. Polymer cell culture substrates with combined nanotopographical patterns and micropatterned chemical domains. J. Vac. Sci. Technol. B 23, 3011. https://doi.org/10.1116/1.2127951.

Chen, P.C., Chen, H.T., Qiu, J., Zhou, C.W., 2010. Inkjet printing of single walled carbon nanotube/RuO2 nanowire supercapacitors on cloth fabrics and flexible substrates. Nano Res. 3, 594–603.

Cheng, D., Yang, L., Li, X., Zhou, J., Chen, Q., Yan, S., 2017. An electrochemical DNA sensing platform using carboxyl functionalized graphene as the electrode modified material. J. Electrochem. Soc. 164, 345–351.

Chronakis, I.S., 2005. Novel nanocomposites and nanoceramics based on polymer nanofibers using electrospinning process—a review. J. Mater. Process. Technol. 167, 283–293. https://doi.org/10.1016/j.jmatprotec.2005.06.053.

Chu, W., Kim, S., Jung, W., Kim, H., Ahn, S., 2007. Fabrication of micro parts using nano composite deposition system. Rapid Prototyp. J. 13, 276–283. https://doi.org/10.1108/13552540710824779.

Chua, C.K., Leong, K.F., Lim, C.S., 2004. Rapid Prototyping: Principles and Applications. World Scientific Publishing, Singapore.

Chung, H., Das, S., 2008. Functionally graded Nylon-11/silica nanocomposites produced by selective laser sintering. Mater. Sci. Eng. A 487, 251–257.

Colvin, V.L., 2003. The potential environmental impact of engineered nanomaterials. Nat. Biotechnol. 21, 1166–1170. https://doi.org/10.1038/nbt875.

Cui, Y., Wei, Q., Park, H., Lieber, C.M., 2001. Nanowire nanosensors for highly sensitive and selective detection of biological and chemical species. Science 293, 1289–1292. https://doi.org/10.1126/science.1062711.

Dalby, M.J., Riehle, M.O., Sutherland, D.S., Agheli, H., Curtis, A.S.G., 2004. Changes in fibroblast morphology in response to nano-columns produced by colloidal lithography. Biomaterials 25, 5415–5422. https://doi.org/10.1016/j.biomaterials.2003.12.049.

Dalla Pria, P., 2007. Evolution and new application of the alumina ceramics in joint replacement. Eur. J. Orthop. Surg. Traumatol. 17, 253–256. https://doi.org/10.1007/s00590-006-0181-1.

Das, B., Mandal, M., Upadhyay, A., Chattopadhyay, P., Karak, N., 2013. Bio-based hyperbranched polyurethane/Fe3O4 nanocomposites: smart antibacterial biomaterials for biomedical devices and implants. Biomed. Mater. 8, 035003.

De Gans, B.J., Schubert, U.S., 2003. Inkjet printing of polymer micro-arrays and libraries: instrumentation, requirements, and perspectives. Macromol. Rapid Commun. 24, 659–666.

Demidov, W., 2004. Nanobiosensors and molecular diagnostics: a promising partnership. Expert. Rev. Mol. Diagn. 4, 267–268. https://doi.org/10.1586/14737159.4.3.267.

Depprich, R., Zipprich, H., Ommerborn, M., Naujoks, C., Wiesmann, H.P., Kiattavorncharoen, S., Lauer, H.C., Meyer, U., Kübler, N.R., Handschel, J., 2008. Osseointegration of zirconia implants compared with titanium: an in vivo study. Head Face Med. 4, 1–8. https://doi.org/10.1186/1746-160X-4-30.

Ding, B., Wang, X., Yu, J. (Eds.), 2019. Electrospinning: Nanofabrication and Applications. Elsevier, https://doi.org/10.1016/C2016-0-01374-8.

Dong, W., Zhang, T., Epstein, J., Cooney, L., Wang, H., Li, Y., Jiang, Y., Cogbill, A., Varadan, V., Tian, Z.R., 2007. Multifunctional nanowire bioscaffolds on titanium. Chem. Mater. 19, 4454–4459.

Dong-Woo, C., Jong Young, K., Jin Woo, L., Seung-Jae, L., Eui Kyun, P., Shin-Yoon, K., 2007. Development of a bone scaffold using HA nanopowder and microstereolithography technology. Microelectron. Eng. 84, 1762–1765.

Ensaff, H., O'Doherty, D.M., Jacobsen, P.H., 2001. The influence of the restoration-tooth interface in light cured composite restorations: a finite element analysis. Biomaterials 22, 3097–3103. https://doi.org/10.1016/S0142-9612(01)00058-8.

Fadhil, N., Saber, D., Cox, P., Vanashi, K., Patra, P., 2014. Energy Harvesting Using Nanofibers PVDF\Graphene Composite for Medical Implanted Devices.

Ferracane, J.L., 2011. Resin composite—state of the art. Dent. Mater. 27, 29–38. https://doi.org/10.1016/j.dental.2010.10.020.

Fong, H., 2004. Electrospun nylon 6 nanofiber reinforced BIS-GMA/TEGDMA dental restorative composite resins. Polymer 45, 2427.

Freitas, S.C., Correa-Uribe, A., Martins, M.C.L., Pelaez-Vargas, A., 2018. Self-assembled monolayers for dental implants. Int. J. Dent. 2018. https://doi.org/10.1155/2018/4395460, e4395460.

Gaitán, C.G., Rosas, R.R., Morallón, E., Amorós, D.C., 2017. Effects of the surface chemistry and structure of carbon nanotubes on the coating of glucose oxidase and electrochemical biosensors performance. RSC Adv. 7, 26867–26878.

Gepreel, M.A., Niinomi, M., 2013. Biocompatibility of Ti-alloys for long-term implantation. J. Mech. Behav. Biomed. Mater. 20, 407–415. https://doi.org/10.1016/j.jmbbm.2012.11.014.

Greco, A., Licciulli, A., Maffezzoli, A., 2001. Stereolithography of ceramic suspensions. J. Mater. Sci. 36, 99–105.

Griffith, M.L., Chu, T.M., Wagner, W., Halloran, J.W., 1995. Ceramic stereolithography for investment casting and biomedical applications. In: Solid Freeform Fabrication Conference, University of Texas At. Austin, USA, pp. 31–38.

Griffith, M.L., Halloran, J.W., 1996. Freeform fabrication of ceramics via stereolithography. J. Am. Ceram. Soc. 79, 2601–2608.

Gu, Y., Chen, X., Lee, J.H., Monteiro, D.A., Wang, H., Lee, W.Y., 2012. Inkjet printed antibiotic- and calcium-eluting bioresorbable nanocomposite micropatterns for orthopedic implants. Acta Biomater 8 (1), 424–431. https://doi.org/10.1016/j.actbio.2011.08.006.

Guo, Q., Mather, J.P., Yang, P., Boden, M., Mather, P.T., 2015. Fabrication of polymeric coatings with controlled microtopographies using an electrospraying technique. PLoS One 10, 0129960.
Hao, L., Savalani, M.M., Zhang, Y., Tanner, K.E., Harris, R.A., 2006. Selective laser sintering of hydroxyapatite reinforced polyethylene composites for bioactive implants and tissue scaffold development. Proc. Inst. Mech. Eng. H J. Eng. Med. 220, 521–531.
Hasirci, V., 2006. Nanobiomaterials: a review of the existing science and technology, and new approaches. J. Biomater. Sci. Polym. Ed. 17, 1241–1268.
Hayashi, K., Uenoyama, K., Matsuguchi, N., Sugioka, Y., 1991. Quantitative analysis of in vivo tissue responses to titanium-oxide- and hydroxyapatite-coated titanium alloy. J. Biomed. Mater. Res. 25, 515–523.
Hench, L.L., 1995. In: Brook, R.J. (Ed.), Ceramics and Society. Techna Srl.
Heo, S.J., Kim, S.E., Wei, J., Hyun, Y.T., Yun, H.S., Kim, D.H., Shin, J.W., Shin, J.W., 2009. Fabrication and characterization of novel nano and micro-HA/PCL composite scaffolds using a modified rapid prototyping process. J. Biomed. Mater. Res. A 89A, 108–116.
Hinczewski, C., Corbel, S., Chartier, T., 1998. Ceramic suspensions suitable for stereolithography. J. Eur. Ceram. Soc. 18, 583–590.
Ho, C.H., Odermatt, E.K., Berndt, I., Tiller, J.C., 2013. Long-term active antimicrobial coatings for surgical sutures based on silver nanoparticles and hyperbranched polylysine. J. Biomater. Sci. Polym. Ed. 24, 1589–1600. https://doi.org/10.1080/09205063.2013.782803.
Hon, K.K.B., Li, L., Hutchings, I.M., 2008. Direct writing technology-advances and developments. CIRP Ann. Manuf. Technol. 57, 601–620.
Hosseini Zori, M., Soleimani-Gorgani, A., 2012. Inkjet printing of micro-emulsion TiO2 nanoparticles ink on the surface of glass. J. Eur. Ceram. Soc. 32, 4271–4277.
Hung-Jen, Y., Ching-Shiow, T., Shan-Hui, H., Ching-Lin, T., 2009. Evaluation of chondrocyte growth in the highly porous scaffolds made by fused deposition manufacturing (FDM) fi lled with type II collagen. Biomed. Microdevices 11, 615–624.
Jakus, A.E., Secor, E.B., Rutz, A.L., Jordan, S.W., Hersam, M.C., Shah, R.N., 2015. Three-dimensional printing of high-content graphene scaffolds for electronic and biomedical applications. ACS Nano 9, 4636–4648. https://doi.org/10.1021/acsnano.5b01179.
Jensen, K., Mickelson, W., Kis, A., Zettl, A., 2007. Buckling and kinking force measurements on individual multiwalled carbon nanotubes. Phys. Rev. 76, 195436.
de Jonge, L.T., Leeuwenburgh, S.C.G., van den Beucken, J.J.J.P., Wolke, J.G.C., Jansen, J.A., 2009. Electrosprayed enzyme coatings as bioinspired alternatives to bioceramic coatings for orthopedic and oral implants. Adv. Funct. Mater. 19, 755–762. https://doi.org/10.1002/adfm.200800819.
Joshi, A., Singh, N., Verma, G., 2016. Chapter 2—Preparation and applications of self-assembled natural and synthetic nanostructures. In: Grumezescu, A.M. (Ed.), Fabrication and Self-Assembly of Nanobiomaterials. William Andrew Publishing, pp. 29–55, https://doi.org/10.1016/B978-0-323-41533-0.00002-7.
Joung, Y.-H., 2013. Development of implantable medical devices: from an engineering perspective. Int. Neurourol. J. 17, 98–106. https://doi.org/10.5213/inj.2013.17.3.98.
Kai, D., Prabhakaran, M.P., Jin, G., Ramakrishna, S., 2011. Polypyrrole-contained electrospun conductive nanofibrous membranes for cardiac tissue engineering. J. Biomed. Mater. Res. A 99, 376–385.
Kellomäki, M., Niiranen, H., Puumanen, K., Ashammakhi, N., Waris, T., Törmälä, P., 2000. Bioabsorbable scaffolds for guided bone regeneration and generation. Biomaterials 21, 2495–2505. https://doi.org/10.1016/S0142-9612(00)00117-4.
Kim, S.G., Chu, W.S., Jung, W.K., Ahn, S.H., 2007. Evaluation of mechanical and electrical properties of nanocomposite parts fabricated by nanocomposite deposition system (NCDS). J. Mater. Process. Technol. 187–188, 331–334. https://doi.org/10.1016/j.

jmatprotec.2006.11.209. 3rd International Conference on Advanced Forming and Die Manufacturing Technology.
Kim, W., Lee, H.H., Knowles, J.C., 2006. Electrospunpoly (L-lactide-co-ε-caprolactone)/polyethyleneoxide/hydroxyapatite nanofibrous membrane for guided bonere generation. J. Biomed. Mater. Res.
Kim, J., Park, S.-Y., Kim, S., Lee, D.H., Kim, J.H., Kim, J.M., Kang, H., Han, J.-S., Park, J.W., Lee, H., Choi, S.-H., 2016. Precise and selective sensing of DNA-DNA hybridization by graphene/Si-nanowires diode-type biosensors. Sci. Rep. 6, 31984. https://doi.org/10.1038/srep31984.
Ko, S.H., Chung, J., Hotz, N., Nam, K.H., Grigoropoulos, C.P., 2010. Metal nanoparticle direct inkjet printing for low-temperature 3D micro metal structure fabrication. J. Micromech. Microeng. 20, 125010. https://doi.org/10.1088/0960-1317/20/12/125010.
Kokubo, T., Kim, H.M., Kawashita, M., 2003. Novel bioactive materials with different mechanical properties. Biomaterials 24, 2161–2175.
Kumawat, M.K., Thakur, M., Gurung, R.B., Srivastava, R., 2017. Graphene quantum dots for cell proliferation, nucleus imaging, and photoluminescent sensing applications. Sci. Rep. 7, 15858.
Lee, G., Barlow, J.W., 2003. Selective laser sintering of bioceramic materials for implants. In: Proceedings of the Solid Freeform Fabrication Symposium. Austin, TX, pp. 376–380.
Lee, Y.K., Ha, Y.C., Yoo, J.I., Jo, W.L., Kim, K.C., Koo, K.H., 2017. Mid-term results of the biolox delta ceramic-on-ceramic total hip arthroplasty. Bone Joint J. 99B, 741–748. https://doi.org/10.1302/0301-620X.99B6.BJJ-2016-0486.R3.
Li, X., Liu, X., Huang, J., Fan, Y., Cui, F.-Z., 2011. Biomedical investigation of CNT based coatings. Surf. Coat. Technol. 206, 759–766.
Li, Y., Yang, C., Zhao, H., Qu, S., Li, X., Li, Y., 2014. New developments of Ti-based alloys for biomedical applications. Materials (Basel), 1709–1800. https://doi.org/10.3390/ma7031709.
Lin, Y., Lu, F., Tu, Y., Ren, Z., 2004. Glucose biosensors based on carbon nanotube nanoelectrode ensembles. Nano Lett. 4.
Liu, Y., Dong, X., Chen, P., 2017. Biological and chemical sensors based on graphene materials. Chem. Soc. Rev. 41, 2283–2307.
Magesh, S., Vasanth, G., Revathi, A., Geetha, M., 2018. 19—Use of nanostructured materials in implants. In: Narayan, R. (Ed.), Nanobiomaterials. Woodhead Publishing, pp. 481–501, https://doi.org/10.1016/B978-0-08-100716-7.00019-2.
Maiti, D., Tong, X., Mou, X., Yang, K., 2019. Carbon-based nanomaterials for biomedical applications: a recent study. Front. Pharmacol. 9, 1401.
Manickam, L.P., Bhatt, A., Rana, D., Ostrovidov, S., Pasricha, R., Wang, X., Ramalingam, M., 2017. Nanopatterning techniques. In: Nanobiomaterials. John Wiley & Sons, Ltd, pp. 189–210, https://doi.org/10.1002/9783527698646.ch8.
Mattson, M.P., Haddon, R.C., Rao, A.M., 2000. Molecular functionalization of carbon nanotubes and use as substrates for neuronal growth. J. Mol. Neurosci. 14, 175.
McDonnell, G., 2012. Gas plasma sterilization. In: Russell, Hugo & Ayliffe's: Principles and Practice of Disinfection. Preservation and Sterilization. vol. 333–34.
McKenzie, J.L., Waid, M.C., Shi, R., Webster, T.J., 2004. Decreased functions of astrocytes on carbon nanofiber materials. Biomaterials 25, 1309–1317.
Menezes, A.J., Kapoor, V.J., Goel, V.K., Cameron, B.D., Lu, J.-Y., 2001. Mechanical Engineering Magazine. Online.
Migliaresi, C., Nicolais, L., 1980. Composite materials for biomedical applications. Int. J. Artif. Organs 3, 114–118. https://doi.org/10.1177/039139888000300213.
Nakamura, H., Karube, I., 2003. Current research activity in biosensors. Anal. Bioanal. Chem. 377, 446–468. https://doi.org/10.1007/s00216-003-1947-5.

Niinomi, M., 2011. Creation of functionality by ubiquitous elements in titanium alloys. Nippon Kinzoku Gakkaishi 75, 21–28. https://doi.org/10.2320/jinstmet.75.21.

Niinomi, M., Nakai, M., Hieda, J., 2012. Development of new metallic alloys for biomedical applications. Acta Biomater. 8, 3888–3903. https://doi.org/10.1016/j.actbio.2012.06.037.

Niyogi, S., Hamon, M.A., Hu, H., Zhao, B., Bhowmik, P., Sen, R., Itkis, M.E., Haddon, R.C., 2002. Chemistry of single-walled carbon nanotubes. Acc. Chem. Res. 35, 1105.

Patino, M.G., Neiders, M.E., Andreana, S., Noble, B., Cohen, R.E., 2002. Collagen as an implantable material in medicine and dentistry. J. Oral Implantol. 28, 220–225. https://doi.org/10.1563/1548-1336(2002)028<0220:CAAIMI>2.3.CO;2.

Ping, J., Vishnubhotla, J.R., Vrudhula, A., Johnson, A.T.C., 2016. Scalable production of high-sensitivity, label-free DNA biosensors based on backgated graphene field effect transistors. ACS Nano 10, 8700–8704.

Polizu, S., Savadogo, O., Poulin, P., Yahia, L.H., 2006. Applications of carbon nanotubes-based biomaterials in biomedical nanotechnology. J. Nanosci. Nanotechnol. 6, 1883–1904.

Popov, V.N., 2004. Carbon nanotubes: properties and application. Mater. Sci. Eng. R. Rep. 43, 61–102. https://doi.org/10.1016/j.mser.2003.10.001.

Porter, A.E., Hobbs, L.W., Rosen, V.B., Spector, M., 2002. The ultrastructure of the plasma-sprayed hydroxyapatite-bone interface predisposing to bone bonding. Biomaterials 23, 725–733.

Prabowo, B.A., Alom, A., Secario, M.K., Masim, F.C.P., Lai, H.-C., Hatanaka, K., Liu, K.-C., 2016. Graphene-based portable SPR sensor for the detection of mycobacterium tuberculosis DNA strain. Procedia Eng. 168, 541–545. https://doi.org/10.1016/j.proeng.2016.11.520. Proceedings of the 30th anniversary Eurosensors Conference—Eurosensors 2016, 4-7. Sepember 2016, Budapest, Hungary.

Price, R.L., Waid, M.C., Haberstroh, K.M., Webster, T.J., 2003. Selective bone cell adhesion on formulations containing carbon nanofibers. Biomaterials 24, 1877–1887.

Puperi, D.S., Kishan, A., Punske, Z.E., Wu, Y., Cosgriff-Hernandez, E., West, J.L., Grande-Allen, K.J., 2016. Electrospun polyurethane and hydrogel composite scaffolds as biomechanical mimics for aortic valve tissue engineering. ACS Biomater. Sci. Eng. 2, 1546–1558.

Puranik, A.S., Dawson, E.R., Peppas, N.A., 2013. Recent advances in drug eluting stents. Int. J. Pharm. 441, 665–679. https://doi.org/10.1016/j.ijpharm.2012.10.029.

Rack, H.J., Qazi, J.I., 2006. Titanium alloys for biomedical applications. Mater. Sci. Eng. C 26, 1269–1277. https://doi.org/10.1016/j.msec.2005.08.032.

Ravichandran, R., Venugopal, J.R., Mukherjee, S., Sundarrajan, S., Ramakrishna, S., 2015. Elastomeric core/shell nanofibrous cardiac patch as a biomimetic support for infarcted porcine myocardium. Tissue Eng. A 21, 1288–1298.

Sachlos, E., Czernuszka, J.T., 2003. Making tissue engineering scaffolds work: review on the application of solid freeform fabrication technology to the production of tissue engineering scaffolds. Eur. Cell. Mater. 5, 29–40.

Sandoval, J.H., Soto, K.F., Murr, L.E., Wicker, R.B., 2007. Nanotailoring photocrosslinkable epoxy resins with multi-walled carbon nanotubes for stereolithography layered manufacturing. J. Mater. Sci. 42, 156–165.

Sawicka, K., Gouma, P., Simon, S., 2005. Electrospun biocomposite nanofibers for urea biosensing. Sensors Actuators B Chem. 108, 585–588.

SCENIHR (Scientific Committee on Emerging and Newly Identified Health Risks), 2015. Final Opinion on the Guidance on the Determination of Potential Health Effects of Nanomaterials Used in Medical Devices.

Schindhelm, K., Milthorpe, B.K., 2003. An overview of biomaterials. Australas. Phys. Eng. Sci. Med. 9, 29–32.

Shekhawat, G., Tark, S.-H., Dravid, V.P., 2006. MOSFET-embedded microcantilevers for measuring deflection in biomolecular sensors. Science 311, 1592–1595. https://doi.org/10.1126/science.1122588.

Shikinami, Y., Okuno, M., 2001. Bioresorbable devices made of forged composites of hydroxyapatite (HA) particles and poly L-lactide (PLLA). Part II: Practical properties of miniscrews and miniplates. Biomaterials 22, 3197–3211. https://doi.org/10.1016/S0142-9612(01)00072-2.

Shor, L., Guceri, S., Wen, X.J., Gandhi, M., Sun, W., 2007. Fabrication of threedimensional polycaprolactone/hydroxyapatite tissue scaffolds and osteoblast scaffold interactions in vitro. Biomaterials 28, 5291–5297.

Sotiropoulou, S., Chaniotakis, N.A., 2003. Carbon nanotube array-based biosensor. Anal. Bioanal. Chem. 375, 103–105. https://doi.org/10.1007/s00216-002-1617-z.

Stradiotto, N.R., Yamanaka, H., Zanoni, M.V.B., 2003. Electrochemical sensors: a powerful tool in analytical chemistry. J. Braz. Chem. Soc. 14, 159–173. https://doi.org/10.1590/S0103-50532003000200003.

Talha, M., Behera, C.K., Sinha, O.P., 2012. Potentiodynamic polarization study of Type 316L and 316LVM stainless steels for surgical implants in simulated body fluids. J. Chem. Pharm. Res. 4, 203–208. 2012, 4 (1): 203–208 Research Article.

Talha, M., Behera, C.K., Sinha, O.P., 2013. A review on nickel-free nitrogen containing austenitic stainless steels for biomedical applications. Mater. Sci. Eng. C 33, 3563–3575. https://doi.org/10.1016/j.msec.2013.06.002.

Tang, L., Wang, Y., Li, J., 2015. The graphene/nucleic acid nanobio interface. Chem. Soc. Rev. 44, 6954–6980.

Tellis, B.C., Szivek, J.A., Bliss, C.L., Margolis, D.S., Vaidyanathan, R.K., Calvert, P., 2008. Trabecular scaffolds created using micro CT guided fused deposition modeling. Mater. Sci. Eng. C Biomim. Supramol. Syst. 28, 171–178.

Teo, A.J.T., Mishra, A., Park, I., Kim, Y.J., Park, W.T., Yoon, Y.J., 2016. Polymeric biomaterials for medical implants and devices. ACS Biomater. Sci. Eng. 2, 454–472.

US FDA, 2020. 3D Printing of Medical Devices [WWW Document]. US Food & Drug Administration. https://www.fda.gov/medical-devices/products-and-medical-procedures/3d-printing-medical-devices. (Accessed 10.2.20).

Vaezi, M., Yang, S., 2014. 2—Freeform fabrication of nanobiomaterials using 3D printing. In: Narayan, R. (Ed.), Rapid Prototyping of Biomaterials. Woodhead Publishing, pp. 16–74, https://doi.org/10.1533/9780857097217.16.

Vozzi, G., Ahluwalia, A., 2007. Microfabrication for tissue engineering: rethinking the cells-on-a scaffold approach. J. Mater. Chem. 17, 1248–1254.

Vozzi, G., Flaim, C., Ahluwalia, A., Bhatia, S., 2003. Fabrication of PLGA scaffolds using soft lithography and microsyringe deposition. Biomaterials 24, 2533–2540.

Vozzi, G., Previti, A., Ciaravella, G., Ahluwalia, A., 2004. Microfabricated fractal branching networks. J. Biomed. Mater. Res. A 71A, 326–333.

Wang, F., Shor, L., Darling, A., Khalil, S., Sun, W., Guceri, S., Lau, A., 2004. Precision extruding deposition and characterization of cellular poly-epsilon caprolactone tissue scaffolds. Rapid Prototyp. J. 10, 42–49.

Webster, T.J., 2006. Nanostructured biomaterials for tissue engineering bone. Adv. Biochem. Eng. Biotechnol. 103, 275–308.

Xian, Y., Hu, Y., Liu, F., Xian, Y., Wang, H., Jin, L., 2006. Glucose biosensor based on Au nanoparticles-conductive polyaniline nanocomposite. Biosens. Bioelectron. 21, 1996–2000.

Xiong, Z., Yan, Y.N., Zhang, R.J., Sun, L., 2001. Fabrication of porous poly(L-lactic acid) scaffolds for bone tissue engineering via precise extrusion. Scr. Mater. 45, 773–779.

Yan, Y., Neville, A., Dowson, D., 2007. Tribo-corrosion properties of cobalt-based medical implant alloys in simulated biological environments. Wear 263, 1105–1111. https://doi.org/10.1016/j.wear.2007.01.114.

Yang, S., Evans, J.R.G., 2004. Acoustic control of powder dispensing in open tubes. Powder Technol. 139, 55–60.

Yang, S., Evans, J.R.G., 2005. On the rate of descent of powder in a vibrating tube. Philos. Mag. 85, 1089–1109.

Yang, S.F., Leong, K.F., Du, Z.H., Chua, C.K., 2002. The design of scaffolds for use in tissue engineering. Part II. Rapid prototyping techniques. Tissue Eng. 8, 1–11.

Yoshida, M., Prasad, P.N., 1996. Sol-gel-processed SiO2/TiO2/poly(vinylpyrrolidone) composite materials for optical waveguides. Chem. Mater. 8, 235–241. https://doi.org/10.1021/cm950331o.

Yu, C., Ma, X., Zhu, W., Wang, P., Miller, K.L., Stupin, J., Koroleva-Maharajh, A., Hairabedian, A., Chen, S., 2019. Scanningless and continuous 3D bioprinting of human tissues with decellularized extracellular matrix. Biomaterials 194, 1–13. https://doi.org/10.1016/j.biomaterials.2018.12.009.

van der Zande, M., Walboomers, X.F., Brännvall, M., Olalde, B., Jurado, M.J., Álava, J.I., Jansen, J.A., 2010. Genetic profiling of osteoblast-like cells cultured on a novel bone reconstructive material, consisting of poly-l-lactide, carbon nanotubes and microhydroxyapatite, in the presence of bone morphogenetic protein-2. Acta Biomater. 6, 4352–4360. https://doi.org/10.1016/j.actbio.2010.06.013.

Zhao, Q., Gan, Z., Zhuang, Q., 2002. Electrochemical sensors based on carbon nanotubes. Electroanalysis 14, 1609–1613.

Zheng, X.T., Ananthanarayanan, A., Luo, K.Q., Chen, P., 2015. Glowing graphene quantum dots and carbon dots: properties, syntheses, and biological applications. Small 11, 1620–1636.

Zheng, G., Patolsky, F., Cui, Y., Wang, W.U., Lieber, C.M., 2005. Multiplexed electrical detection of cancer markers with nanowire sensor arrays. Nat. Biotechnol. 23, 1294–1301. https://doi.org/10.1038/nbt1138.

Zhu, L., Deng, C., Chen, P., Dong, X., Su, Y.H., Yuan, Y., 2014. Glucose oxidase biosensors based on carbon nanotube non-woven fabrics. Carbon 67, 795–796.

Index

Note: Page numbers followed by *f* indicate figures and *t* indicate tables.

N

O

P

Q

R

S

X

Y

Z

FSC
www.fsc.org
MIX
Papier | Fördert gute Waldnutzung
FSC® C083411

Kolibri 360 GmbH
Ferdinand-Jühlke-Straße 7
99095 Erfurt, Deutschland
produktsicherheit@kolibri360.de